Baltie
W9-DII-071

Critical Pathways in Therapeutic Intervention

UPPER EXTREMITIES

Critical Pathways in Therapeutic Intervention

UPPER EXTREMITIES

DAVID C. **Saidoff,** BS, PT

Physical Therapist,
Private Practice,
West Hempstead, New York

ANDREW L. **McDonough,** EdD, PT

Chairman and Clinical Associate Professor,
Department of Physical Therapy,
New York University,
New York, New York

with 216 illustrations

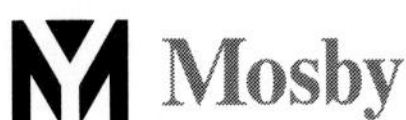

St. Louis Baltimore Boston
Carlsbad Chicago Naples New York Philadelphia Portland
London Madrid Mexico City Singapore Sydney Tokyo Toronto Wiesbaden

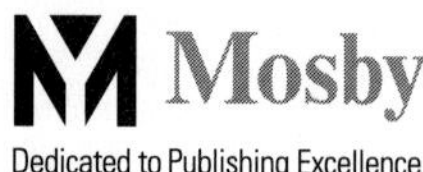

Dedicated to Publishing Excellence

A Times Mirror Company

Vice President and Publisher: Don Ladig
Executive Editor: Martha Sasser
Developmental Editor: Kellie F. White
Project Manager: Dana Peick
Production Editor: Dottie Martin
Manuscript Editor: Carl Masthay
Designer: Amy Buxton
Manufacturing Supervisor: Karen Boehme

Copyright © 1997 Mosby–Year Book, Inc.

All rights reserved. No part of this publication may be reproduced, stored in a retrieval system, or transmitted, in any form or by any means, electronic, mechanical, photocopying, recording, or otherwise, without written permission of the publisher.

Permission to photocopy or reproduce solely for internal or personal use is permitted for libraries or other users registered with the Copyright Clearance Center, provided that the base fee of $4.00 per chapter plus $.10 per page is paid directly to the Copyright Clearance Center, 27 Congress Street, Salem, MA 01970. This consent does not extend to other kinds of copying, such as copying for general distribution, for advertising or promotional purposes, for creating new collected works, or for resale.

Printed in the United States of America
Production and composition by Shepherd, Inc.
Printing/binding by R.R. Donnelly & Sons Company

Mosby–Year Book, Inc.
11830 Westline Industrial Drive
St. Louis, Missouri 63146

Library of Congress Cataloging-in-Publication Data
Saidoff, David C.
Critical pathways in therapeutic intervention: upper extremities/ David C. Saidoff, Andrew McDonough.
p. cm.
Includes bibliographic references and index.
ISBN 0-8151-4486-5
1. Arm—Diseases. 2. Medical protocols. 3. Diagnosis. Differential. I. McDonough, Andrew. II. Title.
[DNLM: 1. Arm Injuries—rehabilitation. 2. Physical Therapy. WE 805 S132c 1997]
RC951.S25 1997
617.5'7—dc20
DNLM/DLC
for Library of Congress 96-33067
CIP

96 97 98 99 00 / 9 8 7 6 5 4 3 2 1

*I wish to dedicate this volume to my best friend,
my lovely wife Debby, and to my son Elisha for their
sacrifice and support over the many hours I spent
away from them while working on this project.*

D.C.S.

Foreword

With *Critical Pathways in Therapeutic Intervention: Upper Extremities,* problem-based educational programs will find a refreshing new approach to presenting and expounding on the types of clinical problems regularly encountered in physical therapy. David Saidoff and Dr. Andrew McDonough have gathered particularly relevant scenarios that provide diverse, yet regularly encountered clinical challenges.

"I have painful tingling in my right hand, especially at night," exemplifies the patient-centered focus of this text. The wording of each chapter utilizes terminology expressed by patients when presenting complaints in the clinical setting. It is important for you as a therapist to focus on hearing what the patient is trying to tell you because the patient seeks to have you focus on what is most important to him or her.

After the case in each chapter is presented, the problem is expanded to provide you with up-to-date information on the diagnosis of the problem, the design of the therapeutic intervention, and evidence of the clinical effectiveness of the approaches that have been employed. The discussion is couched in terms that facilitate deductive reasoning. To further the reasoning process, a rich reference list is provided after each chapter.

Pertinent and most frequently asked questions are posed to the reader in a structured discussion that provides an enlarged view of the problem at hand. The authors do not take a reductionist approach, but rather they use one that expands your insight. By outlining a series of subordinate problems or concerns, the clinician's train of thought is structured somewhat, thereby providing a framework upon which to work on similar clinical problems not covered in the text.

Illustrations add the visualization that is essential for a complete understanding of the clinical problem. The anatomic detail is accurately depicted and provides a ready and quick guide for you.

My compliments to the authors on a most provocative and timely presentation of current and relevant problems encountered by physical therapists. This textbook will provide a model for authors to emulate.

Arthur J. Nelson, PhD, PT, FAPTA

This is what I call a learning experience! Using a case presentation format, this book is the next best thing to going on "rounds" with a mentor who probes just how much you really know about theory and practice. By also supplying the answers to the questions, the authors have devloped a broad-based text that will introduce students to the real complexity of understanding clinical situations, while challenging even experienced clinicians. This is no multiple-choice or true-false format. Put on your thinking caps and enjoy.

Neil Spielholz, PhD. PT

Preface

This book was written to address the needs of those health professionals who attempt to treat their patients with conservative methods before resorting to referral for surgical intervention. To many professionals, the requisite knowledge base so necessary to approaching given maladies becomes foreign and forgotten in direct proportion to the time since their schooling or their last exposure to the pathologic conditions in question.

The scope of this book is generally restricted to those disorders that are amenable to conservative management. We have further narrowed our scope to include the more common maladies and have intentionally left out some of the more unlikely or occult disorders. Moreover, the story line beginning many of the chapters is not always the most classic presentation, especially with regard to the age and sex distribution of the given disorder. The cases have been intentionally structured to veer somewhat away from the standard clinical patient presentation. This is in keeping with our didactic philosophy that the student must learn to think rather than try to memorize simple-fit solutions to a subject as complex as the pathologic process. It is in this spirit that therapy is very much an art, despite its firm grounding in science.

This text will serve as a bridge of sorts, bringing together ideas and concepts from fields as diverse as anatomy, kinesiology, orthopedics, rheumatology, neurology, sports medicine, physiatry, ergonomics, and geriatrics. Although the information presented is not new, the organization and format of this material are novel in that they permit both student and clinician to hone in on the relevant information necessary for an understanding of each disorder. Although students generally view textbooks as something adversarial to conquer, the nature in which information is presented here is considerably nonthreatening. Each chapter is a self-contained study, thus not requiring the reading of the previous chapter. The story line of each chapter is followed by a paradigm of information and an occasional imperative to the clinician's arrival at a conclusive diagnosis. This model has been followed except for these disorders, such as anterior shoulder dislocation, in which many of the acute signs and symptoms are omitted here, since the management of such an acute disorder is best treated by a physician.

Together, the chapters compose a volume that may be used as a guide, review, and reference for professionals and students alike. The actual ratiocination relevant to the encounter with each disorder is laid out for the benefit of the student, with each question and answer in a sequence that encourages critical thinking. We have tried to make the chapters as eclectic as they are focused, so that they stimulate and provoke thought and perhaps even be entertaining. Throughout this volume, we have attempted to be concise and, in the tradition of the late E.B. White, not obfuscate the topics with excessive embellishment. We have deliberately tried to stay away from lofty "medicalese," when possible, and to replace intimidating terms with simple, yet accurate explanations.

The idea of critical path thinking is used in this book in the same way Buckminster Fuller defined this term in his magnum opus *Synergetics 2,* and *Critical Path.* Much more than a simple list of linear thoughts required to arrive at a given objective or conclusion, the use of *critical pathways* implies complexes of thoughts and concepts that come together to create something new that is much more the mere sum of its parts.

I have long felt a yawning gap in professional literature created by the absence of a source book or compendium of the many rheumatologic, orthopedic, and neurologic maladies that are responsive to therapeutic intervention. There is a need for a text that contains a detailed description of the clinical presentation, pathokinesiology, and differential diagnosis. The latter is particularly important because therapists are increasingly assuming the role of primary care providers.

We have chosen some of the most common disorders encountered in outpatient clinics and private practice, recognizing full well that variations of pathologic conditions are all too common and that the responsible clinician must learn not to pigeonhole his or her patients into preassumed disorders. Each patient is unique and must be looked upon anew during the initial evaluation in terms of his or her own unique history and clinical presentation.

In the words of the late Isaac Asimov, "Originality consists in the organization and expression of facts, not the facts themselves" (Opus 200). Although the format and spirit of this book are unique, the information it contains is entirely derivative and has been compiled from the many sources listed at the end of each chapter. The last chapter deals with muscle injuries of the upper and the lower extremities and serves as a bridge introducing the content of a companion volume on the lower extremity that will follow.

The immense effort that went into preparing this volume is payback to the Creator on that precious altar of life. I thank God for a mind that understands, a heart that feels the pain of others, and hands that have learned to heal their wounds.

David C. Saidoff
West Hempstead, N.Y.

I first came to know David Saidoff as one of the students in the physical therapy program at New York University. Early on in his studies, David told me of his interest in writing, and soon after his graduation from NYU, we began to correspond and discuss the articles he had started writing. With each completed article came David's growing sense of enthusiasm for writing and the physical therapy profession in general. It was perhaps a year or more after our first discussions that David began to consolidate his work into a planned book that, from my perspective, seemed years from the reality of publication. I should have known that the amount of energy and interest David displayed would make his dream to write and publish a significant book a reality sooner rather than later. And thus we formally entered into a collaboration that has produced what follows. I have enjoyed seeing David's thoughts and ideas put to paper in what I believe to be an important text that will make a significant contribution to the knowledge base of student therapists and established clinicians. It has been gratifying to see the maturation of a young writer in such a short period of time. One is easily overwhelmed by David's energy and drive, and given his enthusiasm, it is not hard to be impressed with the final product that awaits you. As such, I would like to thank David for asking me to contribute to this book. This has been a rewarding experience for me as well, and I look forward to our continued collaboration.

Andrew L. McDonough
New York, N.Y.

Acknowledgments

The primary motivation for writing this textbook originated in my wishing that such a book were available to me when I began my studies in physical therapy. The temerity to undertake the writing of such a book at a relatively early stage in my career stemmed from the intuition that it was essential to do this before I became too remote from the initial learning process and had forgotten the problems that had caused me difficulty. All this could not have been possible without the efforts of several colleagues whose encouragement and review contributed in the making of this volume. Foremost, I thank Andy McDonough, EdD, for his collaboration and editorial comments. I wish to take this opportunity to thank Sid Hershkowitz for his many helpful suggestions, Yocheved Jacob for proofreading many chapters, and Janet Fink for support of this project. Their encouragement and the valuable time they devoted to clarification of the many topics herein is much appreciated. I thank David Nussbaum for the many hours we discussed and clarified minutiae regarding many kinesiologic topics. I also thank my colleagues at the Bi-Y special education program.

Many thanks to the editorial staff at Mosby, Martha Sasser, Kellie White, Amy Dubin, and Laura MacAdam, and to the production staff, Dottie Martin and Carl Masthay. My deep thanks to Martha Sasser for believing in the premise of this book and in helping define its approach.

I thank Laura Duprey for her expert and beautiful illustrations. I consider myself fortunate to have worked together with so talented an artist. I would also like to thank Barbara Shelly and Steven Maryles for helping prepare the final typescript. Thanks to Menachem Altaras for computer technical assistance.

I wish to acknowledge the many individuals who over the years have contributed to my personal and professional growth. I hope this endeavor serves as a source of satisfaction and pride to my teachers and mentors. I offer thanks as a token of gratitude and appreciation toward their effort.

Above all, I am indebted to my wife Debby for bearing with me during the long and arduous effort involved during the conception, gestation, and birth of this book.

D.C.S.

Contents

Part One Hand and Wrist

Part Two Elbow and Forearm

Part Three Shoulder

Part One

Hand and Wrist

Chilly Fingertips

1

An 18-year-old white woman is referred by your friend, a rheumatologist, with complaints of bilateral chilly index and middle fingers lasting for up to 10 minutes and precipitated by cold, vibration, or even emotional upset. The patient cannot remember when her symptoms started exactly but states that they have become more frequent over the past 4 months. At your request, the patient subjects herself to voluntary cold exposure by placing her hands flat up against the cold window pane in your office. Over the next 10 minutes, you notice how the color of her hands dramatically change from white to blue and finally to red. During this time the patient complains of numbness and cold. Upon communicating with the referring physician you learn that his associate, a vascular surgeon, has ruled out any vessel-obstructing disease. The presence of a cervical rib has also been ruled out. There is no history of injury or diabetes, though the patient reports that her mother occasionally suffers from the same malady. The patient smokes regularly, drinks three cups of coffee daily, and uses oral contraceptives.

OBSERVATION There are no trophic changes observed.

PALPATION The patient's hand (or hands) felt cold and then very warm over the course of 20 minutes.

RANGE OF MOTION Within functional limits.

STRENGTH Within normal limits.

FLEXIBILITY Normal.

SENSATION Normal to light touch, pressure, and proprioception as well as to two-point discrimination.

PULSES Normal.

SPECIAL TESTS Negative Allen test, negative Adson test and costoclavicular maneuver, negative compression or distraction of the cervical spine.

1. **What is most likely causing this young woman's symptoms?**
2. **What is the body's reaction to cold exposure?**
3. **What stimuli may provoke an attack of symptoms?**
4. **What circulatory changes occur during an attack of Raynaud's syndrome?**
5. **What are the differences between primary and secondary Raynaud's syndrome?**

6. **What is the differential diagnosis?**
7. **What treatment strategy is indicated in Raynaud's syndrome?**

1. What is most likely causing this young woman's symptoms?

Raynaud's syndrome (pronounced ray-NOZE) was first described in 1862 by the French physician Maurice Raynaud who postulated that exaggerated sensitivity to cold stemmed from an overly sensitive nervous system. Defining it as *cold-induced reflex digital vasoconstriction and ischemia,* Raynaud proposed a pathophysiology involving an exaggerated reflex sympathetic vasoconstriction.[2] This syndrome, mildly affecting 5% to 10% of the population, causes considerable discomfort and inconvenience and comes in two forms: (1) primary Raynaud's syndrome, or *Raynaud's disease,* and (2) secondary Raynaud's syndrome, or *Raynaud's phenomenon.*[4] An attack may occur after even the slightest provocation such as reaching into the refrigerator momentarily to remove an item or even grasping a cold metal doorknob. Arteriole spasm will follow, resulting in *pallor,* even *cyanosis,* and then *redness* of the digits, and this cycle may also occur in other acral parts such as the toes, nose, ears, or tongue when exposed to cold because these areas are located at the outer reaches of the circulatory system.

2. What is the body's reaction to cold exposure?

Physiologic thermoregulation is governed by the autonomic nervous system and responds to cold fingers by shunting blood to the core by means of a *countercurrent heat-exchange mechanism.*[1] This results in blood vessel constriction of distal, outlying areas of the body so as to divert blood away from the extremities, preventing heat loss by way of exposed hand and feet surfaces. Raynaud's syndrome more frequently involves the fingers than it does the toes.[2]

3. What stimuli may provoke an attack of symptoms?

In the majority of patients symptoms are precipitated by exposure to cold as insignificant as a cool breeze on a hot day, or just from sitting in a drafty room. Some patients' symptoms are triggered by emotional upset. Raynaud's is also common to individuals whose occupations subject hands to unusual wear and tear, such as typists, pianists, and meat cutters, and especially affects those persons using vibrating tools such as jackhammers, chain saws, pneumatic drills, riveting equipment, and mining, quarrying, and grinding machines. Exposure to certain chemicals such as vinyl chloride, commonly used in the rubber industry, may also increase susceptibility. Certain medications are potentially troublesome, and included in this category are oral contraceptives, ergot-containing drugs used to treat migraine headaches by way of vessel constriction, beta-adrenergic receptor blockers used in the treatment of high blood pressure, arrhythmias, or angina, as well as drugs used to treat cancer such as cisplatin, vinblastine, and bleomycinonicotine.[2]

4. What circulatory changes occur during an attack of Raynaud's syndrome?

Circulatory changes may be biphasic or triphasic. In the first stage an exaggerated shutdown in the form of sudden vasoconstriction, experienced as tingling, occurs as the body attempts to conserve heat and causes the fingers to turn pale or *white* (pallor). This is followed by *blueness* (cyanosis) resulting from sluggish flow of poorly oxygenated darker blood and is experienced as numbness. This is then followed by overwarming of the area at the end of the attack as the body overcompensates by way of exuberant blood flow rushing back into the fingers, manifesting as *redness* (rubor), throbbing, swelling, and a sensation of warmth (Fig. 1-1). When circulatory changes occur in a biphasic fashion, the fingers may seemingly bypass the middle cyanotic stage. This sequence may, in addition to cold exposure, be caused by stress, which triggers the release of hormones that initiate constriction. Regardless of the cause of this disorder, color changes do not occur above

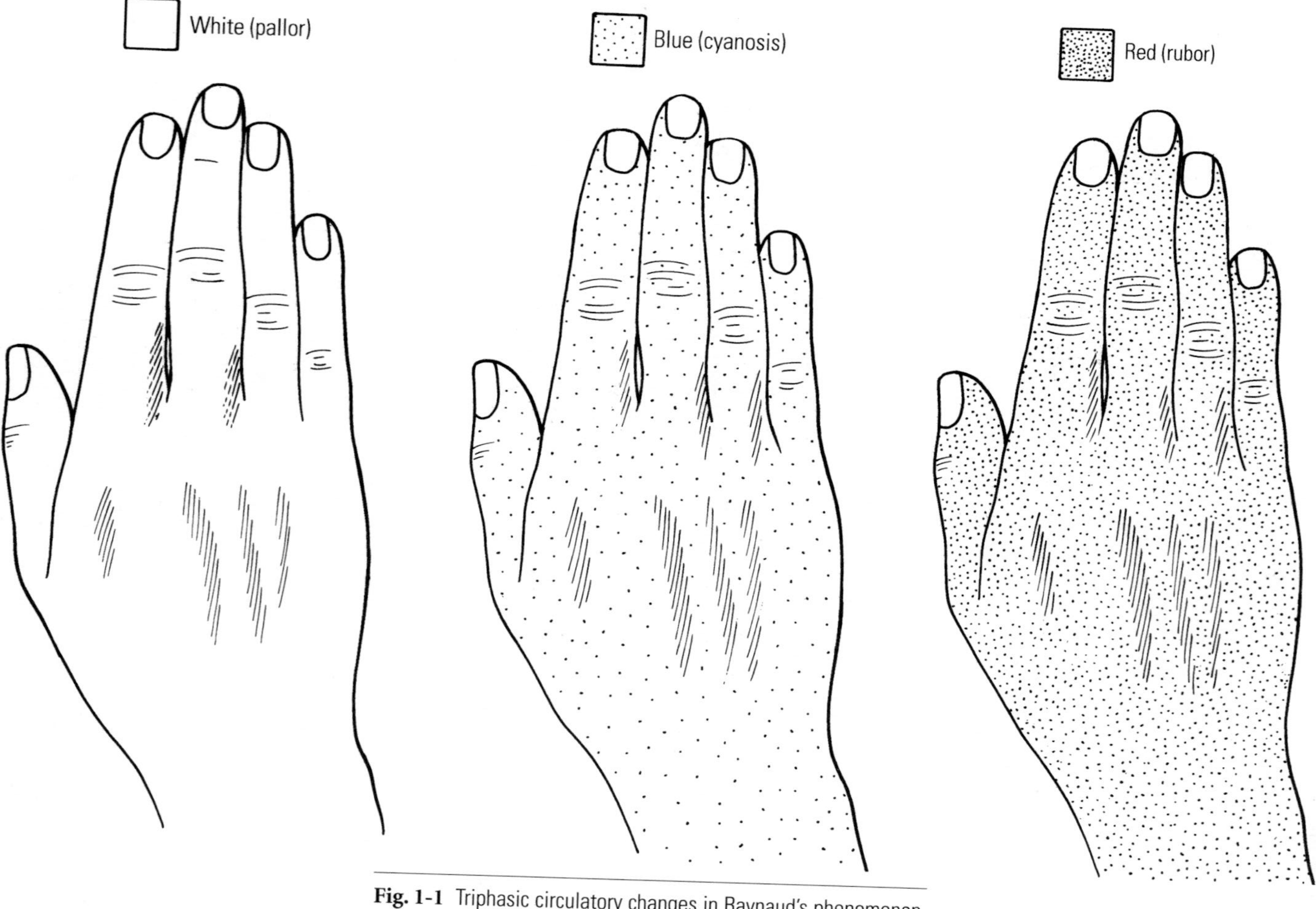

Fig. 1-1 Triphasic circulatory changes in Raynaud's phenomenon.

the metacarpophalangeal joints and rarely involve the thumb. This sharply demarcated pallor is reflective of spasm of the digital arteries. Usually, all digits are symmetrically affected. Although pain may occur, paresthesias are frequent during the attack, which typically lasts 20 to 30 minutes.

5. What are the differences between primary and secondary Raynaud's syndrome?

Primary Raynaud's syndrome (Raynaud's disease) is idiopathic and is five times more common in young women than in men,[2] with symptoms starting in females between 13 and 40 years of age. It occurs frequently in people who have migraine headaches or variant angina.[2] Most patients cannot precisely date the onset of symptoms. Mild symptoms may have been overlooked for years and recognized only in retrospect. Onset is gradual because the patient notices only an occasional mild and short-lasting attack during the winter season.[6] Over the subsequent years, the duration and severity of attacks may increase. Familial cases are not infrequent and this condition is not considered to be symmetric (such as involving the same fingers in both hands).

A diagnosis of primary Raynaud's is pronounced after a history of symptoms for at least 2 years without progression, no evidence of underlying cause, and absent or only minimal trophic changes.

The physical examination is often entirely normal, as are the radial, ulnar, and pedal pulses. Between attacks, however, the fingers and toes may be cool and perspire excessively. Sclerodactyly is thickening and tightening of the digital subcutaneous tissue and develops in 10% of patients. Digital angiography for diagnostic purposes is not indicated as part of the medical work-up.[2]

The prognosis for Raynaud's disease is good. Some 50% of patients show improvement of this disorder, which may completely disappear after several years.

Secondary Raynaud's syndrome (Raynaud's phenomenon) may start in later years, usually after 50 years of age. It may also start more abruptly, occur on one side or one finger only, and be more severe. Here, signs and symptoms of the underlying disease occur within 2 years of the onset of symptoms, and painful ulcerations of the fingers and toes are more common and more troublesome because they may eventually become gangrenous and require amputation. Raynaud's disease in males is most often of this second variety. Secondary Raynaud's is associated with what were previously described as collagen vascular diseases (such as scleroderma, rheumatoid arthritis, and lupus). These diseases have in common vasculitis, a process that thickens the walls of blood vessels thus reducing blood flow. Raynaud's in such patients is attributable to both vessel disease and vessel spasm, a combination that may account for why the secondary form is more severe than the primary. Secondary Raynaud's may also be caused by diseases causing arterial blockage.

6. What is the differential diagnosis?

The differential diagnosis of Raynaud's syndrome includes thoracic outlet compression syndromes (see Chapter 18), primary pulmonary hypertension, acrocyanosis, a history of drug ingestion or exposure, and atherosclerosis. Although the former condition may be excluded by appropriate maneuvers, the latter is a frequent cause of Raynaud's disease in men over 50 years old. Thromboangiitis obliterans is an uncommon cause but should be considered in young men who smoke cigarettes. Approximately 15% of patient's exhibiting Raynaud's symptoms eventually develop a connective tissue disorder, particularly scleroderma. In fact, Raynaud's may be the only symptom for many years before the full-blown manifestation of systemic sclerosis. Prognosis of Raynaud's disease stemming from the latter condition is unsatisfactory, especially when the condition has progressed to ischemic digital ulceration. Gangrene and autoamputation may then follow.[2,6]

A diagnosis of primary Raynaud's is pronounced after a history of symptoms for at least 2 years without progression, no evidence of underlying cause, and absent or only minimal trophic changes.

7. What treatment strategy is appropriate in Raynaud's syndrome?

The following rehabilitative treatment strategy suffices for a patient with mild or infrequent attacks:

- Biofeedback teaches patients to "think" their fingers are warm by consciously wresting out of the unconscious autonomic regulation of finger temperature so as to prevent and abort future attacks of Raynaud's syndrome. Training sessions typically last 30 to 60 minutes and are repeated twice a week for a total of 10 sessions. At each session the temperature of the patient's fingertips is recorded with the results visually displayed so that the patient can visually detect tiny increases in finger temperature.[5]

- Circulatory conditioning involves "teaching" the arteries to remain open despite the fact that the person is out in the cold. Treatment involves sitting outdoors in cool weather while placing one's hands in a pail of warm water. This is repeated several times a day, 10 minutes at a time, every other day over a period of 3 to 4 weeks.[3]
- One should eat a good breakfast. Skipping breakfast results in low blood glucose, which triggers epinephrine (adrenaline) release, which in turn causes small-vessel constriction.
- Keeping the chest warm is important because the body reacts to central warmth by shifting blood from the core to cooler peripheral areas.
- Mittens are better than lined gloves and are to be used when the patient is opening a refrigerator or freezer door, taking out the trash, or reaching for the outdoor mailbox.
- Use of earmuffs, muffler, and scarf.
- Use of electrically heated socks or mittens.
- Wearing layered clothing.
- Avoidance of nicotine and caffeine.
- Avoidance of smoking because smoking causes cutaneous vasoconstriction.
- Use of tepid water to wash vegetables or dishes, or while washing laundry by hand.
- Placement of rubber caps on keys and outside doorknobs.
- Letting the car warm up before driving.
- Fitting the steering wheel with an insulated cover, such as a fleece.
- Use of fabric seat covers.
- Use of cup warmers to hold cold drinks.
- Wearing of reflective inner soles in shoes.
- Learning stress-reducing relaxation techniques.

When Raynaud's syndrome is more frequent or severe, especially when trophic changes or ulcerations have occurred, conservative treatment is supplemented by drug therapy. Of the calcium-channel blockers, nifedipine is the drug of choice. Reserpine, a drug that interferes with sympathetic nerve activity, and topical nitroglycerin or prostaglandin ointment have also been found to be helpful in relieving ischemia during attacks. Preganglionic sympathectomy may be initially beneficial, but the long-term benefits have been disappointing.[6]

References

1. Arms K, Camp PS: *Biology,* ed 2, Philadelphia, 1982, Saunders College Publishing.
2. Isselbacher KJ, editor: *Harrison's principles of internal medicine,* vol 1, ed 13, New York, 1994, Health Professions Div/McGraw-Hill.
3. Jobe JB et al: Home treatment for Raynaud's disease, *J Rheumatol* 12:953-956, 1985.
4. *The Merck Manual,* ed 15, Rahway, N.J., 1987, Merck Sharp & Dohme Research Laboratories.
5. *The New York Times:* HEALTH, B2, Thursday, Dec 4, 1989.
6. Wyngaarden JB, Smith LH, Bennet JC: *Cecil textbook of medicine,* vol 1, Philadelphia, 1992, Saunders.

Recommended reading

Jobe JB et al: Home treatment for Raynaud's disease, *J Rheumatol* 12:953-956, 1985.

Volar Nodule and Flexion Contracture of Ring Finger

2

A 51-year-old jovial white man with a thick Scottish accent complains of no longer being able to clap his hands, put on his gloves, shake hands, or wash his face without sticking his right ring finger in his eye. His past medical history includes bouts of gout, non-insulin dependent diabetes, and a childhood history of epilepsy, and he mentions that his father was plagued by trigger finger and carpal tunnel syndrome. He also discloses that he had pulmonary tuberculosis approximately 18 years previously. He exhibits normal strength to all fingers including his involved ring finger, which is 70° flexed at the right metacarpophalangeal joint of the fourth finger without interphalangeal joint involvement. When asked, the patient reports that his finger remains flexed all day and all night. When questioned further, the patient admits to drinking three to four glasses of scotch vermouth per day since his wife was accidentally killed during a motor vehicle accident 7 years previously. He denies any other such manifestation elsewhere on his person.

OBSERVATION Pitting, fissuring, puckering, and dimpling of skin over right distal palmar crease on the ulnar side of the hand, with the area corresponding to the ring finger drawn into pits and folds.

PALPATION Prominent nodules are felt at the ring and little fingers of both hands, and the involved finger cannot be passively straightened.

MUSCLE STRENGTH Normal.

1. **What is most likely this gentleman's diagnosis?**
2. **What is the evolution of this disease?**
3. **What is the pathogenesis of this disease?**
4. **What is the epidemiology of this disorder?**
5. **Is there a genetic component to this disorder?**
6. **Where else in the body does a similar disorder manifest?**
7. **Which fingers are most commonly involved?**
8. **How rapidly does this disease progress?**
9. **What conservative treatment is attempted for milder cases before surgical intervention?**
10. **What are two indications for surgery, and what is the therapist's responsibility for monitoring the progression of contracture?**
11. **What are the risks of surgery?**
12. **What type of operations are used in the surgical correction of this disease?**

13. What postoperative therapy is indicated?

14. What other pathologic condition affecting the fingers involves nodular development?

1. What is most likely this gentleman's diagnosis?

In 1832 the Parisian surgeon Baron Dupuytren described a progressive nonpainful benign flexion deformity of the fingers caused by a contracture of the palmar and digital fasciae (that is, aponeurosis) as well as the adjacent digital flexor tendon sheaths. The *palmar aponeurosis* consists of four broad divergent bands that extend to the base of the fingers (Fig. 2-1). Early in the course of this disease there is painless proliferation of fibroblasts, histologically manifesting as a low-grade inflammatory fibrosis that results in the transformation of noncontractile tissue into contractile tissue. Diagnosis is made by visual inspection and palpation (Fig. 2-2).

2. What is the evolution of this disease?

The stages in the evolution of this disease are not distinct and begin as a tender[6] nodular thickening at the distal palmar crease of the ring finger that may spread to involve the middle finger. With the passage of time the nodules enlarge and spread longitudinally toward the proximal palmar crease as cordlike bands. As the tenderness subsides,[5] fibrosis expands to involve the surrounding adjacent digital flexor tendon sheaths; contracture develops in the form of subcutaneous cords that extend proximally to the base of the palm and, of greatest concern, distally to encompass the *natatory ligament*[4] (Fig. 2-3) at the base of the fingers.[6] Once the disease has migrated this far, it is only a matter of time before it involves the digital fascia. Subcutaneous cords are not to be confused with the more deeply located flexor tendons, since active finger flexion remains unaffected. The natatory ligament extends across the distal part of the palm, supporting each web space and ending in the first web at the base of the thumb. When this ligament is diseased, the digits cannot be separated.

As the flexion deformity continues, secondary contractures occur in the skin, nerves, blood vessels, and adjacent joint capsules,[6] with eventual articular cartilage destruction.[8] Extension of the involved fingers

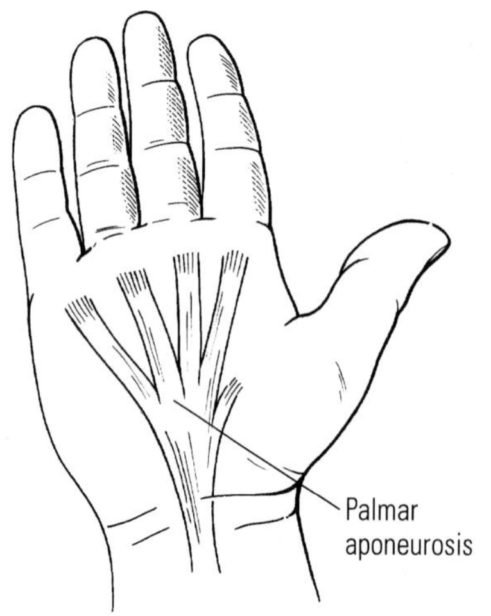

Fig. 2-1 The palmar aponeurosis is composed of four broad and divergent bands that extend to the base of the fingers.

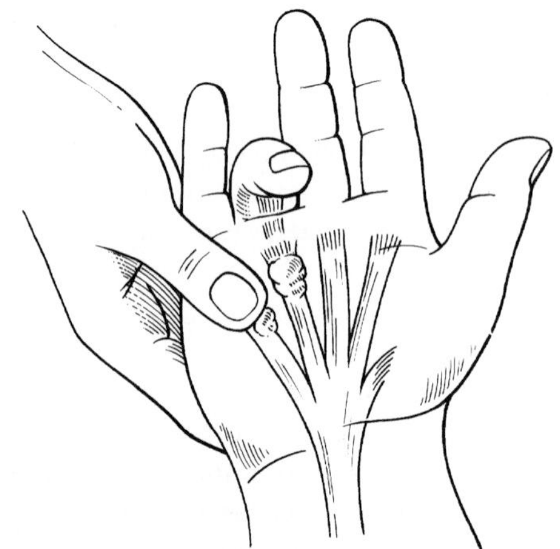

Fig. 2-2 In Dupuytren's contracture the fascia (comprising the palmar aponeurosis and natatory ligament) has palpable thickenings or nodules.

becomes impossible in advanced cases. The underlying fascia is normally attached to the skin so that gripping or pinching an object will occur without the skin or the grasped object sliding away. With Dupuytren's disease there is puckering and dimpling of the overlying skin in the area of the distal palmar crease on the *ulnar* side of the hand caused by adhesion of the skin to the underlying fascia.

3. What is the pathogenesis of this disease?

The cause of this disease remains unclear, though an association exists between Dupuytren's contracture and chronic alcoholism with liver cirrhosis or chronic use of anticonvulsant medication, suggestive of a hormonally affected enzyme abnormality permitting overactivity of myofibroblasts.[5] Gout and diabetes are also associated with this condition, as are tuberculosis, liver disease, chronic invalidism, epilepsy, and patients with pulmonary tuberculosis.[1] Repeated microtrauma may play a role. It is not understood why the ring or little fingers are most commonly involved or why thickening may be quiescent for years and then within a brief time cause symptomatic digital contracture.[5] This disorder may appear as a late sequel to shoulder-hand syndrome after myocardial infarction.

4. What is the epidemiology of this disorder?

Victims tend to be northern Europeans, particularly of Celtic descent.[5] This disorder is common to middle-aged white males to the extent that four out of every five patients are male.[2] However, after menopause the sex

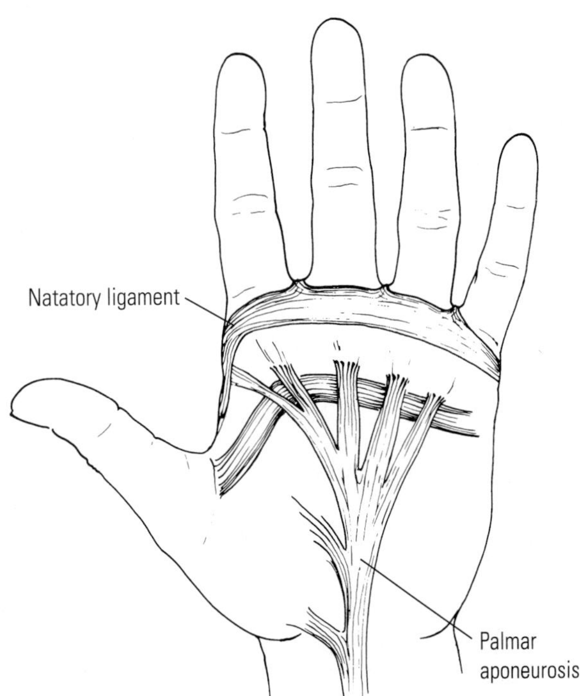

Fig. 2-3 The natatory ligament and palmar aponeurosis. Once the natatory ligament becomes fibrotic, fibrosis will soon spread to the adjacent fascia of the digital flexor tendon sheaths. Additionally, natatory ligament involvement precludes separation of the digits. (From McFarlane RM, Albion U: Dupuytren's disease. In Hunter JM, Schneider LH, Mackin EJ, Callahan AD, editors: *Rehabilitation of the hand: surgery and therapy,* ed 3, St. Louis, 1990, Mosby.)

ratio tends to equalize. In 5% of patients similar contractures occur in the feet.[6] One or both hands may be affected, whereas the right hand is more frequently affected when involvement is unilateral.

5. Is there a genetic component to this disorder?

The genetic profile of this condition implies mendelian dominance with incomplete penetrance. This means that family members may or may not be similarly affected.[5]

6. Where else in the body does a similar disorder manifest?

A similar pathologic process in the plantar fascia of the foot in which fascial thickening develops in the sole of the foot *(Lederhose disease)* as well fibrous plaques within the fascia of the shaft of the penis *(Peyronie's disease)*.[4]

7. Which fingers are most commonly involved?

The disease affects the ulnar side of the hand with the ring finger most commonly affected; the fifth, third, second, and first fingers are then affected in decreasing order of frequency.[7] The latter two are more rarely involved.

8. How rapidly does this disease progress?

Some contractures develop quickly over a matter of weeks, whereas others may progress for years. Long remissions followed by exacerbation with increasing deformity may occur.[6] Thus, although it is a progressive disease, one cannot predict how rapidly the disease will progress from the appearance of the initial nodule to full-blown finger-joint contracture.

9. What conservative treatment is attempted for milder cases before surgical intervention?

Therapeutic intervention focuses on prevention of secondary joint contractures by means of:

- Orally administered vitamin E.[4]
- Iontophoresis over nodule with Iodex (iodine with methyl salicylate) using the negative pole.
- Ultrasound to follow iontophoresis so as to disperse Iodex within soft tissue, applied during passive stretch into extension.
- Posterior extension splints.[9]
- In the early stage of this disease teach the patient to stretch palm and fingers vigorously out into extension in an attempt to elongate the palmar fascia as fast as it contracts.[2]
- Moist heat before stretching, followed by cold application.[9]

10. What are two indications for surgery, and what is the therapist's responsibility for monitoring the progression of contracture?

The only way to alter the course of the disease process is to surgically remove diseased tissue.[4] However, surgical repair should not be performed before contractures develop.[6] Indications for surgery revolve around whether contracture has occurred at the metacarpophalangeal (MP) joint or the interphalangeal (IP) joint. MP joint contractures, regardless of severity, are usually correctable because the collateral ligaments and capsule of the MP joints are stretched taut when the joint is in flexion and therefore without restriction to full extension once the offending fascia is released.[4] Because of this, there is no urgency to operate when the MP joint alone is affected, and it is best to leave it alone until functional limitations have developed[5] for fear of leaving the patient with a worse hand than before.[5] It is best to wait to advise the patient to operate until the *MP joint contractures are at least 30°*.

Additionally, the collateral ligaments stabilizing the IP joints are such that any position of flexion will cause their quick foreshortening. *Fifteen degrees of proximal interphalangeal joint (PIP) contracture* is a definite indication for surgery,[4] whereas procrastination until contracture reaches 50° is too late because the joint will respond poorly to surgery.[5] Distal interphalangeal joint (DIP) flexion contracture is rare and, similar to the situation of contracture greater than 15° of the PIP, it is difficult to correct. In contrast, DIP hyperextension is more common, is most frequently seen in the little finger, and is compensatory to severe PIP flexion.[4]

11. What are the risks of surgery?

The shortcomings of surgery include:

- A triad of skin necrosis, skin infection, and hematoma.[4]
- Surgical injury that may itself generate scarring and joint stiffness.
- Risk of laceration of digital nerves because their course is frequently distorted by contracted fascia.
- Disease recurrence in operated areas or extension into previously undisturbed portions of the hand.[5]

12. What type of operations are used in surgical correction of this disease?

Surgical procedures

Partial palmar fasciectomy. Removal of only the diseased fascia without excision of the uninvolved portion and effective in most instances. It should be made clear to the patient that the disease may indeed recur elsewhere in the palm. This procedure permits full correction of MP joint deformity.

The more radical complete fasciectomy. Removal of all palmar fascia in the palm and finger so as to preclude any source of recurrent contracture. Here maximum correction of the PIP joints is attempted, though with this procedure there is a greater risk for complications as well as prolonged if not permanent disability.[4]

By the time the finger is flexed down into the palm the joint has usually become frozen and uncorrectable. In some cases, the affected digit is amputated through the neck of the metacarpal.[3]

13. What postoperative therapy is indicated?

Prolonged postoperative care may be required for several months and is necessary to obtain optimal results. Recovery time is variable. With most patients, hand function will be incapacitated for 6 to 8 weeks.[4]

Treatment

- Initially record edema at same anatomic landmarks with circumferential measurements and progress to volumetric measurements once wounds have healed.
- Accurately measure the range of motion with a finger goniometer.
- Reassure patients that healing will progress over the coming weeks because patients are often startled by the horrible wound appearance.
- Active range of motion exercises begin the first postoperative day and include the following regimen performed for three or four sets of 10 repetitions per day:
  1. Thumb opposition to each fingertip, abduction, and extension
  2. Finger blocking (DIP joint flexion with the PIP joint and MP joint held in extension with the uninvolved hand, followed by PIP joint flexion with MP joint extension)
  3. Flexion of each finger to the thenar eminence
  4. Fist making
  5. Finger abduction and adduction
  6. Finger extension
  7. Full wrist motion and thumb range of motion
- Caution patient against overdoing his or her exercises, so as not to cause edema and pain.
- Tendon-gliding exercises may be begun by the second postoperative week.
- Instruct patients in gentle passive range of motion of all joints.

- Posterior extension splint fabricated at initial therapy session and necessary adjustments made with frequent visits. Splint removal is permitted only for wound care and exercise. Remember that the MP capsule and ligaments are taut in flexion, whereas the IP capsule and ligaments are taut in extension. In the event that a digit shows early signs of recurring contracture (most frequently seen in the little finger's PIP joint) a splint with a Velcro loop over the outrigger serves to provide extension force instead of a finger loop and rubber band. The Velcro provides a static pull and may be adjusted to provide increased tension as tolerated by the patient between treatments.
- If flexion is a problem, flexion splinting may be necessary and is worn by day; night splinting is reserved for extension.
- Scar management is by lanolin massage to both palm and digits with small, deep, circular strokes over the scar for 10 minutes before each exercise session. After massage, excess lanolin should be removed to prevent skin maceration.
- Desensitization is appropriate in the occasional patient experiencing hypersensitivity beginning with fur and progressing to vibration for 10 minutes each waking hour.
- Remove Velcro straps three or four times per day to flex fingers to distal phalanx crease actively or with active assistance, as well as full extension, fist making, finger blocking, finger abduction and adduction, flexion of each finger to thenar eminence, as well as wrist and thumb circumduction for 10 repetitions per set.
- Whirlpool bath.
- Progress to more difficult exercises (such as crossing fingers, passing coin from finger to finger, using handgrips and putty, and functional exercises).
- Having regained full flexion and extension of the fingers, the patient is advised to continue to wear the night splint for 3 months. Despite this supervised splinting, scar contracture may cause 10% to 15% flexion contracture at the PIP joint.[4]

14. What other pathologic condition affecting the fingers involves nodular development?

Trigger finger is another disorder involving nodules as well as the digital flexor tendon sheaths and, unlike Dupuytren's disease, may also involve the synovial sheaths enveloping those tendons.[6] With Dupuytren's disease, active finger flexion remains complete but not so for trigger finger.[6]

The function of the digital flexor tendon retinacular sheath (that is, the *annular ligament*) is to tightly restrain the tendon as it crosses the flexed MP joint, serving as a simple pulley to prevent bowstringing from origin to insertion during contraction.

Repetitive gliding of the tendon under the restraining sheath as from excessive repetitive handwork or unconscious fist clenching may exceed the lubricating capacity of synovial fluid. This may be worsened by the presence of a sesamoid bone, osteoarthritis,[7] or rheumatoid arthritis.[6] The resulting friction generates localized inflammation at the point where the tendon enters the sheath, causing swelling of the tendon[3] *(tendinitis),* which over time irritates the opening of the sheath causing inflammation and thickening *(tenosynovitis)* (see p. 16). This further restricts tendon gliding, and a vicious cycle is established in which swelling aggravates constriction, and the constriction aggravates the swelling.

Trigger finger progresses to the development of a fusiform swelling—a *nodule* in either the deep or the superficial flexor tendon or tendons at a *metacarpal head*[6] (Fig. 2-4). Palpation over the metacarpal head reveals a tender nodule that moves with the tendon. Early on, this thickened portion may pop in and out of the constricted sheath with a slightly painful click or grating when the finger is *flexed* or *extended,* akin to pulling a knotted rope through a narrow stretch of pipe[5] (Fig. 2-5). Although the *sensation is subjectively perceived at the proximal interphalangeal joint,* the nodule may be palpated just proximal to the metacarpophalangeal joint. The digit often locks in flexion when the patient arises from sleep.[7] As pathologic changes in the tendon and sheath progress, intermittent locking gives way to flexion of the IP joint on the

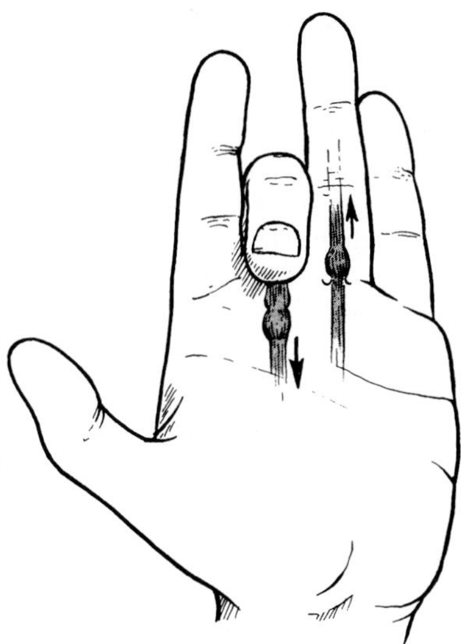

Fig. 2-4 Trigger finger. Locking may occur in either finger flexion or finger extension. (From Dandy DJ: *Essential orthopaedics and trauma,* Edinburgh, 1989, Churchill Livingstone.)

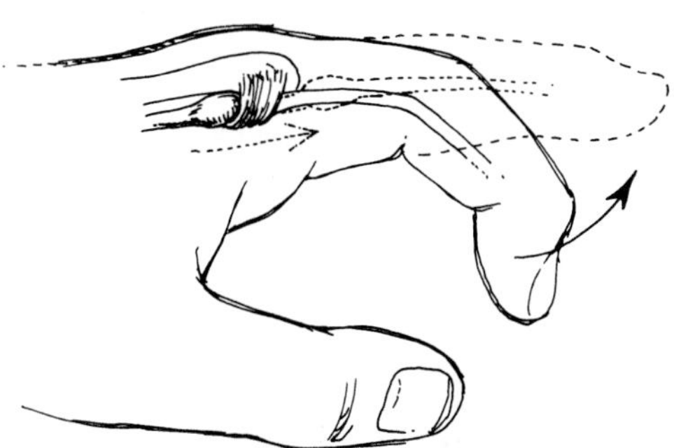

Fig. 2-5 The nodule within the tendon is restrained by the flexor retinaculum sheath on attempted extension. Persistent extension will result in a click sound as the nodular portion of the tendon is forced past the stricture. (From Meals RA: *One hundred orthopaedic conditions every doctor should understand,* St. Louis, 1992, Quality Medical Publishing.)

MP joint arrested in midrange, since the flexors are stronger than the extensors. Extension becomes possible only when performed passively as when the nodule is forced through the stricture. The finger then extends with a click, imparting a crepitation to the examiner's hand.[6]

Early treatment consists in splinting the finger in extension at night along with nonsteroidal anti-inflammatory medication. When more chronic, a steroid injection with a local anesthetic may be indicated. In recalcitrant cases surgical release of the tendon by longitudinal incision of the thickened sheath is indicated.

References

1. Berkon R: *The Merck manual of diagnosis and therapy,* Rahway, N.J., 1987, Merck Sharp & Dohme.
2. Cyriax J: *Textbook or orthopaedic medicine,* vol 1: *Diagnosis of soft tissue lesions,* ed 8, London, 1988, Bailliere-Tindall.
3. Dandy DJ: *Essential orthopaedics and trauma,* Edinburgh, 1989, Churchill Livingstone.
4. McFarlane RM, Albion U: *Dupuytren's disease: rehabilitation of the hand: surgery and therapy,* ed 3, St. Louis, 1990, Mosby.
5. Meals RA: *One hundred orthopaedic conditions every doctor should understand,* St. Louis, 1992, Quality Medical Publishing.
6. Netter FH: *The CIBA collection of medical illustrations,* vol 8: *Musculoskeletal system,* part 2, Summit, N.J., 1990, CIBA-Geigy Corp.
7. Rodnan GP, Schumacher HR: *Primer on the rheumatic diseases,* ed 8, Atlanta, 1983, The Arthritis Foundation.
8. Salter RB: *Textbook of disorders and injuries of the musculoskeletal system,* ed 2, Baltimore, 1990, Williams & Wilkins.
9. Saunders HD: *Evaluation, treatment, and prevention of musculoskeletal disorders,* Bloomington, Minn., 1985, Educational Opportunities.

Recommended reading

Hill N: Current concepts review: Dupuytren's contracture, *J Bone Joint Surg* 67A:1439-1443, 1985.

Hueston JT, Tubicra R: *Dupuytren's disease,* Edinburgh, 1985, Churchill Livingstone.

McFarlane RM, Albion U: Dupuytren's disease. In Hunter JM, Schneider LH, Mackin EJ, Callahan AD, editors: *Rehabilitation of the hand: surgery and therapy,* ed 3, St. Louis, 1990, Mosby. See also McFarlane RM, MacDermid JC: Dupuytren's disease. In Hunter JM, Mackin EJ, Callahan AD, editors: *Rehabilitation of the hand: surgery and therapy,* ed 4, St. Louis, 1995, Mosby.

3

Painful Thumb after Intense Bout of Hammering

An aspiring carpenter spent his first day of apprenticeship atop the roof of a refurbished two-family house, laying down precut planks in slanted fashion across the roof and hammering them down every 4 inches around their periphery using 5-inch nails. He would spend the next 5 months doing this work on six adjacent homes whose roofs were gutted by a fire that had spread from one to the other because of the proximity of homes in that neighborhood. Eager to impress his employer, he worked with gusto for 6 hours at a time without rest except for a quick 15-minute lunch break toward the end of each day. At the end of 1 week's work he was awakened at night by a searing hot pain at the base of his right thumb that came on gradually and partially abated when he wrung his hand. During the following week the same pain would occur after hammering for 2 hours and intensified as he attempted to ignore it.

PAST MEDICAL HISTORY Unremarkable, as was family history. No medications aside from aspirin. When asked, patient could not remember falling and landing on an outstretched hand in recent or past history.

SUBJECTIVE Patient reports decrease in pain upon resting from work and upon taking one or two aspirins per day as needed. When asked, patient reported no numbness, excess sweating, hand color changes, tingling, or paresthesia. The patient was right handed.

OBSERVATION No swelling, color changes, or atrophy.

PALPATION Point tenderness at base of thumb. The skin was not excessively moist. Fine crepitus was noted over the length of tendons in the anatomical snuffbox.

RANGE OF MOTION Grossly the range of motion was within functional limits though touching the tips of the thumb and small finger was slow and painful. Passive thumb extension and abduction beyond midrange was painful. All other fingers were within functional limits.

STRENGTH TESTING All thumb movements were painful, and designation of muscle grade was deferred. All other fingers tested normal.

SENSORY Intact to light touch, pinprick, and temperature to entire hand.

VOLUMETRIC MEASUREMENT No edema.

PULSES Normal.

UPPER QUARTER SCREENING No evidence of double-crush phenomenon, or of different site as cause of symptoms.

SPECIAL TESTS Positive Finkelstein's test.

1. **Based on the history and examination what is most likely wrong with this patient?**
2. **What is the difference between tendinitis, tenosynovitis, and tenovaginitis, and why are the latter two appropriate in describing this patient's condition?**
3. **What are three separate yet related sources of friction causing inflammation in this patient?**
4. **Which segments of the population are more prone to this condition?**
5. **Which predisposing movements identify the mechanism causing this overuse syndrome?**
6. **What signs and symptoms are common to this malady, and what provocative tests or movements elicit the latter?**
7. **How is concomitant inflammation of the tendon of the third dorsal compartment evaluated?**
8. **What other conditions must be ruled out upon eliciting pain and tenderness at the snuffbox?**
9. **Which metabolic abnormalities, though not causative, are associated with this condition?**
10. **What medical management is typical for this patient, and what, if any, are deleterious effects of this management?**
11. **What surgical management is appropriate for this patient, and what complications are associated with surgery?**
12. **What therapeutic intervention will best rehabilitate this patient?**

1. **Based on the history and examination what is most likely wrong with this patient?**

De Quervain's disease is tenosynovitis and tenovaginitis[5,19] at the base of the thumb involving the tendons of the first dorsal compartment (the abductor pollicis longus and the extensor pollicis brevis)[17] and forming the radial border of the anatomic snuffbox. The tendon of the extensor pollicis longus passing through the third dorsal compartment and defining the ulnar border of the snuffbox is less commonly involved (Fig. 3-1).

2. **What is the difference between tendinitis, tenosynovitis, and tenovaginitis, and why are the latter two appropriate in describing this patient's condition?**

Tendinitis occurs in sheath-lacking structures such as the Achilles tendon, supraspinatus tendon, or the bicipital aponeurosis on the ulna. Tendinitis is an inflammation of the tendon with subsequent scarring either (1) within the substance of the tendon or (2) at the insertion of tendon into bone (i.e., tenoperiosteal junction, TPJ).[5]

Tenosynovitis is an inflammation of synovial membrane with subsequent scarring (1) anywhere along the tendinosynovial complex or (2) at the insertion of tendon into bone, the tenoperiosteal junction; this may occur in the peroneal tendons, posterior tibialis tendon, or the distal biceps attachment on the radial tuberosity. Synovial sheaths are like bursae except that they are (1) tubular structures and (2) are found around superficial tendons and provide decreased friction in potentially high-friction areas; thus they are found mostly in hands and feet because these distal areas contain an excess of long superficial tendons.[8]

In addition, certain synovial sheath-tendon complexes are bound down and anchored by fibrous sheaths, or tunnels, and prevent bowstringing when the wrist is flexed.[8] These sheaths act as simple pulleys to divert the line of pull from the long axis of the arm to the plane of the long axis of the hand. This ensheathment may be a source of additional inflammation and thickening *(tenovaginitis)*.

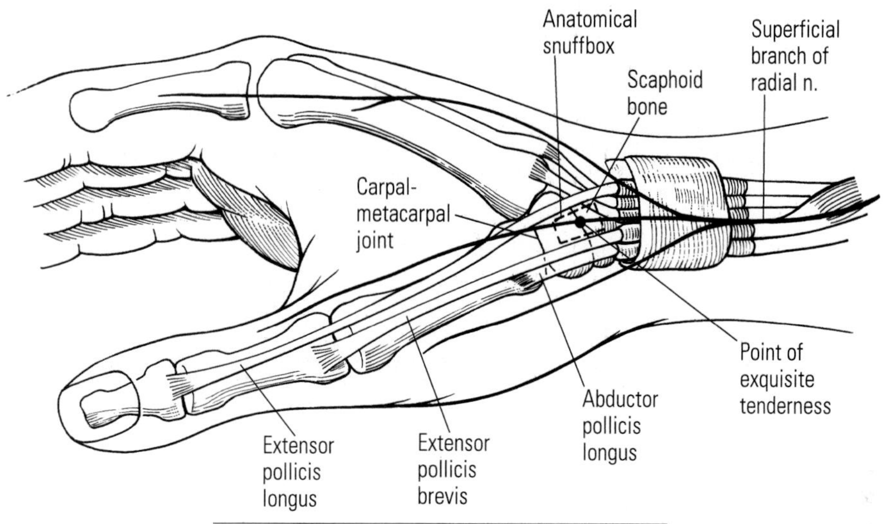

Fig. 3-1 Pertinent anatomy of de Quervain's disease.

3. What are three separate yet related sources of friction causing inflammation in this patient?

In de Quervain's disease there is an additional factor contributing to friction: a fibro-osseous canal. The tendons of the abductor pollicis longus (APL) and of the extensor pollicis brevis (EPB) pass through a shallow groove on the lateral aspect of the radial styloid.[1] If movement through this tunnel as well as against other structures is constant and repetitive, a vicious cycle of inflammation leading to synovitis is encouraged by friction (1) between the tendons, (2) between the tendons and their common tendon sheath, and (3) between the sheath and the bony groove of the radius.[1] A loss of blood flow may affect the nutritional status of the area[18] and contribute to a self-perpetuating cycle of inflammation. Since these structures are additionally roofed by the fibrous extensor retinaculum of the first dorsal compartment, inflammation may spread causing thickening[17] and eventual stenosis[8] of that tunnel.

4. Which segments of the population are more prone to this condition?

During wrist motion the tendons of the first dorsal compartment undergo approximately 105° of angulation as they course over several joints to their distal attachment. These angulations are greatest in females and may be viewed as an anatomic predisposing factor.[3] In addition, as much as 20% of the general population have an additional tendon passing through the first dorsal tunnel and attaching to a carpal bone.

5. Which predisposing movements identify the mechanism causing this overuse syndrome?

The most frequently documented occurrences of de Quervain's disease are in manual laborers who combine wrist motion and forearm rotation.[1,11] The classic case involves the carpenter who continuously hammers many nails, an action that involves repetitive and forceful ulnar deviation and flexion after radial deviation and extension of the wrist. Human tendons will not tolerate more than 1500 to 2000 manipulations per hour.[4] Bilaterally de Quervain's disease may occur in jackhammer operators[14] and is caused by bilateral symmetric trauma to both hands. A high incidence of de Quervain's disease occurs in women between 30 and 50 years of age,[17] three to 10 times more frequently than in men.[9,14,21]

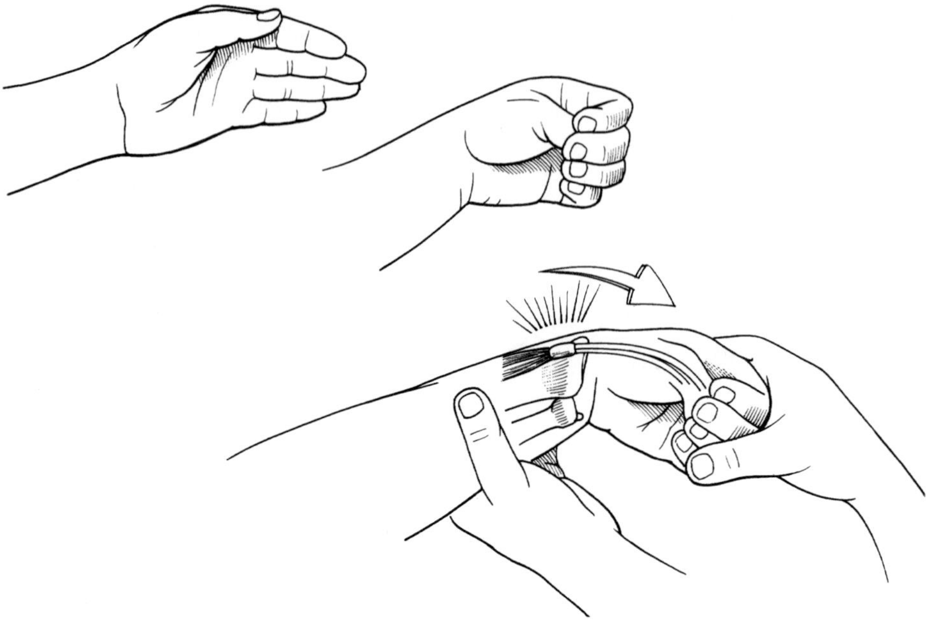

Fig. 3-2 Finkelstein's test. The wrist is sharply deviated ulnarly, provoking severe, sudden pain.

6. What signs and symptoms are common to this malady, and what provocative tests or movements elicit the latter?

Symptoms include hot searing pain over the radial aspect of the wrist that may radiate up the forearm or distally to the fingers.[13] By mimicking the motion that caused the pain in the first place, *Finkelstein's test* (Fig. 3-2) elicits pain by passively stretching the inflamed tendons. All thumb motion, in particular active or resisted extension and abduction of the thumb is painful, with resistance of the former regarded as the result of the hitchhiker's thumb test.[8] Supination is reported to be more painful than pronation. The patient may feel weakness and may demonstrate diminished grip and pinch strength. Since the radial styloid forms the proximal wall of the snuffbox, tenderness is elicited just proximal to the radial styloid. The area of the extensor sheath may also appear or feel thickened. Triggering of the thumb, not to be confused with trigger finger of the flexor sheath, secondary to increased involvement of the first dorsal compartment has been reported.[6] Fine crepitus may result from excessive overuse and resultant tenosynovitis.[5]

7. How is concomitant inflammation of the tendon of the third dorsal compartment evaluated?

Sometimes involvement of the extensor pollicis longus is found to accompany inflammation of the first dorsal compartment and is evaluated by testing the resisted thumb extension while stabilizing the proximal and distal joints. Discomfort with selective tension dictates rest and immobilization of this tendon.[10]

8. What other conditions must be ruled out upon eliciting pain and tenderness at the snuffbox?

Although excruciating pain in the area of the radial styloid is helpful in diagnosis, it is not pathognomonic of de Quervain's disease. Other causes must be ruled out and include the following:

- *Scaphoid fracture.* Since the scaphoid lies at the base of the anatomic snuffbox, pain in the hollow just distal to the radial styloid is characteristic of scaphoid fracture when followed by a history of falling forward on outstretched hands. When the hand is laid palm down against a flat surface, the bony resting points on the heel of the hand are the scaphoid tubercle radially and the pisiform tubercle ulnarly. When one falls on an outstretched arm and an extended wrist, the scaphoid tubercle is more vulnerable to fracture than the pisiform because the scaphoid is trapped against the distal end of the radius whereas the pisiform is free to move and usually escapes injury (see Fig. 5-2 and p. 43).

- *Radial nerve neuritis.* The superficial radial nerve (SRN) is purely sensory and supplies cutaneous innervation to the dorsoradial aspect of the thumb and thenar eminence, as well as the dorsum of the index, long, and ring fingers as far as the proximal interphalangeal joints. This nerve branches off the radial nerve at the level of the lateral epicondyle and travels under cover of the brachioradialis to emerge distally in the distal third of the forearm between the extensor carpi radialis longus and brachioradialis tendons where it becomes subcutaneous. Entrapment of the SRN may occur when the forearm is pronated, compressing the nerve by the scissors-like action of the two tendons.[7] Patients may complain of dysesthesia, numbness, and tingling in the radial nerve distribution, possibly with pain radiating proximally to the elbow or shoulder. A positive Tinel's sign may be elicited over the radial nerve and the junction of the middle and distal forearm. Wrist flexion, ulnar deviation, and forearm supination will increase symptoms because these positions place traction on the nerve.

  Compressive neuritis may also occur from a tight-fitting wristwatch, bangle, or handcuff, or from a tight cast.[6] Finkelstein's test will be positive. SRN neuritis is differentiated from de Quervain's disease by a maneuver that tenses the radial nerve. Beginning distally with thumb flexion, wrist ulnar deviation, and forearm pronation, one subjects the proximal upper extremity to the following sequence of postures: elbow flexion, shoulder depression, medial rotation, abduction, or extension as well as cervical lateral flexion.[2] Regardless of the cause of nerve damage, an electrophysiologic test with diminished amplitude of the sensory action potentials confirms the suspected diagnosis. Compression of the radial nerve secondary to de Quervain's disease is unlikely. Carpal tunnel syndrome in which the median nerve is compressed may occur secondary to acute and chronic flexor tenosynovitis.

- *Basal joint arthritis.* The carpometacarpal (CMC) joint of the thumb is the articulation of trapezium and the first metacarpal. Osteoarthritis has a predilection for the CMC joint of the thumb and is known as basal (or CMC) joint arthritis. This condition may yield painful thumb motion and a positive Finkelstein's test with pain not at the snuffbox but at the involved joint. Basal joint arthritis may be further distinguished from de Quervain's disease by a *positive axial compression test* (such as passive grinding and rotation of the metacarpal against the trapezium), resulting in pain, tenderness, and swelling over the site of the CMC joint. Unlike true de Quervain's disease, pain is not elicited on resisted thumb extension and abduction. Nor is pain experienced in that position that places the tendons and sheath on stretch (that is, ulnar wrist deviation while the thumb is fixed in flexion). Additionally, joint play movements at the CMC joint will be painful and restricted. Basal joint arthritis may be viewed on an x-ray film. Involvement of the interphalangeal joint of the thumb is more common in rheumatoid and psoriatic arthritis.

- There is a syndrome involving tenosynovitis of the tendons of the second dorsal compartment as that compartment is crossed over by the muscle bellies of the abductor pollicis longus (APL) and the extensor pollicis brevis (EPB) of the first dorsal compartment (Fig. 3-3). The significance of the term "outcropping muscles" describing the muscles of the first dorsal compartment is that although they lie within the deep layer of the forearm their tendons rise to the surface by "outcropping" so as to allow the extensor carpi radialis longus and brevis of the second dorsal compartment to pass through. The tendons of the second dorsal compartment may be stressed to elicit pain, swelling, and crepitus on wrist movement more proximal to that of de Quervain's disease. These tendons become palpable when the fist is clenched. This syndrome goes by many names such as *tenosynovitis crepitans, intersection syndrome, peritendinitis crepitans,* and *abductor pollicis longus bursitis.*

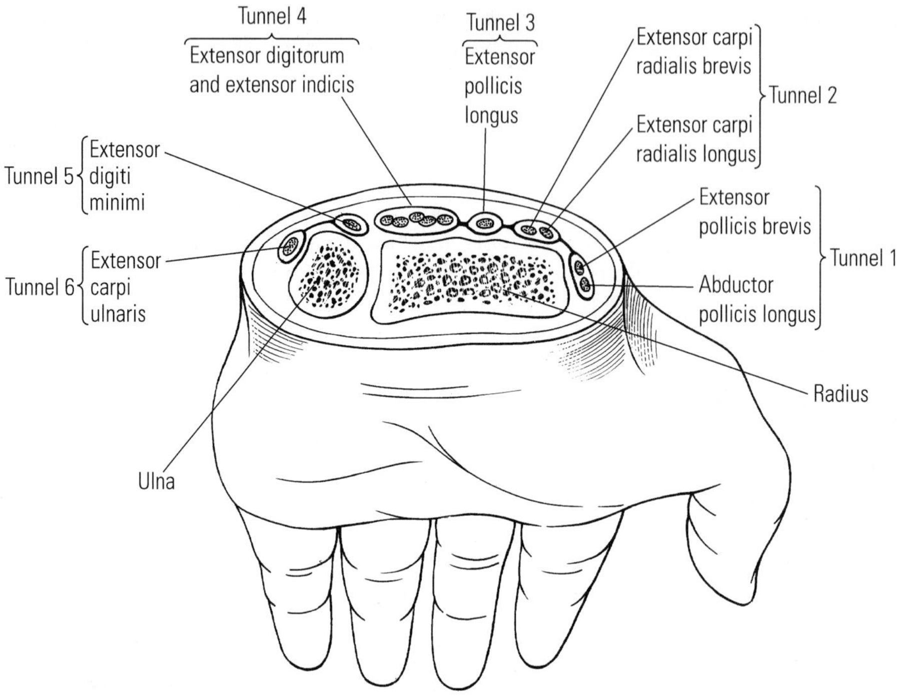

Fig. 3-3 The six tunnels on the dorsum of the wrist that transport the extensor tendons to the hand.

- *Double-crush phenomenon.* The double-crush phenomenon in which proximal disorders ranging from tennis elbow, shoulder capsulitis, or cervical spondylosis frequently coexist with de Quervain's disease (see p. 32).

9. Which metabolic abnormalities, though not causative, are associated with this condition?

Metabolic abnormalities, though not demonstrated to be causative, are at times associated with de Quervain's disease and include diabetes, hyperuricemia, hypothyroidism, rheumatoid arthritis, and gonococcal arthritis. De Quervain's disease may also, as in carpal tunnel syndrome, occur during pregnancy and may occasionally persist until nursing is terminated.[20] Patients who do not respond to simple therapeutic measures should be suspected of secondary medical conditions and be ruled out as causative factors.

10. What medical management is typical for this patient, and what, if any, are deleterious effects of this management?

Several steroidal injections are made directly into the fibrous sheath of the first dorsal compartment. The problems of steroids are well documented and may cause subcutaneous fat atrophy, tendon deterioration, and skin depigmentation.

11. What surgical management is appropriate for this patient, and what complications are associated with surgery?

If the second or third steroidal injection provides no relief, surgical decompression may be considered. De Quervain's tenosynovectomy involves slitting open the tendon's fibrous sheath of the first dorsal compartment by a transverse incision; this is favored over the longitudinal incision because it minimizes scar and keloid formation.[12,16] This is then followed by a longitudinal incision of the overlying retinaculum. After surgery the thumb is immobilized in a spica splint applied with the wrist in slight extension for 3 to 5 days, after which early mobilization is begun. Some surgeons prescribe immediate early active range of motion without mobilization.[16]

Complications after surgery primarily includes superficial radial nerve injury either from direct nerve laceration, vigorous retraction of the superficial radial nerve when the surgical field is exposed, or neuroma from scar hypertrophy. These problems may be caused when surgeons unaccustomed to the anatomy of the region.[6] These complications may not result in sensory loss but, rather, in extremely painful paresthesias such that some sensitive patients may not even tolerate anything touching their skin. This may be accompanied by reflex sympathetic dystrophy.[15] Another complication is tendon subluxation from overaggressive incision of too extensive a portion of the retinaculum overlying the first compartment structures.

12. What therapeutic intervention will best rehabilitate this patient?

Ninety percent of nonsevere cases of de Quervain's disease may expect relief with conservative management. Treatment may be divided into two phases.

Phase I (weeks 1 to 4)

- Rest.
- Iontophoresis or phonophoresis of anti-inflammatory agents into area of first dorsal compartment.
- Ice massage, with avoidance of prominences, for a maximum duration of 5 minutes.
- Nonsteroidal anti-inflammatory medication.
- Thumb spica splint is a forearm-based splint fabricated from a volar or radial approach; its design immobilizes the wrist, carpometacarpal, and metacarpophalangeal joints of the thumb and serves to rest both the radial wrist extensors and the proximal thumb. The following positions are prescribed: wrist in a 15° extension, carpometacarpal joint in a 40° to 50° palmar abduction, and the metacarpophalangeal joints in 5° to 10° of flexion to allow for light prehensile and opposition activities. The interphalangeal joint is left free to perform active motion unless the pollicis longus extensor is involved. It is very important to ensure that the superficial radial nerve and ulnar digital nerve of the thumb are not compromised. The splint is worn at all times except for removal for hygiene and exercise. Upon removal of the splint the patient is reminded not to exacerbate symptoms by "testing out his hand."
- Gentle active range of motion exercises for short periods lasting 10 to 20 minutes within the pain-free range are performed to prevent joint stiffness and adhesion formation between tendons and sheath, enhance circulation, and minimize protective posturing.
- Performing overhead finger pumping every few hours and encouraging the patient to elevate the involved hand above the heart as much as possible.
- Hygienic activities of daily living should be performed by gentle stabilization of the thumb against the lateral aspect of the index finger.
- Towel gathering and unfolding with the thumb initially actively splinted against the index finger and becoming actively involved as treatment progresses.
- Grasp and release of small objects emphasizing a wide variety of prehensile patterns that avoid overuse of first dorsal compartment tendons.[10]

Phase II (weeks 4 to 12)

In this stage the patient is gradually weaned from the protective splint during daylight hours but still wears it at night.

- Incorporate adaptive equipment, such as built-up handles for writing, or the use of a hammer and a bent handle.
- After beginning strengthening with isometric exercises, because this involves little or no tendon excursion, by pushing a dowel through putty with the thumb initially stabilized laterally on the proximal

phalanx of the index finger, the patient then progresses to placing the thumb around (such as medial to) the dowel and finally atop the dowel. Frequency is 5 minutes for three times per day. The patient is progressed to the subsequent position when multiple repetitions are pain free.
- Patient then progresses to isotonic strengthening by (1) moving the thumb up and down the length of a pencil while the fingers are wrapped transversely around the length of the pencil to provide graded resistance, (2) syringe use, (3) link belt fabrication, and (4) putty pinching.
- Isokinetic strengthening of thumb in liquid, as during daily bath.[10]

References

1. Boyes JH: *Bunnel's surgery of the hand,* Philadelphia, 1970, Lippincott.
2. Butler D: *Mobilization of the nervous system,* Melbourne, 1991, Churchill Livingstone.
3. Calliet R: *Hand pain and impairment,* Philadelphia, 1982, FA Davis.
4. Conklin JE, White WL: Stenosing tenosynovitis, *Surg Clin North Am* 40(2):531, 1960.
5. Cyriax J: *Textbook of orthopedic medicine,* vol 2, London, 1987, Bailliere-Tindall.
6. Dawson DM, Hallet M, Millender LH: *Entrapment neuropathies,* ed 2, Boston, 1990, Little, Brown & Co.
7. Dellon AL, Mackinnon SE: Susceptibility of the superficial sensory range of the radial nerve to form painful neuromas, *J Hand Surg* 9B:42-45, 1984.
8. Goldberg S: *Clinical anatomy made ridiculously simple,* Miami, 1988, MedMaster.
9. Hall CL: Chronic stenosing tenovaginitis of the wrist, *J Int College Surg* 14(1):48, 1950.
10. Hunter JM, Schneider LH, Mackin EJ, Callahan AD, editors: *Rehabilitation of the hand: surgery and therapy,* ed 3, St. Louis, 1990, Mosby.
11. Hymovich L, Lindholm M: Hand, wrist and forearm injuries, *J Occup Med* 8(11):573, 1966.
12. Keon-Cohn B: de Quervain's disease, *J Bone Surg* 33B(1):96, 1951.
13. Kilgore E, Graham W: *The hand: surgical and nonsurgical management,* Philadelphia, 1977, Lea & Febiger.
14. Leaao L: De Quervain's disease, *J Bone Joint Surg* 40A(5):1063, 1958.
15. Lee VH: The painful hand. In Moran C, editor: *Hand rehabilitation,* New York, 1986, Churchill Livingstone.
16. Muckart RD: Stenosing tenovaginitis of abductor pollicis longus and extensor pollicis brevis at the radial styloid (de Quervain's disease), *Clin Orthop* 33:201, 1964.
17. Netter FH: *The CIBA collection of medical illustrations,* vol 8: *Musculoskeletal system,* part 2, Summit, N.J., 1990, CIBA-Geigy Corp.
18. Poole B: Cumulative trauma disorder of the upper extremity from occupational stress, *J Hand Ther* 1(4):172, 1988.
19. Salter RB: *Textbook of disorders and injuries of the musculoskeletal system,* ed 2, Baltimore, 1987, Williams & Wilkins.
20. Schumacher HR, Bomalski JS: *Case studies in rheumatology,* Philadelphia, 1990, Williams & Wilkins.
21. Strandell G: Variations of the anatomy in stenosing tenosynovitis at the radial styloid process, *Acta Chir Scand* 113:234, 1957.
22. Viegas SF: Trigger thumb of de Quervain's disease, *J Hand Surg* 11A(2):235, 1986.

Recommended reading

Armstrong TJ, Fine LJ, Goldstein SA, et al: Ergonomics consideration in hand and wrist tendinitis, *J Hand Surg* [AM] 12A(5):830-837, 1987.

Conklin JE, White WL: Stenosing tenosynovitis, *Surg Clin North Am* 40:531, 1960.

Hunter JM, Schneider LH, Mackin EJ, Callahan AD, editors: *Rehabilitation of the hand: surgery and therapy,* ed 3, St. Louis, 1990, Mosby, p. 305.

Pick RY: de Quervain's disease: a clinical trial, *Clin Orthop* 143:165, 1979.

Saplys R, Mackinnon SE, Dellon AL: The relationship between nerve entrapment versus neuroma complications and the misdiagnosis of de Quervain's disease, *Contemp Orthop* 15:51-57, 1987.

Nocturnal Wringing of Painful Tingling Right Hand

4

A 51-year-old female pianist complains of annoying nighttime numbness of 6 weeks in duration to her entire right hand that is relieved by placing her hand under cold running water for 5 minutes. The patient is ambidextrous and admits to having recently performed intense calligraphy of some 300 invitations in preparation for her daughter's wedding with her left hand, which, she admits, "also feels funny." Numbness and tingling are prominent to her right index finger when driving her automobile or playing piano. She states that she had entered menopause 3 years previously. When asked, the patient also reveals that she is a non-insulin dependent diabetic of 6 years in duration but denies any paresthesias to the feet, loss of balance, history of injury, or any neck and shoulder pain.

OBSERVATION No swelling, trophic changes, atrophy, or deformity observed.

PALPATION No tenderness or swelling are present at hand, wrist, or cubital fossa; there is good capillary refilling.

RANGE OF MOTION Within functional limits to both hands.

MOTOR TESTS Good minus muscle strength in thumb opposition and abduction in right hand compared to a normal grade for left hand.

SENSATION Normal to light touch, two-point discrimination and vibration to all fingertips except for the thumb.

SELECTIVE TENSION Resisted pronation and supination, as well as all other resistive tests are negative.

SPECIAL TESTS Negative Allen test, positive Phalen test, negative Tinel sign, negative axial compression test of the spine, and negative hyperabduction test.

CLUE Nerve conduction velocities are as follows:

	Right	Left	Normal
Sensory latency across wrist	3.7	3.6	<3.5 msec
Motor latency across wrist	4.5	4.4	<4.5 msec

1. **What is most likely causing this woman's symptoms?**
2. **What is the cause of carpal tunnel syndrome (CTS)?**
3. **What anatomy is relevant to understanding this disorder?**
4. **What are the functions of the flexor retinaculum?**
5. **What is the clinical presentation?**
6. **What is the clinical course of the disorder?**
7. **What is the differential diagnosis?**
8. **What is anterior interosseous syndrome?**
9. **What are the electrophysiologic findings in CTS?**
10. **What other pathologic conditions are associated with CTS?**
11. **How is motor function best tested?**
12. **Which provocative tests elicit symptoms?**
13. **What disorders of the workplace are implicated as possible causes of CTS?**
14. **What chronic, rheumatologic, or metabolic disorders are associated with CTS?**
15. **What is the double-crush phenomenon?**
16. **What nonsurgical treatment or treatments are appropriate before surgical decompression?**
17. **What are indications for surgery, and what does surgery involve?**
18. **What is postsurgical management?**
19. **What sequelae may follow surgery?**

1. What is most likely causing this woman's symptoms?

Carpal tunnel syndrome (CTS) is one of the most common, best defined, and most carefully studied entrapment neuropathy. CTS commonly affects middle-aged females between 40 and 60 years of age,[6] that is, menopausal women, a characteristic suggestive of a hormonal aberration as a cause in the development of this disorder.[16] The most common cause of CTS is an idiopathic nonspecific flexor tenosynovitis[6] that may simply arise from chronic repetitive occupational stress.[16] CTS may occur acutely after lunate bone dislocation or from a Colles fracture and requires immediate medical attention so as to prevent acute nerve ischemia.[6]

2. What is the cause of carpel tunnel syndrome (CTS)?

The causes of CTS may be subdivided into one of four categories:

1. An increase in volume or tunnel contents secondary to nonspecific tenosynovitis of the flexor tendons within the carpal tunnel.
2. Thickening (fibrosis) of the transverse carpal ligament.
3. Alteration of the osseous margins of the carpus caused by fractures, dislocations, or arthritic joint changes.
4. Tumor or systemic disease.

3. What anatomy is relevant to understanding this disorder?

The median nerve enters the hand through an osseofibrous carpal tunnel that is bounded dorsally and laterally by the convex bony carpus and volarly by the thick transverse carpal ligament, otherwise known as the *flexor retinaculum*.[6] The corners of this tunnel are the pisiform, hamate, scaphoid tubercle, and trapezium tubercle.[17] The transverse carpal ligament spans between the scaphoid tubercle radially and the hamate bone ulnarly. The median nerve shares the tunnel with nine other flexor tendons, each of which is covered with two layers of synovium (Fig. 4-1). The radial and ulnar arteries, the ulnar nerve, and flexor palmaris longus do *not* pass through the carpal tunnel and are referred to as extracarpal structures. After its passage through the carpal tunnel, the median nerve divides into five digital branches,[6] the

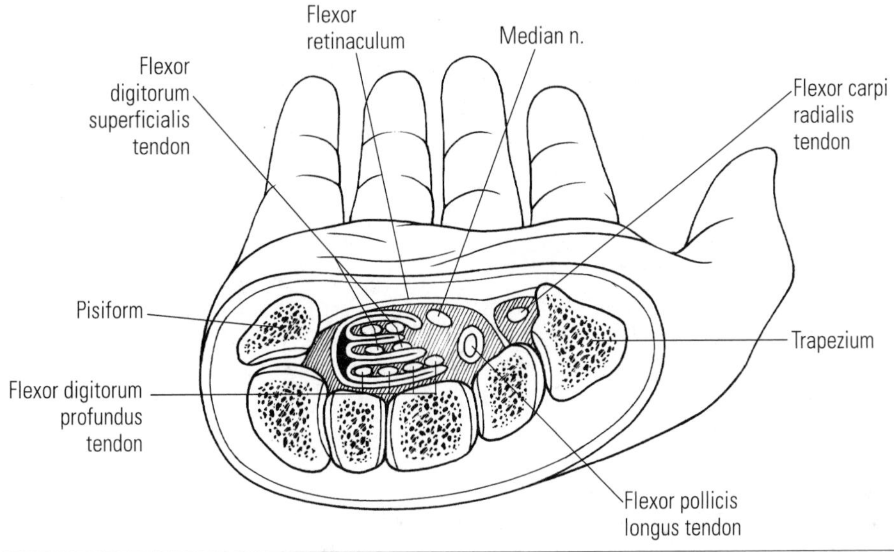

Fig. 4-1 Cross-sectional view of the carpal tunnel and its contents. The median nerve lies adjacent to the tendons of the flexor digitorum superficialis tendons.

most radial of which supplies the thenar musculature and the latter two finger lumbricales; the other four (ulnar) branches supply sensation to the palmer aspect of the lateral (that is, radial) three and a half digits and their dorsal fingertips. The palm itself is spared of sensory loss in CTS because the palmer cutaneous sensory branch takes leave of the median nerve before that nerve enters the carpal tunnel.[5] This cutaneous branching occurs approximately 3 cm proximal[6] to the transverse carpal ligament between the tendons of the palmaris longus and flexor carpi radialis muscles, beyond which the nerve travels superficially toward the palm (Fig. 4-2). The essential concept is that there is little if any spare space within the carpal tunnel, and so anything that decreases volume within the tunnel such as swollen tendons will occupy more space and will do so at the expense of the median nerve suffering ischemia.

4. What are the functions of the flexor retinaculum?

Forming the roof of the carpal tunnel, the stout transverse carpal ligament offers attachment for the thenar and hypothenar muscles, helps maintain the transverse carpal arch of the hand, prevents bowstringing of the extrinsic flexor tendons, and offers protection to the median nerve.

5. What is the clinical presentation?

Some patients will merely complain of numbness *(hypoesthesia)*, without much pain, in the median nerve distribution.[16] Many patients complain of nocturnal pain that may occur from the flexed position the body's extremities assume during sleep. Patients may be awakened by tingling *(paresthesia)* or burning[16] pain and will wring or fling the hand up and down in an attempt to alleviate symptoms. Because of variable innervation of the median nerve as well as subjective difficulty interpreting symptoms while half asleep, some patients will complain of dysesthesia of the entire hand and not of just the thumb, index, middle, and radial half of the fourth digit.[17] The patient often returns to sleep by hanging the affected limb over the edge of the bed[11] in the loose-packed position. During the day, functional activities such as driving, sewing, or hammering precipitate symptoms. As this condition progresses, symptoms may spread above the wrist to the forearm and, less commonly, to the upper arm. Sensory testing may demonstrate diminishment or absence of tactile sensation

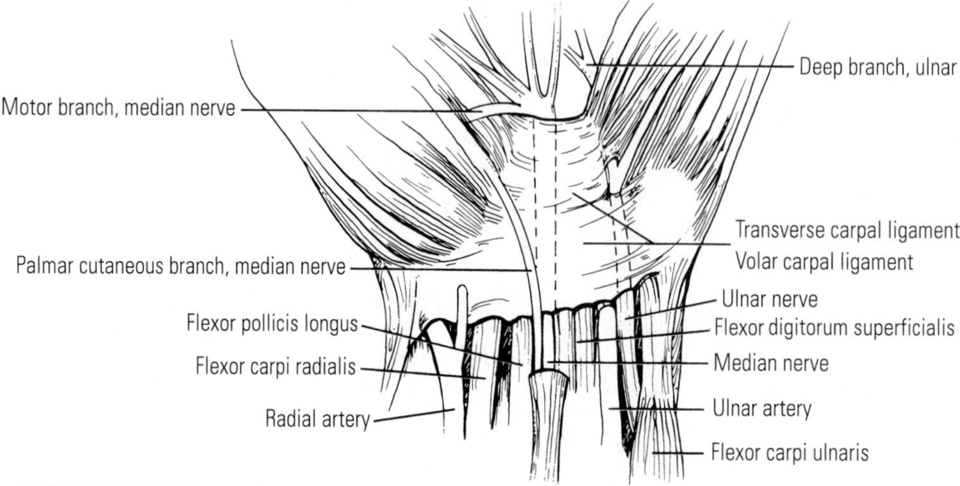

Fig. 4-2 Anterior view of the wrist and palm showing extracarpal course of the palmar cutaneous branch of the median nerve. (Redrawn from The American Society for Surgery of the Hand: *Regional review course in hand surgery,* Aurora, Colo., 1985.)

(anesthesia).* Motor symptoms, that is, loss of thumb opposition and abduction, as well as thenar atrophy generally appear late in the course of CTS.[11] Bilateral upper extremity CTS is common.[16] In long-standing cases the thumb metacarpal bone may become fixed in supination because of muscle imbalance.

6. What is the clinical course of the disorder?

Patients with CTS can be grouped into three categories (or stages outlined by Sunderland) convenient not only for diagnosis but also as a guide to treatment and prognosis. These groupings may be said to correspond to neuropraxia, axonotmesis, and neurotmesis, respectively. It is helpful to bear the following two items in mind before reading on:

- The median nerve has both sensory and motor branches. During median nerve compression at the carpal tunnel sensory abnormalities usually occur first[17] only to progress to motor involvement as the pathology evolves.
- Clinical findings are proportional to the degree of nerve damage, which in turn is related to the severity of compression and not to the duration of compression.[6]

Group I presents with the mildest symptoms of weakness or clumsiness brought on by drawing, holding a newspaper, or performing manual labor. Symptoms are initially sporadic only to increase in frequency over time. No abnormal findings may occur during the initial examination. Physiologic changes include progressive obstruction of venous return resulting in circulatory slowing, hence impaired nutrition to the nerve fibers.

Group II is characterized by pain, often of a burning quality, and is often a major complaint during this stage, with some thenar weakness or atrophy, skin changes, sensory loss, realization of clumsiness, loss of pinch, and loss of dexterity. The patient requires longer periods of hand wringing, rubbing, or placing of the hand under running water so as to help alleviate symptoms. There may be a positive Phalen test or Tinel sign.[6] Pain may be referred as proximally as the shoulder. Physiologic changes include slowing of capillary circulation so severely that anoxia damages the endoneurium.

*Moore KL: *Clinically Oriented Anatomy,* 2nd ed. Baltimore, 1984, Williams and Wilkins.

Group III is characterized by pronounced thenar wasting and sensory loss, skin atrophy, and significant loss of dexterity; there is often loss of two-point discrimination and significant functional impairment. Pain may have either subsided or become severe. Here the prognosis is very poor regardless of treatment[6] because the compressed nerve has become a fibrotic cord.

7. What is the differential diagnosis?

- C6 radiculopathy caused by *cervical spondylosis* most commonly occurs in middle-aged or elderly patients and is the root with the greatest degree of nearly identical symptoms to those of median nerve pathosis.[6] Patients with CTS may complain of some mild to moderate diffuse aching pain in the forearm or arm, whereas neck and shoulder pain are distinctly unusual. Pain with coughing, sneezing, or when bearing down (Valsalva maneuver) during a bowel movement are not commonly associated with radiculopathy but are highly specific when reported; these do not occur with CTS. Similarly, pain radiating posteriorly along the medial scapular border is characteristic of radiculopathy. Relief from pain by massaging, shaking, or immersing one's hand in water are common evasive maneuvers in CTS, whereas patients suffering from radiculopathy often find that use of the hand and arm makes the pain even worse. Additionally, patients suffering from cervical root irritation from cervical spondylosis tend to have a quiet night's sleep only to experience morning pain upon awakening, or daytime pain with arm usage, whereas patients with CTS usually experience pain at night.

  If the sixth cervical nerve is affected, there may be weakness of elbow flexion and wrist extension, the biceps reflex may be lost or reduced, and electromyographic (EMG) studies will show denervation out of median nerve territory if the cause of the disorder is nerve root damage;[6] sensory loss of the sixth cervical dermatome differs topographically from that of the median nerve distribution.

  Diminished biceps and brachioradialis (C5, C6) reflexes with increased triceps reflex (C7) is known as the *inverted radial reflex* and is a clinical clue to spondylosis causing C6 nerve root compression. The idea here is that excess tone may be recircuited so as to manifest briskly in nerve roots supplying other deep tendon reflexes (DTR) further distally along the spinal cord, in this case the next immediate DTR.[8]
- With CNS lesions, an intermittent condition affecting one cerebral hemisphere such as a *focal motor seizure* or *transient vascular episode* in the carotid distribution may mimic CTS. Complaints can be surprisingly restricted in their territory, with reports of numbness, tingling, or weakness of one or two fingers of one hand with episodes lasting several minutes, hours, or even permanently in the event of infarction. Absence of pain is a characteristic of such CNS lesions.[6]

  Lesions of the spinal cord such as tumors, *syringomyelia,* and *multiple sclerosis* do not usually yield transient or intermittent symptoms that vary from one hour to the next.[6]
- *Pronator syndrome* (Fig. 4-3) refers to compression of the median nerve (1) by pronator muscle as it passes through the heads of that muscle and (2) to a lesser extent by fibrous bands[16] near the origin of the deep flexor muscles,[16] known as the lacertus fibrosus and flexor digitorum superficialis arcade,[2] and (3) even less commonly by the ligament of Struthers (Fig. 4-4), an anomalous structure found in about 1% of the population.[18] This ligament runs from an abnormal bone spur located on the medial aspect of the distal humerus to the medial humeral epicondyle. This syndrome commonly occurs in patients whose jobs require repetitive pronation-supination motions, or in those who have sustained trauma to the proximal volar part of the forearm.[7,19]

  Although the pronator syndrome may also be expressed with median nerve paresthesias mimicking those of CTS, it differs in several aspects. Night pain, symptoms brought on by wrist movement, intrinsic weakness of opponens and abduction movements, as well as positive Phalen and Tinel wrist signs are not common to this condition. The pronator syndrome is distinguished by exacerbation attributable to resisted pronation and passive supination activities, positive Tinel sign at the proximal forearm overlying the median nerve, tenderness and paresthesias in the median nerve distribution on direct compression over

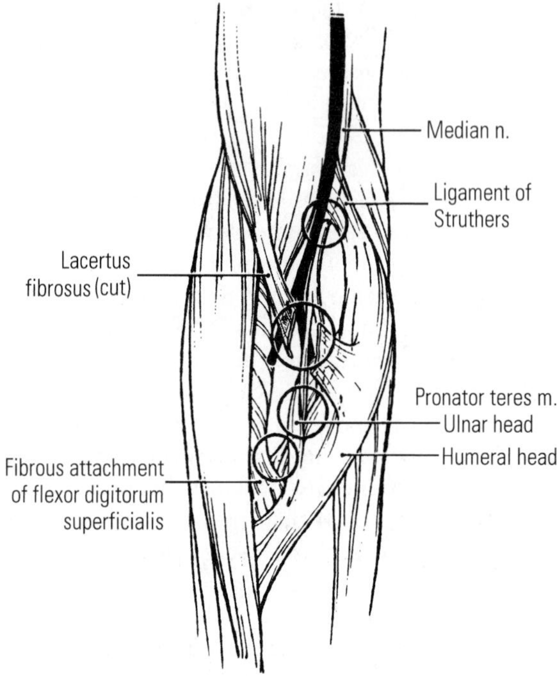

Fig. 4-3 Sites of median nerve compression in pronator syndrome. (From Chabon SJ: *Physician Assistant,* Sept 1990.)

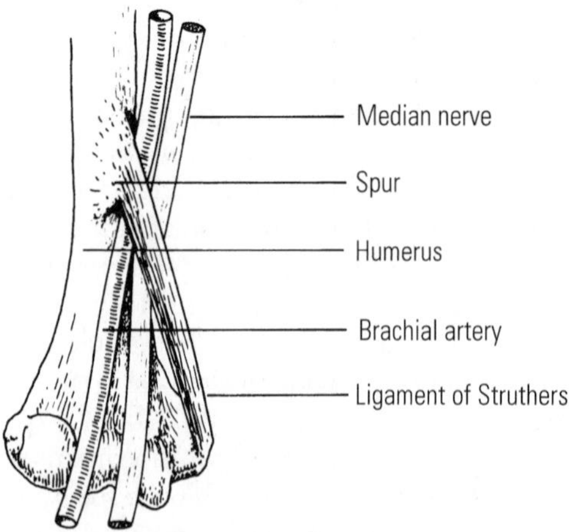

Fig. 4-4 Median nerve compression by the anomalous ligament of Struthers. (From Magee DJ: *Orthopaedic physical assessment,* Philadelphia, 1987, Saunders.)

pronator muscle, and pain and median nerve paresthesias with forced pronation, as well as passive supination at the limit of full extension. Like anterior osseous syndrome, there is also difficulty with pincer movement involving the thumb to the index finger. Nerve conduction velocity (NCV) and EMG studies show slowed conduction velocity across the forearm and denervation potentials of flexor pollicis longus and abductor pollicis brevis. Treatment includes stretching exercises to both pronator and supinator muscles; surgical decompression is appropriate when conservative treatment is ineffective.[4]

- In *Raynaud's phenomenon,* the symptoms caused by local vasospasm are differentiated from CTS in the sense that Raynaud's phenomenon does not involve any distinction between the fingers, with all the fingers and palm being equally affected. This relationship to cold is not observed in patients with CTS.[6]
- *Reflex sympathetic dystrophy* (RSD) (see Chapter 6) is similar to CTS in the sense that pain, paresthesias, trophic changes, puffy hands, and decreased function of flexor tendons are features of both pathoses. In addition, both conditions can show sympathetic abnormalities. However, in patients with true RSD there is more trophic change, redness, cyanosis and atrophy of fingertips, and pronounced variation in color with dependence of the limb.[6]
- *Diabetic neuropathy* can manifest as an asymmetric condition reflecting partial or complete infarction of nerves or nerve trunks, usually occurring in relationship to the lumbosacral plexus or to the sciatic or femoral nerves. The result is sudden onset and often painful asymmetric loss of function with prominent weakness and little sensory loss. The median nerve is rarely affected.[6]

8. What is anterior interosseous syndrome?

The anterior interosseous nerve arises from the median nerve 5 to 8 cm distal to the lateral epicondyle and moves distally to the anterior interosseous membrane. It is the last major tributory branch off the median nerve.[6] Purely a *motor nerve,*[17] the anterior interosseous nerve innervates the flexor pollicis longus, the flexor digitorum profundus to the index and long digits, and the pronator quadratus.

The cause of *anterior interosseous syndrome* is controversial and may be ascribed to one of several causes that include a tendinous origin of the deep head of the pronator teres muscle (Fig. 4-5) or of the flexor digitorum superficialis of the long finger, or from accessory muscles and tendons from the latter muscle, or from the flexor pollicis longus, as well as aberrant vessels, or thrombosed collateral vessels.[6] Spontaneous anterior interosseous nerve paralysis may result from minimal trauma only in the presence of one of the aforementioned preexisting anomalous conditions. Specifically, motions such as excessive and repetitive elbow flexion and pronation are seen in butchers, carpenters, or leather cutters.[15] Strenuous exercise and lifting heavy weights have also provoked this syndrome.[10,12] Provocation of this syndrome may occur directly and not as a function of overuse, in fractures, gunshot wounds, and lacerations, and from drug injections by addicts.[6] Extrinsic pressure causes include wearing a cast and carrying a handbag.

Clinical features of spontaneous anterior interosseous syndrome includes acute pain prodrome in the proximal forearm lasting hours to days. There may be a recent history of heavy muscular exertion or local trauma. With the onset of paresis, patients may notice a loss of dexterity and discover that their pinching is impaired. Physical examination shows characteristic difficulty in flexing the distal interphalangeal joints of the thumb and index finger to form a pincer movement because of weakness (Fig. 4-6). Paralysis of the pronator quadratus is tested with the elbow in flexion to block the contraction from the humeral head of the pronator teres.[6] There may be elbow pain on resisted pronation or while one stretches the pronator quadratus in extreme supination.

Treatment of this relatively common condition[6] includes a 6-month conservative trial of therapy that includes avoidance of movements or the occupation that exacerbates symptoms. An ergonomic analysis of the workplace is appropriate and suggestions should be offered how to perform one's occupation in a nonprovoking manner. Therapy also includes rest, nonsteroidal anti-inflammatory medications, and

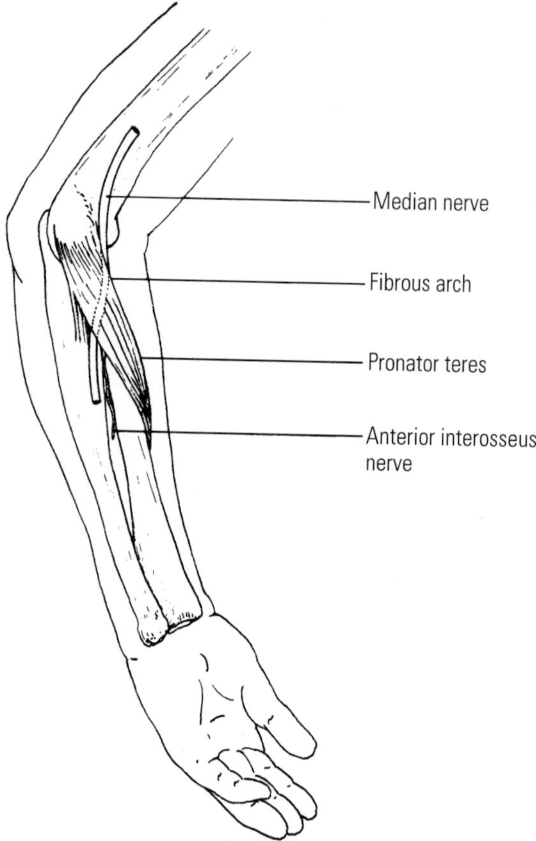

Fig. 4-5 The anterior interosseous nerve, which is a branch of the median nerve, may become entrapped as it passes between the two heads of the pronator teres. (From Magee DJ: *Orthopaedic physical assessment,* Philadelphia, 1987, Saunders.)

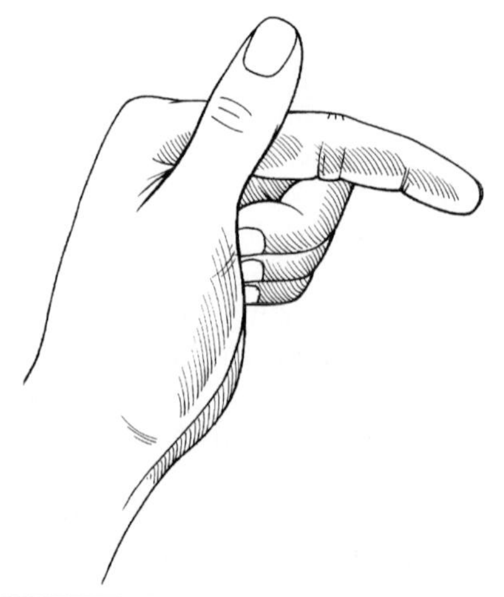

Fig. 4-6 Hand posture associated with anterior interosseous nerve palsy.

immobilization of the forearm in partial supination to relieve pressure on the pronator teres. The physician may inject a steroid in the region of the pronator teres.[6]

9. What are the electrophysiologic findings in CTS?

Electrophysiologic studies are indicated when the clinical diagnosis is uncertain. The first step is to examine the sensory action across the wrist so as to rule out generalized neuropathy. The second step involves motor-conduction studies in the hope of finding a prolonged distal motor latency or, even better, a prolonged residual latency and normal conduction velocity in the forearm that would confirm focality of the lesion. The third step is electromyography, which is mainly useful to rule out coexisting radiculopathy although this test may prove normal in as much as one fourth of patients suffering from CTS.[14]

10. What other pathologic conditions are associated with CTS?

Patients with CTS may have other forms of tendon pathoses such as de Quervain's disease, rotator cuff tendinitis, or trigger finger. CTS is a common complication of chronic renal failure treated by hemodialysis; beta$_2$-microglobulin-derived amyloid can be found deposited in the transverse carpal ligament.[17] Although not a pathologic condition, some women who experience pregnancy may succumb to CTS, with typical time of onset at the sixth month.[6] It may be that changes in hormonal levels or weight gain somehow influence fluid retention.

11. How is motor function best tested?

The abductor pollicis brevis is the easiest of the thenar muscles to be tested. The thumb is brought up perpendicularly to the palm, and the patient resists pressure directed against the distal phalanx (Fig. 4-7). However, the clinician must be on guard against tricky substitution by the abductor pollicis longus, which is innervated by the radial nerve and abducts the thumb radially. Alternatively the patient may flex the

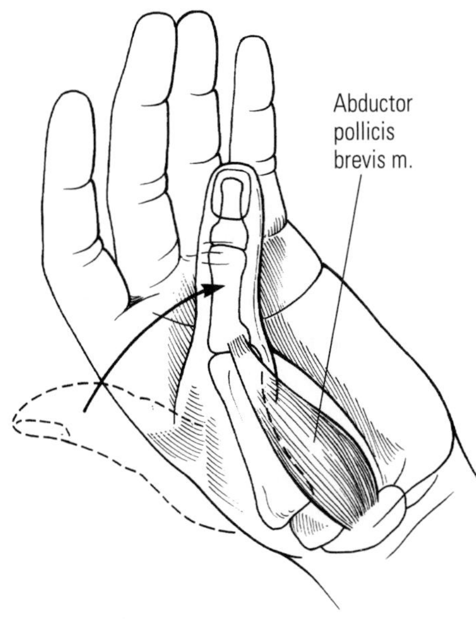

Fig. 4-7 Manual abductor pollicis brevis testing for median nerve injury. Weakness manifests as a decreased ability to abduct the thumb, making it difficult to grasp a large object. Eventually an adduction deformity of the thumb may result (ape hand).

thumb across the palm using the long flexor, which is innervated by the median nerve proximal to the forearm. Either substitution will not yield true 90° abduction.[6]

The significance in choosing to test this muscle becomes apparent when we consider how the other muscles supplied by the median nerve either have dual innervation or may be compensated for by the long forearm muscles.[13] One can best test opposition by requesting the patient to place the tips of the thumb and fifth finger together and resist the examiner's attempt to break this pinch. It is helpful to remember that the dominant hand is normally 10% stronger than the nondominant hand.

12. Which provocative tests elicit symptoms?

In *Phalen's test* or *Tinel's sign* (Fig. 4-8), the median nerve is easily depolarized when mechanically stimulated by direct tapping over the palmaris longus tendon over the flexor retinaculum. However, positive findings occur only in approximately 45% of all cases.[14] Intercarpal pressure is greatest at 90° wrist flexion superimposed on ulnar deviation.

13. What disorders of the workplace are implicated as possible causes of CTS?

Repeated overuse, whether at work or in recreation, will result in swelling of the tendons or of the synovia surrounding those tendons. Occupational variants predisposing CTS may include carpentry, secretarial work, keyboard operators, and jackhammer operators.

14. What chronic, rheumatologic, or metabolic disorders are associated with CTS?

Chronic disorders associated with CTS include trauma, obesity, pregnancy, local tumors, and infection. Rheumatic disorders associated with CTS include rheumatoid arthritis, systemic lupus erythematosus, gout, and pseudogout. Metabolic disorders associated with CTS include hypothyroidism, diabetes mellitus, acromegaly, myxedema, eosinophilic fasciitis, dysproteinemia, amyloidosis, and mucopolysaccharidoses.[17]

15. What is the double-crush phenomenon?

A nerve may be compressed at more than one site (Fig. 4-9), a condition known as *double-crush syndrome.* Since nerve tissue is extremely sensitive to ischemia, pressure on the nerve at the neck, at the thoracic outlet, or at the elbow will make the nerve even more susceptible to even mild pressure in the carpal tunnel. The idea here is that the nerve tract is susceptible to mechanical injury because of either tethering at the intervertebral foramen or proximity to unyielding bone or simply because branching at an abrupt angle involves a diminishing of the nerve's gliding mechanisms. By tautening the nerve along its proximal and distal length in a specific sequence a clinician may confirm a suspected doublecrush. This sequence of postures tenses the brachial plexus, particularly the median nerve trunk, and includes shoulder depression and abduction, elbow extension, forearm supination, wrist extension, and lateral cervical flexion.[3] The idea here is that the nerve tract is susceptible to mechanical injury because of either tethering at the intervertebral foramen or proximity to unyielding bone or simply because branching at an abrupt angle compromises the nerve's gliding mechanisms.[3] Suspicion of a second crush site of the median nerve at a more proximal site may be confirmed if one superimposes a series of upper limb postures that tauten the nerve along its length. Shoulder depression, abduction, elbow extension, forearm supination, and wrist extension may elicit provocation of symptoms and confirm the presence of a suspected additional proximal lesion. Thus, in those patients with new onset of symptoms after surgical release, attention ought to be directed to more proximal sites of possible compression rather than reattempting surgery. Conservative treatment may more likely have positive results, especially when patients readily report relief of hand symptoms after proximal stretching techniques, massage of the upper trapezius area, or other therapeutic modality.

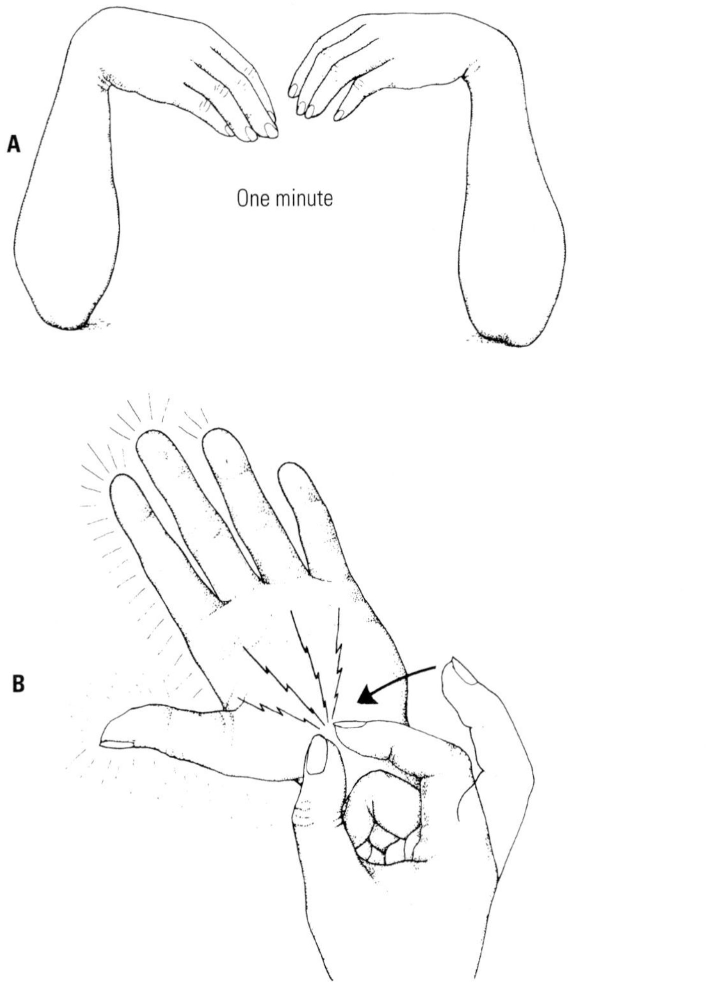

Fig. 4-8 **A,** Phalen's test: The patient is asked to report any sensory changes in the median nerve–innervated area after holding his wrists flexed for 1 minute. **B,** Tinel's sign: The examiner taps the hand from the fingertips proximally to the palm. The patient is asked to report any "electric shocks" or tingling when percussed. (From The American Society for Surgery of the Hand: *The hand examination and diagnosis,* New York, 1983, Churchill Livingstone.)

16. What nonsurgical treatment or treatments are appropriate before surgical decompression?

Nonsurgical treatment is advised for patients with mild or intermittent symptoms and include the following:

- Rest.
- Modification of work condition and habits, wrist posture, and tool design.
- Cock-up volar splint with wrist in loose-packed position (10° to 30° dorsiflexion) to be worn at night as well as by day continually for 4 to 6 weeks and with gradually decreasing splint use over the subsequent 4 weeks.[9]
- A short course of nonsteroidal anti-inflammatory medication or oral steroids.

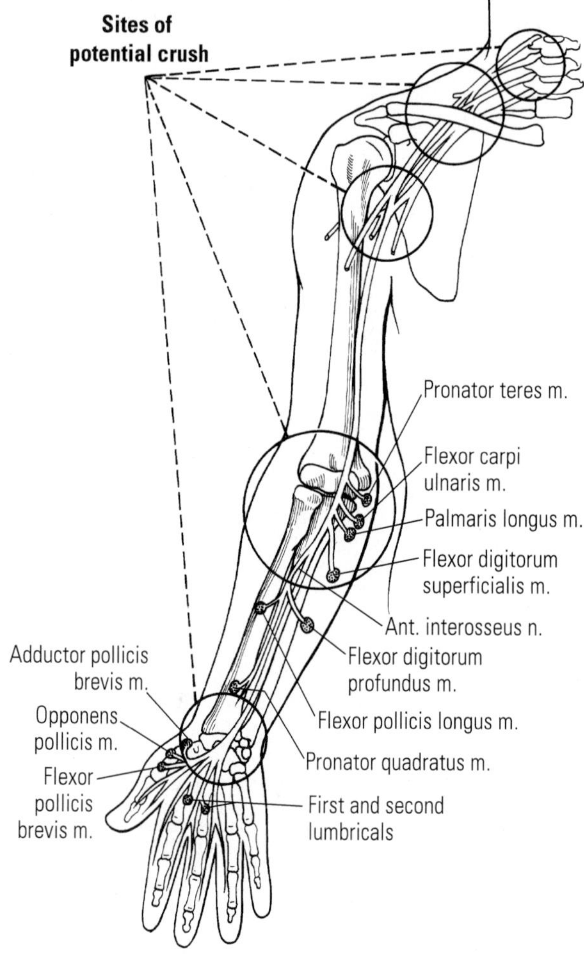

Fig. 4-9 Double-crush phenomenon. After an initial "crush," the involved nerve presumably becomes sensitized and thereby more vulnerable to ischemic injury elsewhere along its length. A second "crush" site may occur proximally where the median nerve exits the spine at the intervertebral foramen, between the first rib and the clavicle (costoclavicular space), or at any of the nerve's multiple branchings in the vicinity of the cubital region.

- A trial of diuretics, especially when symptoms are perimenstrual.
- Avoidance of certain wrist and hand postures and repetitive wrist motions such as gripping or pinching objects while flexing the wrist and performing repetitive wrist flexion-extension exercise motions.
- One hundred to 200 mg of vitamin B_6 per day is sometimes added to the diet despite inconclusive evidence that pyroxidine is beneficial.*
- Local steroid injection proximal to the transverse carpal ligament and into the perineurium but not into the nerve itself, since the latter is quite painful and dangerous. Injection should not be performed

*Merck Manval, Raway N.J.

if significant swelling is present because the presence of additional volume only exacerbates the symptoms. Relief occurs within 1 to 3 days. If there is no change in symptoms, the second injection is not indicated. Repeated injections carry the danger of tendon attrition and rupture as well as permanent median nerve injury; a total of 3 or 4 injections are the maximum allowable number before one should insist on surgical release. Greater than 4 injections are considered only in a patient with a poor surgical risk or in an elderly patient.

- It is imperative to evaluate the work environment and to suggest alternatives such as an ergonomically designed keyboard for a secretary or a bent handle on a hammer for a carpenter.
- *Tendon-gliding exercises* facilitate isolated excursion of each of the two flexor tendons to each finger passing through the carpal tunnel. Each exercise is initiated from a position of full finger and wrist extension. To obtain maximum differential gliding of profundus with respect to superficialis excursion, the patient assumes a hooked-fist position. To obtain maximum flexor digitorum superficialis excursion, the patient is instructed to flex the metacarpophalangeal joints and the proximal interphalangeal joints while maintaining the distal interphalangeal joints in extension. A full fist exercise completes the series of tendon-gliding exercises and provides maximum profundus tendon excursion. These exercises are performed five times each, five times daily.
- For some patients experiencing transient episodes of CTS (as in pregnancy), reassurance and explanation are often all that is needed.

17. What are indications for surgery, and what does surgery involve?

Absolute surgical indications include failure of nonoperative treatment or clinical evidence of thenar atrophy. A relative indication for surgery is the patient with persistent sensory loss, especially if long standing.[6] Decompression, by way of division of the flexor retinaculum, often provides gratifying results[16] with dramatic immediate relief and has a good long-term prognosis in the treatment of CTS.

Before surgery, electrophysiologic studies are performed so as to provide a baseline value in determining the postoperative state of the nerve should surgery fail to relieve the patient of his or her symptoms.[6] Surgery is performed under local anesthesia with sedation, or regional intravenous anesthesia. The most accepted surgical incision is a curved interthenar incision along the bisected line through the fourth digit. Complications reported from using the older transverse incision at the wrist crease involving blind release of the flexor retinaculum include injury to the superficial palmar arch and laceration of the sensory branch of the median nerve.[6]

18. What is postsurgical management?

Postoperatively, because pressure on the median nerve increases with wrist motion, a bulky hand dressing and wrist splint are applied for 1 week after surgery. If the patient is allowed to remove the cast before 1 week, wrist motion may result in prolonged hypersensitivity and early digital motion is encouraged. One week after surgery the volar cast is removed and a volar wrist extension splint is fabricated, positioning the wrist in some 10° to 20° of wrist extension. This splint is worn at night during sleep and during strenuous exercise.[6]

Depending on the preoperative severity of symptoms as well as response to surgery, patients may require few or no therapy sessions, moderate intervention (3 to 8 weeks), whereas others require a comprehensive rehabilitation program (8 to 16 weeks).

The goals of therapy during the first 3 weeks after surgery are edema control, maintaining range of motion, preventing adhesion formation, and protected hand use. This is accomplished by instructing the patient to elevate the involved hand constantly and to do retrograde massage, three sets of 10 repetitions of tendon-gliding exercises and thumb flexion, extension, and opposition exercises, as well as shoulder and elbow exercises.[1]

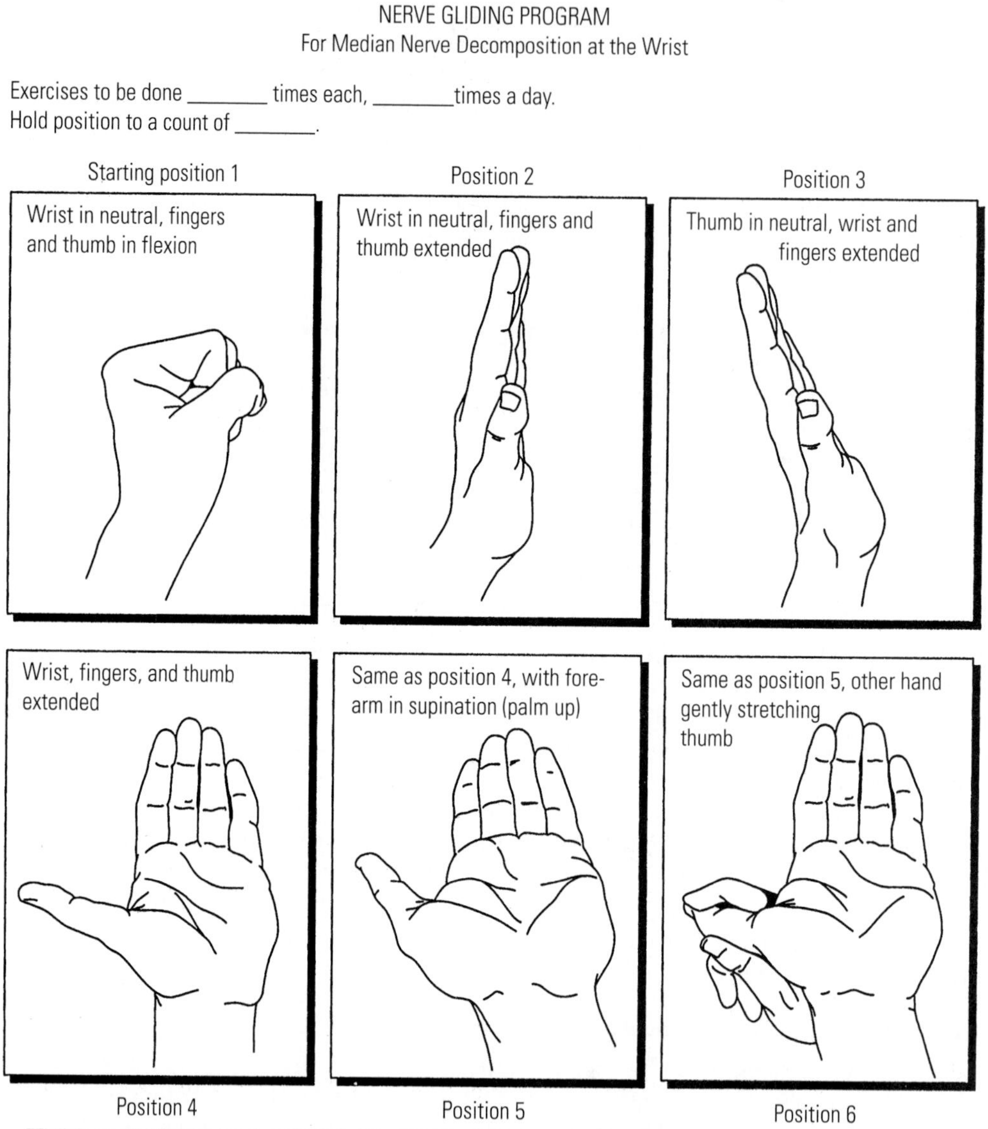

NERVE GLIDING PROGRAM
For Median Nerve Decomposition at the Wrist

Exercises to be done _______ times each, _______times a day.
Hold position to a count of _______.

Starting position 1
Wrist in neutral, fingers and thumb in flexion

Position 2
Wrist in neutral, fingers and thumb extended

Position 3
Thumb in neutral, wrist and fingers extended

Position 4
Wrist, fingers, and thumb extended

Position 5
Same as position 4, with forearm in supination (palm up)

Position 6
Same as position 5, other hand gently stretching thumb

Fig. 4-10 Nerve-gliding exercises permit mobilization of the median nerve. (From Hunter JM, Schneider LH, Mackin EJ, Callahan AD, editors: *Rehabilitation of the hand: surgery and therapy,* ed 3, St. Louis, 1990, Mosby. Exercises developed by Dr. James Hunter; home program designed by Julie Belkin, OTR.)

Therapeutic goals during weeks 3 to 8 include edema reduction, scar modeling, reduction of hypersensitivity, and increasing strength and functional use. If thick hypertrophic scar develops along the incision site, elastomer is applied to the palmar scar to model it. Active and passive exercises are initiated for the digits and wrist if the patient lacks full motion. If edema persists, the patient may be instructed to perform overhead bilateral fisting exercises, one set of 20 repetitions per hour. String wrapping may also be helpful, as are elevated prehension activities, such as macramé, that recruit gravity to assist in edema reduction. *Nerve-gliding exercises* (Fig. 4-10) are initiated to ensure that the median nerve glides through the carpal tunnel and adjacent thenar and hypothenar eminences. Passive stretching of the thumb is necessary to prevent adhesion formation along the palmar cutaneous and motor branch of the median nerve. These exercises are performed for three sets of 10 repetitions daily.[1]

At the eighth week after surgery, graded isometric as well as isotonic strengthening exercises for the hand and wrist are initiated. The patient is cautioned against overexercise that might result in tenosynovitis. Work hardening is initiated at 8 to 12 weeks. Return to sedentary or clerical work is reasonable at this time, as is light house repair and housecleaning chores, but any strenuous activity is best preceded by a work-tolerance program. Premature return to heavy work can cause local pain, tenosynovitis, painful scarring, and local arthritis.[1]

Raynaud's phenomenon may be present in association with CTS and may be related to disordered neurovascular hand function after median nerve decompression.[16]

19. What sequelae may follow surgery?

Reflex sympathetic dystrophy (Chapter 6) can often be forestalled and staved off by being especially on guard for the anxious patient with low pain tolerance who will not actively flex the digits after surgery.

References

1. Baxter-Petralia PL: Therapist's management of carpal tunnel syndrome. In Hunter JM, Schneider LH, Mackin EJ, Callahan AD, editors: *Rehabilitation of the hand: surgery and therapy,* ed 3, St Louis, 1990, Mosby.
2. Beaton LE, Anson BJ: The relation of the median nerve to the pronator teres muscle, *Anat Rec* 75:23, 1939.
3. Butler D: *Mobilisation of the nervous system,* Melbourne, 1991, Churchill Livingstone.
4. Chabon SJ: Uncommon compressive neuropathies of the forearm, *Physician Assistant,* p 57, Sept 1990.
5. Dandy DJ: *Essential orthopaedics and trauma,* Edinburgh, 1989, Churchill Livingstone.
6. Dawson DM, Hallet M, Millender LH: *Entrapment neuropathies,* ed 2, Boston, 1990, Little, Brown & Co.
7. Gessini L, Jandolo B: The pronator teres syndrome: clinical and electrophysiologic features in six surgically verified cases, J *Neurosurg Sci* 31:1-5, 1987.
8. Hauser SL, Levitt LP, Weiner HL: *Case studies in neurology for the house officer,* Baltimore, 1986, Williams & Wilkins.
9. Lillegard WA, Rucker KS: *Handbook of sports medicine: a symptom-oriented approach,* Boston, 1993, Andover Medical Publishers.
10. Nakano KK, Ludergen C, Okihiro MM: Anterior interosseous nerve syndromes, *Arch Neurol* 34:477, 1977.
11. Netter FH: *The CIBA collection of medical illustrations,* vol 1: *Nervous system,* part 2, *Neurologic and neuromuscular disorders,* West Caldwell, N.J., 1986, CIBA-Geigy Corp.
12. O'Brien MD, Upton ARM: Anterior interosseous nerve syndrome: a case report with neurophysiological investigations, *J Neurol Neurosurg Psychiatry* 35:531, 1972.
13. Patton J: *Neurological differential diagnosis,* ed 2, London, 1996, Springer-Verlag.
14. Pianka G, Hershman EB: Neurovascular injuries. In Nicholas JA, Hershman EB, editors: *The upper extremity in sports medicine,* St Louis, 1990, Mosby.
15. Rask MR: Anterior interosseous nerve entrapment (Kiloh-Nevin syndrome), *Clin Orthop* 142:176, 1979.
16. Rodman GP, Schumacher HR: *Primer on the rheumatic diseases,* ed 8, Atlanta, 1983, Arthritis Foundation.
17. Schumacher RH, Bomalski JS: *Case studies in rheumatology for the house officer,* Baltimore, 1990, Williams & Wilkins.
18. Spinner M, Spencer PS: Nerve compression lesions of the upper extremity: a clinical and experimental review, *Clin Orthop Rel Res* 104:46, 1974.

19. Werner CO, Rosen I, Thorngren K: Clinical and neurophysiological characteristics of the pronator syndrome, *Clin Orthop* 197:231-236, 1985.

Recommended reading

Baxter-Petralia PL: Therapist's management of carpal tunnel syndrome. In Hunter JM, Schneider LH, Mackin EJ, Callahan AD, editors: *Rehabilitation of the hand: surgery and therapy,* ed 3, St Louis, 1990, Mosby.

Butler D: *Mobilisation of the nervous system,* Melbourne, 1991, Churchill Livingstone.

Dawson DM, Hallet M, Millender LH: *Entrapment neuropathies,* ed 2, Boston 1990, Little, Brown & Co.

Phalen GS: The carpal-tunnel syndrome: 17 years' experience in diagnosis and treatment of 654 cases, *J Bone Joint Surg* 48A:211-228, 1966.

Schumacher RH, Bomalski JS: *Case studies in rheumatology for the house officer,* Baltimore, 1990, Mosby.

5 Fall Resulting in Wrist Deformity

A 58-year-old white female fractured her wrist after falling and slipping on ice in front of her home and now appears in your office 1 day after cast removal. There is a slight dinner-fork deformity observed. Her skin appears flaky and looks somewhat smaller than the contralateral limb. There is no history of congestive heart failure. Your associate, the orthopod, saw this patient several weeks ago, administered a local anesthetic, and with your help manipulated the wrist and forearm so as to disimpact the fracture and appose the fragment ends. The patient is now referred to your practice for rehabilitation.

1. **What is a Colles fracture, and how does it occur?**
2. **What is the mechanism of injury, the resulting pattern of deformity, and why?**
3. **What requisite kinesiology of wrist biomechanics is necessary to fully appreciate the ramifications of a Colles fracture?**
4. **What are the three different kinds of Colles's fractures?**
5. **Why does deformity tend to recur after setting and immobilization of a displaced Colles fracture?**
6. **When is external fixation appropriate?**
7. **What other disorders may occur from a similar or near-similar mechanism of injury?**
8. **How may a Colles fracture be confused with a Galeazzi fracture-dislocation?**
9. **Describe the important role of the pronator teres in radial fractures and how this determines fragment splinting.**
10. **What are some sequelae of a Colles fracture?**
11. **What potential loss of range of motion may occur from typical bone setting of a Colles fracture in pronation and wrist flexion, and why?**
12. **What rehabilitative therapy is appropriate after cast removal?**

1. What is a Colles fracture, and how does it occur?

A *Colles fracture* is a dorsally angulated fracture of the distal end of the radius with or without accompanying ulnar fracture and was described by the Irish surgeon Abraham Colles in 1814 in the only article he ever wrote.[8] Colles's fracture is the commonest fracture in adults over 50 years of age and more common in white females than in other groups. This fracture has the same sex and age incidence as a femoral neck fracture has and for the same reason: a combination of senile and postmenopausal osteoporosis.[12] There are several components to a Colles fracture:

- Backward (dorsal) angulation of the distal fragment.
- Backward displacement of the distal fragment.
- Radial deviation.
- Transverse fracture pattern with main fracture line within distal 2 cm of the radius. This occurs because the lunate acts as a wedge to shear the distal 2 cm of the radius off in a dorsal direction.[3]

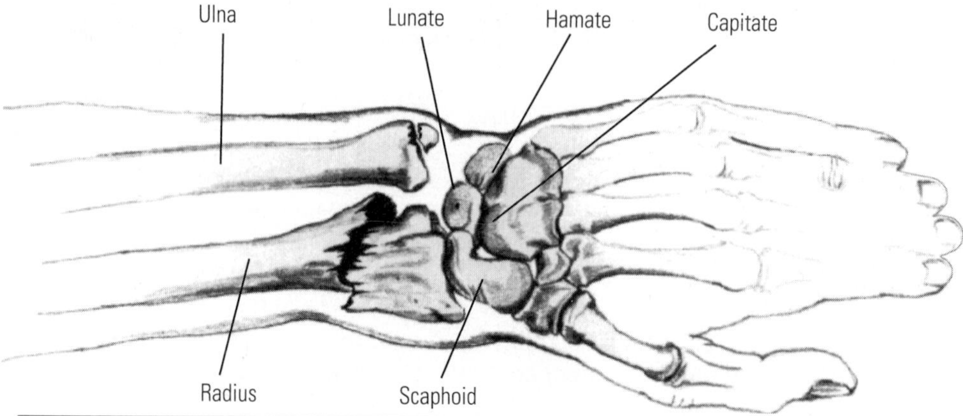

Fig. 5-1 Profile of a Colles fracture. (From Peterson L, Renström P: *Sports injuries: their prevention and treatment,* London, 1986, Martin Dunitz, Ltd.)

- Comminution of the thin cortex, especially in osteoporotic bone of the elderly. A cross section of the radius can show how the thick cortical bone of the shaft thins out to form only a thin layer over the cancellous bone at the distal end. This anatomic design flaw is compounded by the presence of osteoporosis.[6]
- Proximal impaction caused by the jagged ends of bone having been driven one into the other and further causing the distal ends of the radius and ulna to be level,[9] instead of the normal relationship between those two bones in which the radius extends slightly beyond the distal end of the ulna.
- It may be associated with sprain of the ulnar collateral ligament and avulsion fracture of the ulnar styloid. The latter occurs secondarily to displacement of the distal end of the radius because of the concomitant pull of the biconcave articular disk connecting the distal ends of the radius and ulna.[9]
- Subluxation or partial dislocation of the distal radioulnar joint.
- Supination. Since the fracture occurs in conjunction with a supination moment, supination is preserved in the deformity.
- When the pronated arm is laid upon the examining table, its profile resembles a dinner fork lying horizontally with the tines pointing downward, so that the base of the tines forms an upward curve[2] (Fig. 5-1).

2. What is the mechanism of injury, the resulting pattern of deformity, and why?

Typically a patient either slips or trips and attempts to break his or her fall by means of a parachute reflex, landing on the outstretched volar surface of the hand with the forearm pronated.[12] The intended outcome is dissipation of force that is transmitted along the length of the upper extremity, which, unfortunately, does not always occur. Two mechanisms contribute to fracture at the distal end of the radius, as follows:

- In the attempt to break a fall, the hand moves into physiologic extension while the proximal carpal row moves palmarly, locking the radius against the scaphoid and lunate bones (Fig. 5-2). While the hand stops moving once it contacts the ground, that distal end of the arm will continue to move toward the ground, causing a shearing of the distal end of the radius off the main body of bone.[3]
- A supination moment is created by the pronator quadratus and brachioradialis muscles. The latter muscle is a better supinator than the pronator because of the sudden reflexive stretching in the pronator direction, causing maximal stress at the junction of cortical and cancellous bone in the distal radial metaphysis.[5]

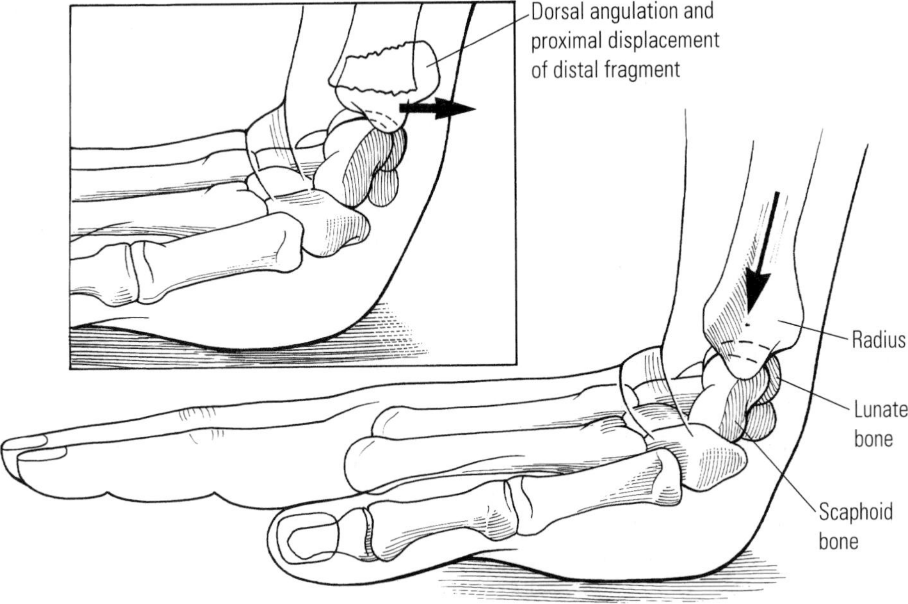

Fig. 5-2 Mechanism of a Colles fracture.

3. What requisite kinesiology of wrist biomechanics is necessary to fully appreciate the ramifications of a Colles fracture?

- At the wrist, the radius is the principal bone in the sense that it and not the ulna articulates with joint of the carpal bones (that is, the radiocarpals). The ulna has no direct contact with the carpus. The wrist is stabilized by the radial and ulnar collateral ligaments.[7]
- The hand moves along with the radius as it pivots about the ulna. The ulna cannot rotate at all because of the nature of the humeroulnar joint. Thus pronation and supination are more the function of the radius than of the ulna and occurs at the proximal and distal radioulnar joints. It is during pronation that the radius rotates and crosses the ulna. In supination both bones lie parallel with each other (see Fig. 5-10).
- With motions of the wrist the (convex) proximal row of carpal bones slides in the direction opposite the physiologic motion of the hand.
- There is an oblique axis between the distal ends of the radius and ulna, much the same as in the distal ends of the tibia and fibula in the lower extremity. In the same way ankle inversion has a greater range of motion than eversion because the fibular malleolus extends more distally, ulnar deviation has slightly greater range than radial deviation, since the radial styloid extends more distally.
- Since the advent of *Homo erectus* the interosseus membrane between the radius and ulna no longer has been needed to prevent splaying, just as the same structure (that is, the tibiofibular syndesmosis) functions in the lower extremity. Rather, the interosseous membrane provides additional surface area for muscle and tendon attachment.
- The principal supinators are the biceps brachii and supinator muscles. The former supinates by virtue of its distal attachment to the posterior radial tuberosity. When the biceps contracts, not only is the forearm flexed, but also the radius unwinds as its tuberosity is anteriorly rotated (that is, forearm supination). The biceps's twin function is best remembered as the twisting of a corkscrew into a bottle (supination) and

then a pulling out of the cork (flexion) (see Fig. 8-3). The chief pronators are the pronator teres and the pronator quadratus.

4. What are the three different kinds of Colles's fractures?

The three kinds of Colles's fractures are:

- Undisplaced fractures, which are uncommon and require immobilization in a below-elbow cast for 4 weeks.
- Displaced fractures, having one main transverse fracture with little cortical comminution.
- Unstable fractures, having gross comminution of cortical bone and pronounced crushing of softer cancellous bone.

The latter two categories may be radiographically differentiated.[12]

5. Why does deformity tend to recur after setting and immobilization of a displaced Colles fracture?

Perfect anatomic alignment is often impossible without the use of skeletal fixation (such as an external bar, intramedullary pin, or bone graft to fill in the defect at the distal part of the radius). Despite successful manipulation and alignment with immobilization, the deformity, in a displaced Colles fracture, tends to recur for two reasons:

- Whereas before the fracture occurred the ulna projected distally slightly less than the radius did, after a fracture the distal parts of the radius and ulna are aligned one with the other. Because the crushed cancellous bone of the distal radial fragment does not return to stay at its proper location on reduction, a cavity is created, and the distal comminuted cortical shell is internally unsupported. Normally, forces arising from muscle pull will produce further shortening with angulation of the distal fragment so that the wrist, particularly in the elderly, will yield a characteristic hump resembling a dinner fork *(dinner-fork deformity)*. Since the blood supply to the distal end of the radius is excellent, bony malunion may occur. The surgeons competence is often called into question despite the resultant good hand function in the patient. As such, patients must be warned of the possible cosmetic deformity caused by closed reduction and plaster immobilization.
- If painful restriction occurs with deformity, excision of the distal end of the ulna will relieve pain, and improve the range of motion and cosmesis, as it recreates the original anatomic alignment.
- Many patients will have bony resorption at the fracture site that, over time, translates into shortening of the radius.

6. When is external fixation appropriate?

External fixators such as the Hoffman frame or the Roger-Anderson frame have two pins proximally through the radius and two pins distally in the second and third metacarpals and are used as anchors because they are immobile. External fixation is appropriate in the extremely comminuted (hence unstable) Colles fracture, particularly in persons under 60 years of age or in those having careers such as modeling where a premium is placed on the aesthetic of near perfect and permanent anatomic alignment. External fixation is also important in persons who must use their hands and cannot wear a cast, such as professional piano players. Other approaches may include percutaneous pinning, or open reduction with internal fixation to achieve the desired result.[12]

7. What other disorders may occur from a similar or near-similar mechanism of injury?

In the years after Colles's description of this fracture an eponym war erupted over other, slightly different fracture patterns at the distal radius. Today the trend is to lump them all as distal radius fractures and simply describe the exact pattern of fracture lines. Listed below are some of the more well-known fractures.[8]

- R.W. Smith succeeded Colles as professor of surgery at Dublin, Ireland, and described the reverse Colles fracture, or *Smith's fracture* (Fig. 5-3), which occurs after a fall onto a flexed wrist. The resulting fracture

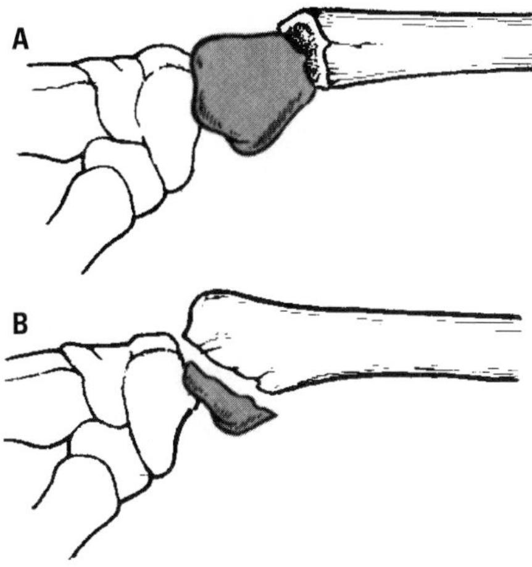

Fig. 5-3 **A,** Smith's fracture. **B,** Barton's fracture, which enters the joint. (From Dandy DJ: *Essential orthopaedics and trauma,* Edinburgh, 1989, Churchill Livingstone.)

pattern, like the mechanism of injury, is reverse from that of a Colles fracture in that the distal fragment is forward (palmar) versus backward (Fig. 5-3). The fracture line is usually obliquely upward and forward. Upon presentation it is observed as a reverse dinner-fork deformity with the tines pointing upward, or more imaginatively as a garden-spade deformity. Pressure applied during traction is the reverse of that of a Colles fracture.[2]

- John R. Barton of Philadelphia, the founding father of American orthopedic surgery, described a fracture in which the fracture line of the distal end of the radius enters the radiocarpal joint and forces (that is, subluxes) the carpal bones upward and backward, causing a fracture dislocation. The resulting deformity, a *Barton's fracture,* also presents as the typical dinner-fork deformity but differs from a Colles fracture in two ways: (1) the anterior and posterior prominences are at a lower level and (2) the radial styloid can be palpated in its normal position. Displacement is corrected with local or general anesthesia and is then casted for 4 to 5 weeks.[1]
- A *wrist sprain* may occur from landing on outstretched hands as well as from hyperflexion and torsion and may damage either one of the ligaments stabilizing the wrist (that is, the radial and ulnar collateral ligaments) as well as the lunate capitate ligament dorsally and the radiocarpal ligament palmarly[6] (Fig. 5-4). Localized swelling after a wrist injury almost never accompanies an isolated ligamentous injury. Every sprain should be radiographed in all views to rule out fracture or dislocation. Pain on radial deviation with tenderness over the scaphoid area implicates the ulnar collateral ligament, whereas pain on ulnar deviation is suggestive of a radial collateral ligament involvement. Pain provocation of the dorsal lunocapitate and palmar radiolunate ligaments are often reproduced when the patient places his or her hand on the examining table and places his or her body weight over the wrist by leaning forward. Passive and active movements may be painless. Resisted movement may be strong and painless. Dorsal palmar glide of the capitate on the lunate and the lunate on the radius may produce pain.

  When in doubt regarding a suspect radial collateral ligament sprain, one should cast the arm for 3 weeks suspecting potential scaphoid fracture. If no tenderness is present in conjunction with normal radiographs, wrist sprain is implicated by the process of elimination.[1] For a lateral collateral ligament injury, follow the same protocol as with any sprain. If pain is severe, immobilization in a cast from the palmar crease to the midforearm area is appropriate, otherwise an elastic bandage may suffice.[1] Management of a sprain to the lunate-capitate and radiocarpal ligaments is by rest and by friction massage

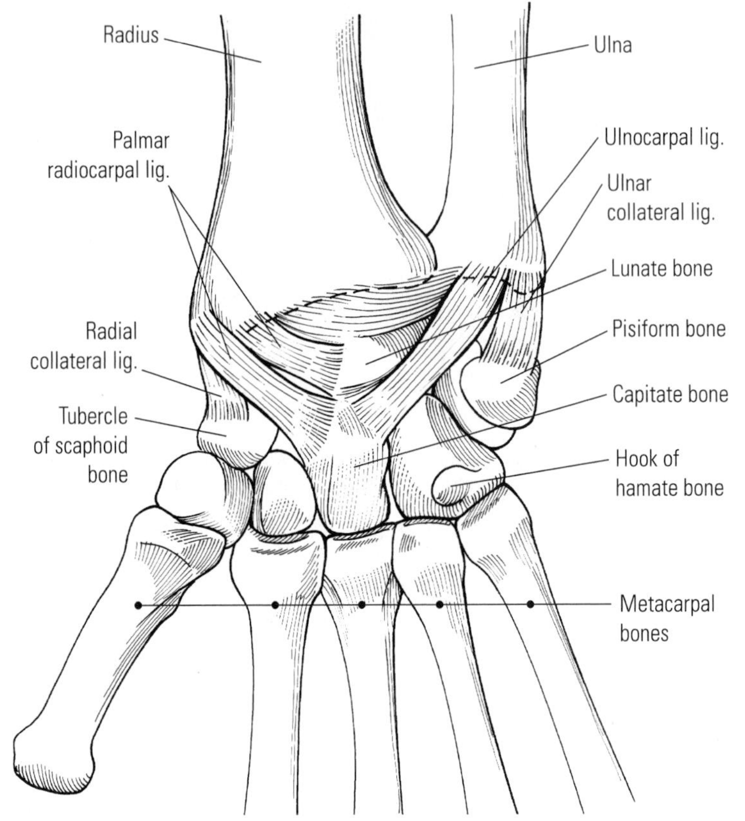

Fig. 5-4 Ligaments of the volar aspect of the wrist with the transverse carpal ligament removed.

to increase mobility of the collagen fibers without longitudinal stressing of the ligament. Ultrasound may be used as an adjunct in the resolution of chronic inflammatory exudates.[6]

- Isolated *fracture of the ulnar styloid* is rare and occurs when one lands on the ulnar side of the radially deviated hand. Although there is little swelling, there is considerable pain. Treatment is by wrist immobilization in ulnar deviation for 3 to 4 weeks. If nonunion occurs, the fragment should be removed.
- *Triquetral fractures* may occur from either one of two possible mechanisms: (1) falling onto a flexed wrist held in radial deviation resulting in an avulsion fracture of the dorsal surface of the bone, or less commonly (2) compression fracture from falling onto a hyperextended wrist. Radial deviation and wrist flexion are painful, with acute tenderness localized over the dorsal surface of the wrist just distal to the ulna. Treatment is by immobilization only until clinical symptoms subside.[4]
- Colles's fractures in children do not occur for one simple reason. Despite an obvious dinner-fork deformity, damage is either in the form of a greenstick fracture (alias buckle or torus fracture) or one of five general patterns of radial epiphyseal growth plate injuries. The reason is that the cartilaginous epiphyseal plate is stronger than bone whereas bone is relatively more supple in children. It is a clinical error to consider children as miniature models of adults. Generally children's bone structure is more resilient and adaptable, whereas their muscles, tendons, and ligaments are relatively stronger and more elastic than those of adults.[2]

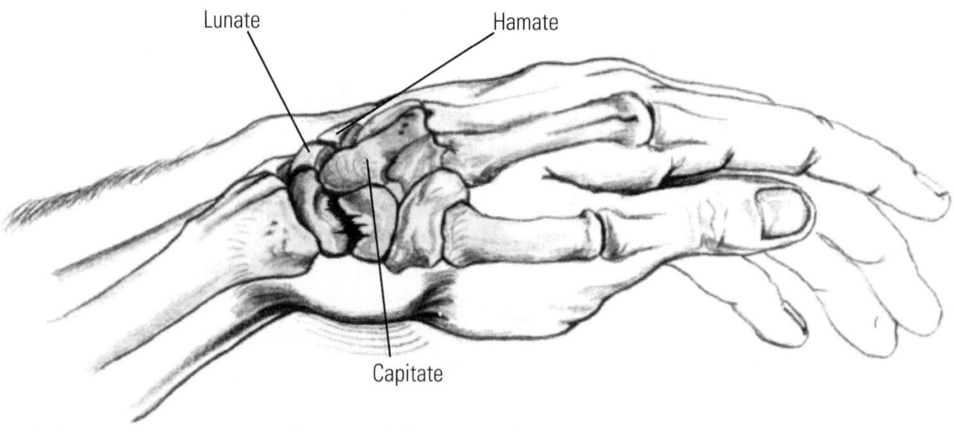

Fig. 5-5 Fracture of the scaphoid. (From Peterson L, Renström P: *Sports injuries: their prevention and treatment,* 1986, Martin Dunitz, Ltd.)

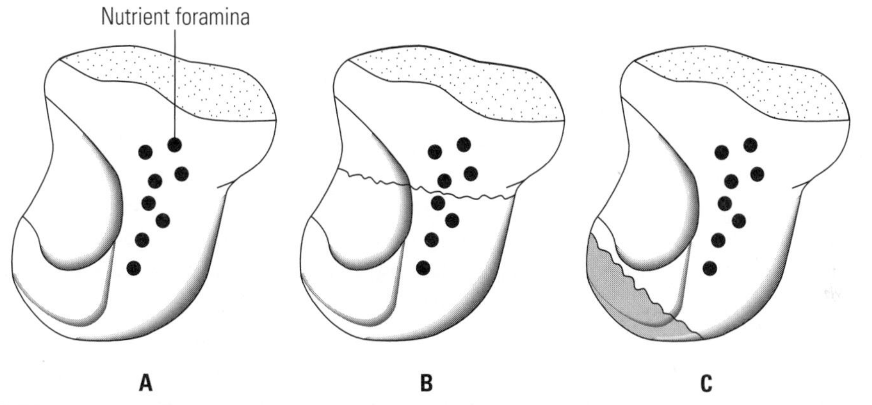

Fig. 5-6 Blood supply of the scaphoid. **A,** Blood enters the bone principally in its distal half. **B,** Fracture through the waist of the scaphoid. Vessels to the proximal scaphoid are preserved. **C,** Fracture near the proximal pole of the scaphoid. In this case there are no vessels supplying the proximal fragment, and aseptic necrosis of bone is therefore inevitable. (From Ellis H: *Clinical anatomy,* ed 7, Oxford, 1983, Blackwell Scientific Publications.)

- *Scaphoid fractures* (Fig. 5-5) are the most common of carpal bone fractures,[5] are often misdiagnosed as a sprained wrist or thumb, and occur when one falls onto a hyperextended and radially deviated wrist. Ironically, despite their relative frequency, they are the most commonly missed fractures of the upper limb.[10] Often, they are passed off as simply a wrist sprain.[12] In this injury the scaphoid bone bears the brunt of injury because, locked between the radius and the capitate, it is the only bony link between the forearm and the hand.[12] Fracture will most likely occur in the middle of the scaphoid (Fig. 5-6). Avascular necrosis and nonunion are a complication of this injury that may occur because the scaphoid is usually supplied by two nutrient arteries, one to the proximal half and then one to the distal half. However both vessels supply the distal segment in most persons, which is the same as

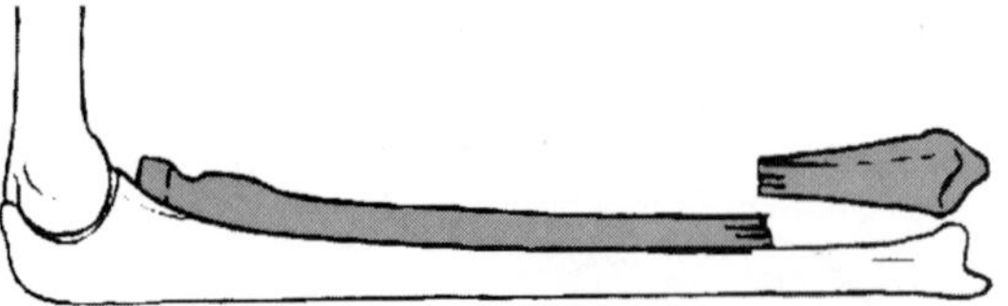

Fig. 5-7 Galeazzi fracture. (From Dandy DJ: *Essential orthopaedics and trauma,* Edinburgh, 1989, Churchill Livingstone.)

saying that the proximal pole is supplied by way of the distal pole. A fracture through the wrist will subsequently cause devitalization of the proximal pole.[4] An oblique radiograph is needed for diagnosis since standard radiographs may miss this fracture. Positive radiographic findings may demonstrate cyst formation at the fracture site as well as sclerosis of fracture surfaces. Continued movement will contribute to nonunion of bone fragments. Thus, even if no fracture is visualized, a scaphoid cast should be applied for several weeks.[11] This below-elbow cast should include the proximal phalanx of the thumb while holding it roughly opposite the ring finger and not in wide abduction, since that interferes with function and may displace fracture fragments.

Minimal immobilization with the wrist in 20° dorsiflexion and slight radial deviation is for 6 weeks but may require several months in the event that no union has occurred. Healing is characteristically slow because the relative absence of periosteal bone covering places the burden of healing on endosteal callus formation. In cases of suspected fracture, scaphoid radiographs should be repeated 10 days after the injury, since a fracture line may more easily be seen because of decalcification (that is, bone resorption) along its length and partly because of the slight separation of fragments. Operative treatment for nonunion varies according to the presence of traumatic arthritis. The clinical signs of scaphoid fracture are tenderness and swelling in the anatomic snuffbox or on the anterior aspect of the wrist over the scaphoid tubercle.[12]

- *Lunate dislocation* may also occur when one falls onto a hyperextended hand, which may push the carpus off the back of the radius, except for the lunate, which remains attached to the radius by the palmar radiocarpal ligament through which it derives its blood supply. Dislocation is easily missed on the anteroposterior radiograph but is obvious on the lateral view. The typical deformity observed is an anterior bulge or swelling just proximal to the volar wrist crease. Wrist flexion is limited and painful. Shortly afterward, dislocation pressure on the median nerve may provoke an acute carpal tunnel syndrome necessitating immediate closed reduction. The lunate bone is relocated under general anesthesia and must be immobilized for at least 4 weeks in 20° of wrist flexion, occasionally in a bivalved cast to allow for swelling. With an early reduction, prognosis is excellent; however, if neglected, closed reduction may be impossible and may necessitate open reduction.[1]

8. How may a Colles fracture be confused with a Galeazzi fracture-dislocation?

A *Galeazzi fracture* (Fig. 5-7) is similar to a Colles fracture in that the radius will fracture, yield deformity, and be accompanied by disturbance of the distal radioulnar joint. It differs, however, in several respects:

- Fracture of the shaft of the radius occurs more proximal than that of a Colles fracture.
- There is more striking clinical deformity, having a wrenched look.
- There is complete disruption and even dislocation of the distal radioulnar joint.
- It usually occurs in young adults.[12]

Like its mirror image, the *Monteggia fracture* (fractured one half of the ulna and dislocated proximal radioulnar joint, Fig. 5-8) requires internal fixation. The reason is that the strong pull of forearm muscles will cause either angulation or longitudinal torsion of fragments and will result in a considerable loss of pronation and supination. Thus a Galeazzi fracture is *not* treated with a short forearm cast as if it were a Colles fracture.[12]

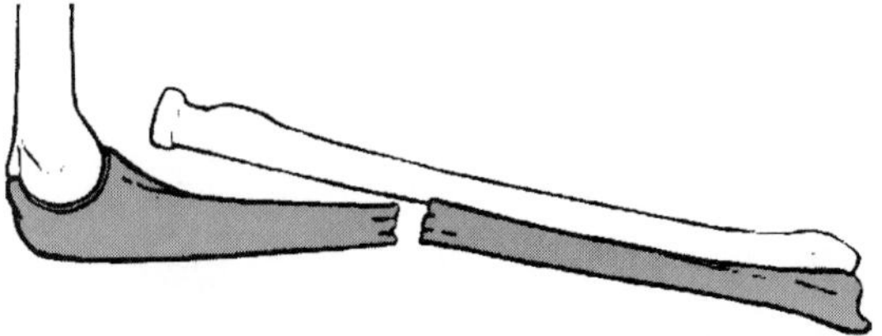

Fig. 5-8 Monteggia fracture. (From Dandy DJ: *Essential orthopaedics and trauma,* Edinburgh, 1989, Churchill Livingstone.)

9. Describe the important role of pronator teres in radial fractures and how this determines fragment splinting.

The important role of the pronator teres in radial fractures is clarified when we consider Fig. 5-9. In proximal fractures (Fig. 5-9, *A*) above the insertion of the pronator teres, the distal fragment is pronated. Such a fracture must be splinted in the supinated position. When the fracture is distal to the pronator teres insertion (Fig. 5-9, *B*), the action of this muscle on the proximal fragment is cancelled by the supinator action of the biceps. This fracture is therefore held reduced in the neutral position, midway between pronation and supination.

10. What are some sequelae of a Colles fracture?

Most persons with a Colles fracture are left with some albeit minor residual dysfunction. Complications after a Colles fracture abound and include the following:

- Malunion occurs because of either imperfect reduction or inadequate immobilization. Malunion secondary to crushed cancellous bone and comminuted cortical bone may be anticipated. Associated with malunion is painful subluxation of the distal radioulnar joint with limitation of wrist motion.

Operations for malunion include the following:

- For the elderly patient, simple excision of the distal ulna improves appearance but may disturb wrist stability.
- Corrective osteotomy of the radius with or without distal ulna excision may be required if the main problem is backward angulation of the radius.
- With Baldwin's procedure a 2 cm long segment of the ulna is excised along with its periosteum while leaving the ulnar styloid intact so that the ulnar head is allowed to move.
- With late rupture of the extensor pollicis longus (EPL) tendon, the EPL moves distally to the hand through the third dorsal tunnel, acting as a simple pulley located at the ulnar side of the radial (that is, Listers) tubercle. In the event of this tubercle's disturbance by a fracture, the EPL tendon will undergo fraying and eventual rupture because of friction against a roughened or sharp shard of bone. This usually develops 1 to 2 months after the fracture and suddenly manifests by the patient's inability to extend the thumb. Surgical repair is ineffective though tendon transfer may be contemplated.
- In median nerve compression and ischemia, the nerve may be compressed by initial bleeding around it or by later bleeding after the cast is removed when the nerve catches against the callus while the wrist moves.
- The sensory branch of the radial nerve supplying the dorsal hand may be stretched or torn. Anesthesias and paresthesias usually resolve after several weeks.
- The extensor carpi ulnaris runs through the sixth dorsal tunnel and is most palpable when the wrist simultaneously ulnarly deviated with wrist extension. If the distal ulnar styloid is fractured during a

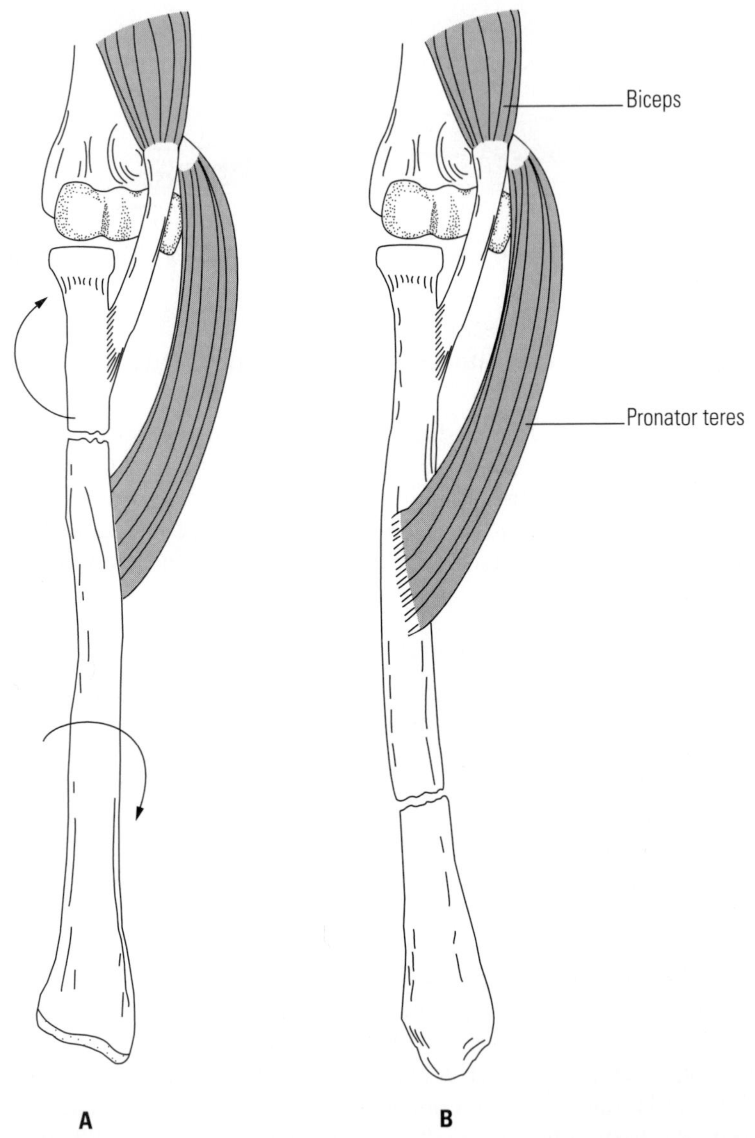

Fig. 5-9 The casting position after a radius fracture depends on whether the fracture occurs proximally, **A,** or distally, **B,** to the insertion of the pronator teres on the radius. (From Ellis H: *Clinical anatomy,* ed 7, Oxford, 1983, Blackwell Scientific Publications.)

Colles fracture, the dorsal carpal ligament may tear, resulting in dislocation of the extensor tendon during pronation, and is accompanied by an audible snap with or without pain.

- Residual finger stiffness may be forestalled by encouragement of active range of motion exercises and elevation of the fingers during immobilization.
- In Sudeck's atrophy anesthetic block of the inferior cervical or stellate ganglion will often relieve this condition if more conservative measures are unsuccessful.
- Nonunion is not considered a complication, since the blood supply to the distal end of the radius is excellent.[2]

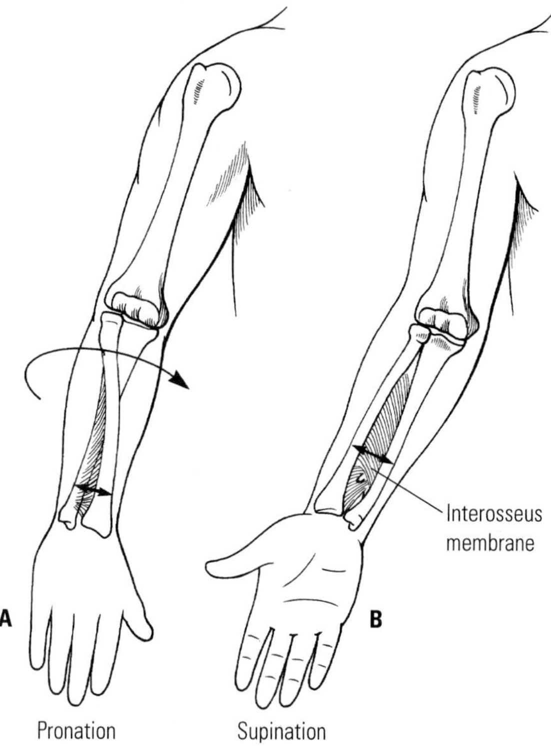

Fig. 5-10 **A,** The attachments of the interosseous membrane are approximated when the forearm is pronated. **B,** When the forearm is supinated, the distance between the radius and the ulna is greatest. Casting the forearm in any position other than supination will predispose shortening of the interosseous membrane, which may limit joint motion once the cast is removed.

11. What potential loss of range of motion may occur from a typical bone setting of a Colles fracture in pronation and wrist flexion, and why?

There is clinical significance to describing the radius and ulna as two bones that have a bow inherent to their anatomic features (Fig. 5-10). When the forearm is pronated, the distance between the two bows is lessened, and the convexity of each bow may be said to face each other (Fig. 5-10, *A*). However, when the forearm is supinated, the transverse distance between the two bones is greatest, and so the bones face away from each other (Fig. 5-10, *B*). The problem with casting in pronation is that any soft tissue spanning from the radius to the ulna will develop a contracture, which leads to difficulty in regaining premorbid forearm supination.

12. What rehabilitative therapy is appropriate after cast removal?

Provided that the bone or bones are well healed:

- During immobilization in a cast it is important to stress full range of motion of the noninvolved joint and muscle groups of the shoulder, elbow, thumb, and other fingers.
- Regular forearm isometric exercises within a cast will stave off muscle atrophy and edema.
- Retrograde massage helps decrease edema once the cast is removed.
- Progressive exercises begin with passive ones and progress to active and resistive exercises, which include the following:
  1. Approximation of thumb pad to each of the finger pads.
  2. Finger flexion, extension, abduction, and adduction.

3. Wrist flexion and extension.
4. Wrist radial and ulnar deviation.
5. Circular wrist motions in clockwise and counterclockwise directions.
6. Passive, active, and resistive pronation/supination exercises in sequential progression.

- If the skin is dry and flaky, use of a whirlpool is appropriate unless the patient has edema as well, in which case a hot whirlpool with the hand in a dependent position will only exacerbate the edema.
- Gentle dorsal and ventral glide (joint mobilization) of distal ends of radius and ulna, respectively, one relative to the other in pronation and especially in the supinated position.
- Shoulder and elbow abduction and adduction range of motion to prevent stiffness.
- Encouragement of the patient to use the wrist and hand in daily living activities so as to stave off neglect of the involved extremity.

References

1. Conwell HE: Injuries to the wrist, *Clin Symp* 22 (1):14, 1982.
2. Dandy DJ: *Essential orthopaedics and trauma,* Edinburgh, 1989, Churchill Livingstone, p 204.
3. De Palma F: *The management of fractures and dislocations: an atlas,* ed 2, Philadelphia, 1990, Saunders.
4. Ellis H: *Clinical anatomy,* ed 7, Oxford, 1983, Blackwell Scientific Publishers, p 209.
5. Gould JA III: *Orthopaedic and sports physical therapy,* ed 2, St Louis, 1990, Mosby, p 452.
6. Hertling D, Kessler RM: *Management of common musculoskeletal disorders,* ed 2, Philadelphia, 1990, Lippincott.
7. Kapit W, Elson LM: *The anatomy coloring book,* New York, 1977, Harper & Row, plate 16.
8. Meals RA: *One hundred orthopaedic conditions every doctor should understand,* St Louis, 1992, Quality Medical Publishing, p 67.
9. Moore KL: *Clinically oriented anatomy,* ed 2, Baltimore, 1985, Williams & Wilkins, p 691.
10. Netter, F: *The CIBA collection of medical illustrations,* vol 8: *Musculoskeletal system,* part 3, Summit, N.J., 1993, CIBA-Geigy Corp, p 61.
11. Peterson L, Renström P: *Sports injuries: their prevention and treatment,* London, 1986, Martin Dunitz, Ltd., pp 224, 404, 407.

Recommended reading

Dandy DJ: *Essential orthopaedics and trauma,* Edinburgh, 1989, Churchill Livingstone, p 204.

Gould JA III: *Orthopaedic and sports physical therapy,* ed 2, St Louis, 1990, Mosby, p 452.

Meals RA: *One hundred orthopaedic conditions every doctor should understand,* St Louis, 1992, Quality Medical Publishing, p 67.

Peterson L, Renström P: *Sports injuries: their prevention and treatment,* London, 1986, Martin Dunitz, Ltd, pp 405 and 407 (distributor in USA: Mosby, St Louis).

Netter F: *The CIBA collection of medical illustrations,* vol 8: *Musculoskeletal system,* part 3, Summit, N.J., 1993, CIBA-Geigy Corp, p 61.

Part Two

Elbow and Forearm

6

Burning Pain, Swelling, and Trophic Changes in Hand, Wrist, and Forearm out of Proportion to a 2-Week-Old Negligible Injury

A 29-year-old woman of average height and ruddy cheeks presents with a constant burning pain of her right hand, wrist, and distal forearm that, she reports, has spread proximally over the preceding 2 weeks. She complains of loss of use of her right extremity, which at times feels alternately cold and hot.

The patient recalls being stung in the right foot by a stingray some 4 months previously while snorkeling in the Caribbean. Subsequently, she developed severe cellulitis in that extremity for which she was hospitalized for a short period until the infection resolved. Upon returning home, she subsequently sustained a deep gash over her right anatomical snuffbox, which necessitated three stitches.

Her physician reveals to you his suspicions regarding the source of her malady over the telephone and mentions that all radiographic and MRI data for the neck, shoulder, and lungs were negative. He also ruled out scleroderma, venous obstruction, and angioedema. Radiographs of the hand demonstrate patchy osteopenia.

The patient offers that she has been seeing a psychologist for counseling over the past 2 years for occasional attacks of anxiety. When inquiring about her occupation, you learn that she is an aspiring actress with a leading role in an off-Broadway play of a patient who feigns a hysterical conversion disorder. There is no history of rheumatoid arthritis.

OBSERVATION There is moderate swelling to the right hand, the wrist, as well as slight fusiform swelling to the fingers of the right hand. Light moisture appears to cover the whole right hand as if it were perspiring. When compared to the contralateral hand, the involved hand appears shiny.

PALPATION Even a slight touch causes the patient to cringe and pull away; the involved hand feels warm. The contralateral palm feels moist. The patient mentions that she has always had sweaty palms.

RANGE OF MOTION There is mild to moderate stiffness of the right wrist and fingers, with the fingers in slight flexion, and flattening of the palmar crease lines over the interphalangeal and metacarpophalangeal joints.

MUSCLE STRENGTH Untested secondary to pain and tenderness.

SPECIAL TESTS Negative compression/distraction tests to the cervical spine.

SENSATION Paresthesia in a glove-and-stocking type of distribution over the distal right extremity.

1. **What is most likely afflicting this woman?**
2. **What is the normal sympathetic reflex?**
3. **What is the course of nerve-impulse transmission generated by the normal reflex sympathetic arc?**
4. **What is the abnormal reflex sympathetic arc?**
5. **What are the five clinical types of reflex sympathetic dystrophy (RSD)?**
6. **What is minor causalgia?**
7. **What are the three most common nerves injured whose sequelae include minor causalgia?**
8. **What is minor traumatic dystrophy?**
9. **What is the shoulder-hand syndrome?**
10. **What is major traumatic dystrophy?**
11. **What is major causalgia?**
12. **What are the signs and symptoms common to RSD?**
13. **What are the stages of RSD?**
14. **What factor does diathesis play in the development of RSD in certain individuals?**
15. **What is the differential diagnosis of RSD?**
16. **What medical intervention is appropriate to management of RSD?**
17. **What are the cardinal and secondary signs and symptoms of RSD, and how does their presence justify trial sympathetic block?**
18. **What therapeutic intervention is appropriate to management of RSD?**

1. What is most likely afflicting this woman?

Reflex sympathetic dystrophy (RSD) is a well known but poorly understood condition of the extremities[1] that was first clearly described by the American Civil War neurologist Silas Mitchell in the last year of that war (1864).[4] Most cases of RSD occur after major or minor trauma to the extremity in question or may also stem from visceral sources of injury such as myocardial infarction, stroke, stomach ulcer, or Pancoast's tumor to the apex of the lung.[3] RSD is now understood to be generated by an abnormal sympathetic reflex that encompasses painful states ranging from mildly uncomfortable vasomotor disorders to the full-blown classic Mitchell type of causalgia. Pain is the outstanding feature of the various clinical types of RSD and is grossly out of proportion to that expected from an injury or surgical insult.[1] The sympathetic nervous system has, of late, been implicated as an important mediator of this disorder,[5] though the exact cause and pathogenesis of RSD remain unknown.[3] Females more commonly suffer from RSD.[3]

2. What is the normal sympathetic reflex?

The normal *sympathetic reflex arc* is the body's reactive mechanism to trauma or disease that works by negative feedback to return the abnormal deranged state to that of normalcy (homeostasis).[3]

3. What is the course of nerve-impulse transmission generated by the normal reflex sympathetic arc?

After trauma, afferent nerve fibers transmit a pain message from the extremity and synapse in the posterior root ganglion projecting to the posterior horn and finally to the lateral horn where the pain message is communicated to the sympathetic nerve cell bodies. The sympathetic reflex (Fig. 6-1) is activated

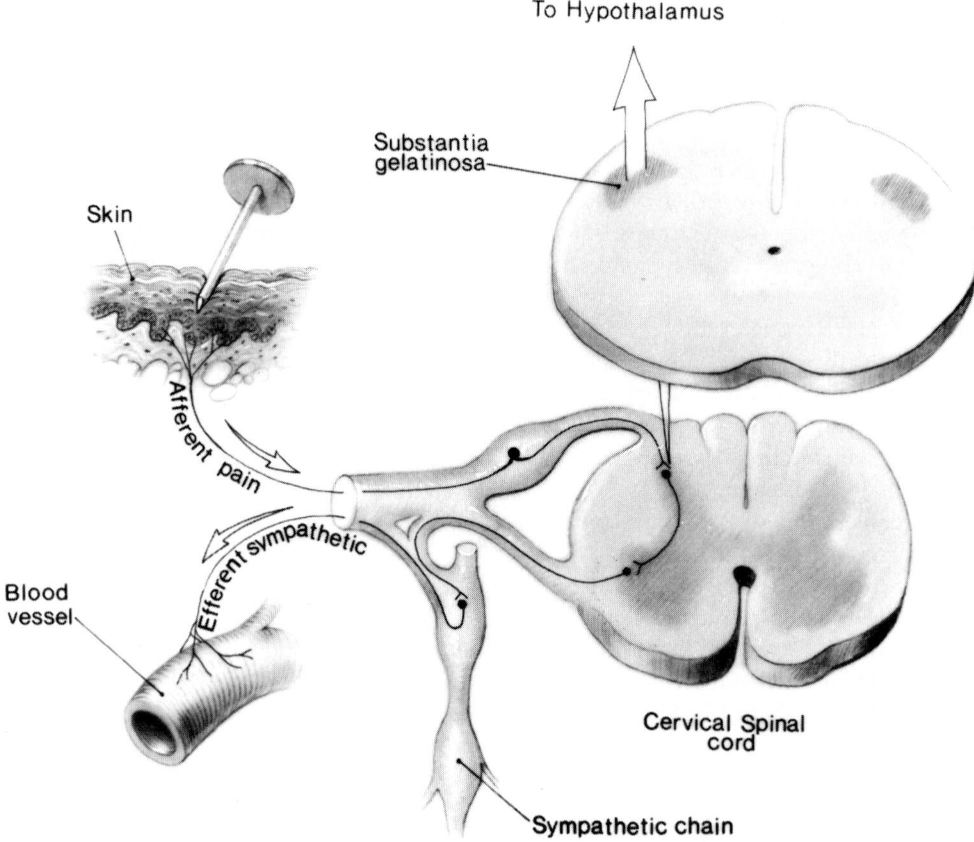

Fig. 6-1 A normal sympathetic nerve reflex arc is set into motion with any painful stimuli; it results in a temporary vasoconstrictive action of the small vessels. However, if this normal sympathetic reflex arc fails to shut down at the appropriate time, an abnormal sympathetic reflex may develop, thus producing one of the etiologic factors of reflex sympathetic dystrophy. (From Lankford LL, Thompson JE: *Reflex sympathetic dystrophy, upper and lower extremity: diagnosis and management.* In American Academy of Orthopaedic Surgeons: Instructional course lectures, vol 26, St. Louis, 1977, Mosby.)

when efferent sympathetic impulses are sent out the anterior horn through the anterior root to sympathetic chains. This reflex is then communicated through the white ramus in the sympathetic ganglion, where a synapse occurs. The postganglionic sympathetic fiber then leaves the ganglia through the gray ramus where it enters the peripheral nerve and travels distally along with it to the extremity to produce small-vessel vasoconstriction. This *vasoconstrictive reflex,* or *sympathetic pain reflex,* is believed to be a protective mechanism necessary to prevent excessive bleeding within injured tissue; this reparative process gives way to vasodilatation after a few hours as part of an orderly stepwise progression culminating in the return to homeostasis.[3]

4. What is the abnormal reflex sympathetic arc?

Occasionally the normal sympathetic reflex arc does not shut down at the appropriate time for unknown reasons. Rather, the reflex continues on in an accelerated fashion, and will ultimately produce an intense degree of sympathetic activity (Fig. 6-2). The increased and persistent vasoconstriction leads to tissue ischemia, which is painful and causes increased afferent pain impulses to be sent centrally. Hence there is initiated a vicious cycle (Fig. 6-3) in which the sympathetic reflex arc is repeatedly propagated resulting in

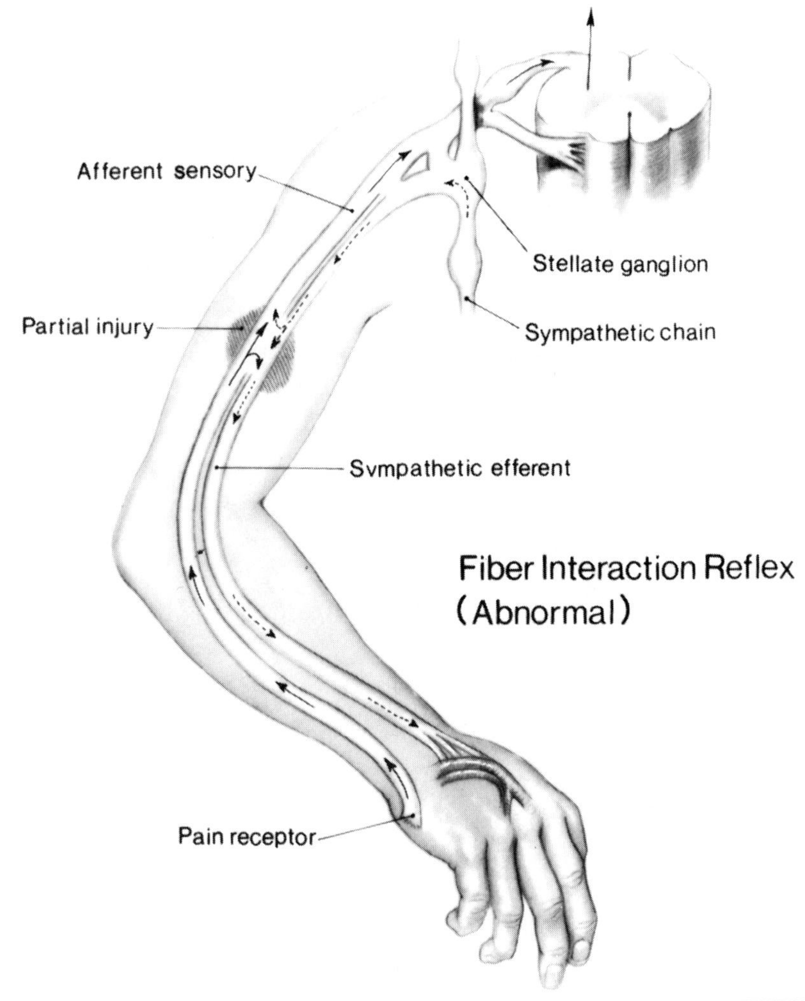

Fig. 6-2 Doupe described a physiologic breakdown of myelin sheath in an area of partial nerve injury that produced a "fiber interaction" of efferent and afferent impulses, which results in increased sympathetic nerve activity and increased pain. (From Lankford LL, Thompson JE: *Reflex sympathetic dystrophy, upper and lower extremity: diagnosis and management.* In American Academy of Orthopaedic Surgeons: Instructional course lectures, vol 26, St. Louis, 1977, Mosby.)

maintenance of sympathetic nerve activity, which, with time, manifests as reflex sympathetic dystrophy. The precise cause of malfunction in the shutdown mechanism of the sympathetic reflex arc is not known.[3]

5. What are the five clinical types of reflex sympathetic dystrophy (RSD)?

Because of its varied vasomotor manifestations, RSD has been described by various nomenclature. However, the common denominator to all forms of RSD is that all share a common mechanism of pathosis: the abnormal reflex arc. Because of this, all forms of this disorder fall under the nomenclature heading of reflex sympathetic dystrophy. These varied manifestations may be reduced to five clinical types: (1) minor causalgia, (2) minor traumatic dystrophy, (3) shoulder-hand syndrome, (4) minor traumatic dystrophy, and (5) major causalgia.

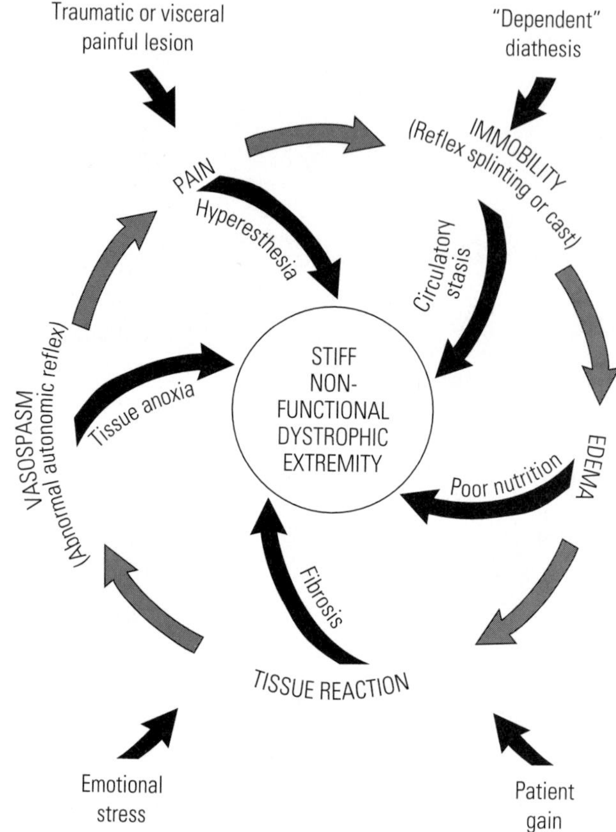

Fig. 6-3 Vicious circle is produced when tissue ischemia produces greater tissue reaction and pain caused by vasoconstrictive action of increased sympathetic nerve activity, resulting in a painful, stiff, swollen, and dystrophic extremity, as seen in reflex sympathetic dystrophy. (From Lankford LL, Thompson JE: *Reflex sympathetic dystrophy, upper and lower extremity: diagnosis and management.* In American Academy of Orthopaedic Surgeons: Instructional course lectures, vol 26, St. Louis, 1977, Mosby.)

6. What is minor causalgia?

Minor causalgia (Kausos: burning heat; algia: pain). Injury to a peripheral nerve, most commonly in the distal part of the extremity, represents the inciting trauma in this type of RSD. Symptoms and signs may be limited to only one or two fingers and are relatively less noxious. Whether the nerve became injured and scarred and underwent repair or the nerve was even cut through, as may occur during amputation, a neuroma may develop. Nerve fibers will sprout from the cut or lacerated nerve into nowhere in particular and are, not surprisingly, abnormally sensitive to pressure, movement, squeezing, or stretching. Many are also sensitive to norepinephrine (noradrenaline), which is emitted all around them by the accompanying sympathetic nerve fiber. Over time these nerve fibers very commonly bind down to surrounding fixed structures with adhesions so that any movement, such as wrist flexion, will produce a painful stretching of the nerve. This stretching, in turn, generates fibrous tissue proliferation (scar tissue), which serves only to further enmesh the nerve. The result of this process is a painful *neuroma,* with additional pain impulses being fired off to the spinal cord after subsequent provocation.[3] The pain of minor causalgia is constant, and other features of RSD such as pain on motion, swelling, stiffness, and osteoporosis are much greater than would be expected from simple neuroma.[3]

7. What are the three most common nerves injured whose sequelae include minor causalgia?

The nerve most commonly injured is the *dorsal superficial sensory branch of the radial nerve*[3] overlying the radial styloid area of the wrist. It may have iatrogenic sequelae to de Quervain's tenosynovectomy, after bone grafting for the carpal scaphoid, or from intravenous lines or shunts for hemodialysis. De Quervain's tenosynovectomy is considered to be minor surgery but is occasionally performed by physicians unaccustomed to the anatomy of that region.[1]

The next most common site of nerve injury is the *palmar cutaneous branch of the median nerve.* This branch takes leave of the median nerve 3 cm proximal to the transverse carpal ligament[1] and enters the hand superficially through the wrist. This nerve offshoot may be inadvertently injured by a surgeon employing the frowned-upon transverse incision of the flexor retinaculum at the volar side of the wrist in the treatment of carpal tunnel syndrome.[1,3]

The next most common sites of nerve injury include the *dorsal superficial sensory branches of the ulnar nerve,* especially over the dorsal ulnar aspect of the wrist and hand, and the common digital and proper digital branches of the median and ulnar nerves.[3]

8. What is minor traumatic dystrophy?

Minor traumatic dystrophy is the most common clinical type of RSD because minor traumas are more common and also because injuries more often do not involve a specific nerve. This type of RSD is also the *most frequently overlooked* form, since it is not common knowledge that RSD can involve only a small segment of the hand. The inciting factor is a minor injury such as a fracture, dislocation, sprain, or even a penetrating wound that does not involve injury to a nerve. Signs and symptoms vary and the degree of involvement may encompass only one or two fingers rather than the entire hand. Redness is characteristically found over the dorsum of the metacarpophalangeal joints and interphalangeal joints as well as over the collateral ligaments. A mild degree of palmar fasciitis may also be present. The digits are usually stiffened in flexion.[3]

9. What is the shoulder-hand syndrome?

The *shoulder-hand syndrome* is incited by a proximal insult, whether external or internal, and typically occurs in patients between 45 and 55 years of age and more commonly affects females than any other form of RSD. Shoulder-hand syndrome usually starts with considerable pain and stiffness in the shoulder, spreads to the distal part of the extremity, and produces moderate to pronounced swelling of the wrist, hand, and sometimes the upper arm. There is often a fusiform swelling of the fingers that are stiffened in extension rather than flexion. Palmar fasciitis with nodules are more commonly found. Redness, when present, is diffuse, and the hand is usually warmer and dryer than normal.[3]

10. What is major traumatic dystrophy?

Major traumatic dystrophy may occur after a major trauma such as a crushed hand, Colles fracture, or a severe fracture dislocation of the wrist. This form of RSD yields the greatest degree of pain, stiffness, swelling, and dysfunction in the non-nerve injury type of RSD. Flexion contractures of the digits are more frequent than extension contractures. Wrist motion is usually severely limited, and flexion deformities may be present. There is often accompanying limitation of rotary forearm motion, especially in pronation.[3]

11. What is major causalgia?

Major causalgia is the classic Mitchell causalgia. It causes the greatest degree of pain and devastation to the patient. The median nerve is most commonly involved in the upper extremity, whereas the sciatic nerve is most commonly involved in the lower extremity. These two nerves possess a greater sympathetic nerve distribution as compared with other nerves of the extremities. Pain is characteristically described as "burning," which may become exacerbated by a light touch of the skin, by becoming emotionally upset, or even by auditory stimulation such as hearing a squeaky noise. Pain may become so severe at times that a patient might consider amputation of the part. The vibration from riding in an automobile or even from another person walking across the floor may aggravate the pain. The patient may seek relief by wrapping his or her hand or extremity in wet towels. At first, pain is confined to the distribution of the injured nerve, but it soon spreads to the hand and entire extremity. Early stages of this form of RSD find the extremity almost always pale or cyanotic in color with sweating and coolness a prominent feature. Flexion contractures of the fingers occur, and, although stiffness is extreme, the degree of contracture is often not so great as in major traumatic dystrophy.[3]

12. What are the signs and symptoms common to RSD?

- *Pain,* characteristically described as having a burning quality, is the most prominent symptom of RSD. Although most forms of trauma and disease states produce pain that eventually abates over time, the distinguishing feature of RSD is that the pain experienced is entirely out of proportion to the original injury and in fact worsens with time and so what began as a burning sensation will intensify into pressure, crushing, binding, searing, cutting, cramping, or aching superimposed on the initial pain. The pain is constant and is aggravated by active or passive attempts at motion, making examination difficult because the patient will often withdraw from the examiner. Initially, pain is limited to a small area, such as the area of distribution of a given nerve at the site of injury, only to soon spread to encompass the entire extremity. In many cases pain may not begin until after a cast to treat a fracture is removed. Tenderness is quite pronounced, especially around the interphalangeal joints of the fingers.[3]
- *Swelling,* usually the first physical sign, occurs initially in the involved area and then slowly spreads to encompass the entire extremity in some cases. Finger swelling, which at first has a fusiform appearance, gradually leads to circumarticular thickening at the joints. At first, the swelling manifests as a soft edema but over time becomes a hard and brawny edema that almost certainly contributes to loss of motion.[3]
- *Stiffness,* like pain, is distinctive in that it increases over time—unlike trauma without the presence of RSD in which stiffness abates as the wound heals. The initial lack of motion is attributable to enforced immobility so as to further escape aggravation of pain. Subsequently, stiffness is attributed to fibrosis of the ligamentous structures and adhesion formation around tendons that causes the adjacent gliding structures to stick to one another. The result is that all fibrous joint structures become thickened, hard, and inelastic. Accompanying palmar fasciitis only serves to add to the severity of flexion contractures in the joints.[3]
- *Discoloration* is an ever-present sign that initially manifests as redness (rubor) and is most commonly located over the dorsum of the metacarpophalangeal and interphalangeal joints of the fingers or may at times diffusely involve the entire hand. Redness occurs as a function of vasodilatation of both the arterial and venous systems. As the disease progresses, the hand may become pale, whereas at other times turn pale to cyanotic. *Pallor* results from simultaneous vasoconstriction of both sides of the vascular tree, whereas blueness occurs from vasoconstriction of the venous system. Purplish discoloration may often be seen in the flexor creases of the fingers and palm, especially if palmar fasciitis has developed. Although redness and vasodilatation occur initially in the disease process, vasoconstriction may be present in the very early stages of RSD.[3]
- *Osteoporosis.* Initial demineralization occurs in the carpal bones producing punched-out areas as well as in the polar regions of the long bones of the metacarpals and phalanges. This spotty involvement evolves, in the untreated condition, to become a diffuse osteoporosis. Demineralization primarily occurs from increased blood flow to the joints and secondarily from immobilization.[2]
- *Sudomotor changes.* Excessive moisture (hyperhidrosis) is more often present in the early stages of RSD. At times the diaphoresis is so great that beads of sweat are observed to drop from the hand. In the later stages of RSD, dryness is the rule.[3]
- *Temperature.* In the early stages of RSD when redness is present, the temperature is more commonly elevated (hyperthermia), whereas when pallor or cyanosis is present, as it commonly is toward the severe

stage of the disease, the temperature is nearly always diminished. In some instances there may be simultaneous increased temperature over the reddened joints and diminished temperature in between the joints where pallor is observed.

- *Palmar fasciitis.* Palmar fasciitis with acute nodules and thickening of the longitudinal bands of palmar fascia in the fingers and hand may be seen in several clinical types of RSD.
- *Vasomotor instability.* Prolonged capillary refill time, indicative of vasoconstriction, is commonly found in RSD and is generally found with pallor, cyanosis, or excessive sweating. In contrast, rapid capillary refill may be seen in the reddened hand, and this is indicative of vasodilatation.
- *Trophic changes.* The characteristic glossy, often shiny skin appearance in RSD is initially attributable to swelling and ironing out of skin wrinkles secondary to lack of joint motion. The skin feels quite tight to the patient. Later on, nutritional (trophic) changes occur resulting in a glossy, shiny skin surface as a result of subcutaneous tissue atrophy. Fingertips may take on a "pencil-pointing" appearance because of atrophy of the finger fat pad or pads and concomitant downward curving of the fingernail or fingernails.[3]

13. What are the stages of RSD?

The course of RSD is usually divided into three stages:

Stage I. Stage I has an average duration of 3 months. Signs and symptoms include painful paresthesia to light touch, pitted swelling over the dorsum of the hand, observed skin tightness, decreased motion in the fingers and wrist, vasoconstriction or peripheral vasospasm resulting in paleness or cyanosis, and increased sweating and coolness. Near the end of stage I pain becomes aggravated by attempts at motion, and redness as well as dryness may manifest. Osteoporosis may be seen by the fifth week.[3]

Stage II. Pain is the most prominent feature in stage II, and swelling changes from that of a soft nature to a brawny, hard edema. It is difficult to reduce swelling by elevation and other standard means during this stage; subsequently, stiffness continues to increase. Additionally, redness, increased heat, and decreased sweating are most commonly observed during this stage. Increasing demineralization appears as a more widespread homogeneous radiographic appearance. The shiny, glossy-looking skin is maintained during this stage and may intensify. The duration of stage II commonly progresses through the ninth month.

Stage III. In stage III the severity of pain has peaked and either remains constant for several months or just slowly improves. In many cases, however, pain continues for up to 2 years and indefinitely in some cases. Swelling changes from brawny edema to periarticular thickening of the joints. The hand becomes pale, dry, and cool, and the glossy appearance peaks at this stage. Skin and subcutaneous tissue atrophy results in "pencil-pointing" of the fingertips. Osteoporosis is profound, and the hand is severely dysfunctional.[3]

14. What factor does diathesis play in the development of RSD in certain individuals?

Diathesis is defined as individual disposition that causes susceptibility to given disease. Two different types of diathesis are recognized in RSD though neither is mutually exclusive of the other.

1. The first diathesis tends to occur in those individuals possessing an increased sympathetic nerve activity that is evidenced by a history of sweaty palms (hyperhidrosis), pallor, or excessive coolness of fingers and toes when exposed to colder temperatures. On physical examination the clinician finds evidence of peripheral vasoconstriction and poor capillary refill of the uninvolved extremity. There may be historical evidence of vasomotor dysfunction such as fainting spells, excessive flushing or blanching, or even migraine headaches.
2. The second diathesis has to do with the psychologic makeup of the individual, which is considerably more difficult to discern than the aforementioned hypersympathetic factor. Psychiatrists have described several psychologic traits present in many RSD patients that include fearful, suspicious, emotionally labile, or inadequate personality; a chronic complainer; a dependent personality, and an insecure and unstable personality. Patients who develop RSD also tend to have a very low pain threshold,

in contrast to the stoic or spartan type of individual. The patient may ask a multitude of irrelevant questions, try to control his or her own treatment, display lack of cooperation, may think up excuses for not doing what he or she is told, seek to place blame for the condition upon others, and try to control and manipulate the treatment. It is important to realize that the patient cannot control this diathesis and therefore cannot willfully cause this to happen to his or her self.[3]

There is speculation that RSD may in fact be a hysterical conversion disorder, highlighting the strong relationship that exists between mind and body. It would seem that patients would probably not benefit greatly from concurrent psychologic counseling, since they would tend to resist the implication that anything might be wrong with them emotionally.[3]

15. What is the differential diagnosis of RSD?

Differential diagnoses of RSD include rheumatoid arthritis, scleroderma, angioedema, and venous obstruction. The last condition may produce hand edema but usually causes more proximal swelling and does not tend to be so painful.[5]

16. What medical intervention is appropriate to management of RSD?

The old axiom that early diagnosis and early treatment produce the best results has never been more correct than in the case of RSD.

Stellate ganglion block is both diagnostic of RSD as well as an effective treatment for RSD because it interrupts the abnormal sympathetic reflex by blockade of all sympathetic efferent impulses to the extremity without anesthesia or paralysis. The stellate ganglion is composed of the fusion of the superior and middle cervical ganglia. Confirmation of successful blockade is provided by an immediate accompanying Horners sign, though effective sympathectomy may occur without the presence of this sign. Patients often react in amazement at the immediate change in the condition of their hands as well as a very prompt and distinct improvement of pain and generalized feeling of well-being. Benefit may last from 1 to 3 days before reassertion of sympathetic nerve hyperactivity and regeneration of the abnormal sympathetic reflex. Because of potential tissue irritation, not more than one or two blocks are administered per week unless the patient is in very severe distress. The usual number of blocks often necessary for the abolition of the abnormal sympathetic reflex is either four or five.

With very severe cases of RSD or if stellate ganglion blocks have not been started early enough, it may not be possible to break adequately the abnormal sympathetic reflex cycle. If definite improvement has accrued from several blocks, although relief is of short duration, surgical sympathectomy involving removal of the first four thoracic sympathetic ganglia may be considered.[3]

17. What are the cardinal and secondary signs and symptoms of RSD, and how does their presence justify trial sympathetic block?

Cardinal signs and symptoms include (1) pain, (2) swelling, (3) stiffness, and (4) discoloration. *Secondary signs and symptoms* are often present, though not inevitable, and include (1) osseous demineralization, (2) sudomotor changes, (3) trophic changes, (4) temperature changes, (5) vasomotor instability, and (6) palmar fibromatosis.

If all four of the cardinal signs and symptoms are present and at least several of the secondary signs and symptoms are found, a presumptive diagnosis of RSD is made. Actual confirmation comes after interruption of the sympathetic nerve reflex. At least three or four blocks with completely negative effects are administered so that one can completely rule out RSD.[3]

18. What therapeutic intervention is appropriate to management of RSD?

- Treatment of RSD requires early aggressive therapy *within and not to or beyond* the limits of pain. The overzealous therapist who ignores this warning is more likely to worsen the patient's condition rather than to improve it. The old adage of pain is gain certainly does not hold true here. Exercise is an important part of the treatment of RSD but only when the protective umbrella of sympathetic blockade has been provided.[3]

- The patient, in many cases, may have a poor self-image and may have given up hope and experienced a psychologic amputation of the limb.[3]
- The patient is administered a highly structured but simplified program of therapy. The therapist must attempt to instill motivation in the patient and communicate that he or she has the power to improve his or her condition.
- Establish a baseline value of perceived pain using a scale for assessing pain before initiating a pain management program.[3]
- Volumetric evaluations before and after treatment modalities for hand and wrist circumference reading are appropriate only when one or two digits are involved.[6]
- Initially, *gentle active exercises* without reaching the point of pain, performed frequently and for short periods, as well as *light massage.*
- TENS (transcutaneous electrical nerve stimulation) treatment sends sensations of light touch, pressure, and proprioception by way of the faster-transmitting, larger-diameter, myelinated, and afferent nerve fibers to bypass pain transmitting C fibers. Thus the normal-sensation impulses flood the sensorium and become a vocal majority that outshout the pain message by virtue of arriving at the T cells in the substantia gelitanosa faster and en masse and thus close the gate to the pain impulse (the gate-control theory of pain).[3] TENS treatment is best performed frequently, and a change of electrode position facilitates maximum benefit.
- *Stress-loading program* of the affected extremity for pain relief and desensitization. This treatment may be instituted as an early intervention strategy when RSD in suspected, whereas invasive techniques cannot. *Scrub*—The patient is positioned in quadruped on the floor. With a coarse bristled scrub brush in the affected hand the patient is instructed to lean on the arm with the shoulder directly over the hand for maximum pressure. The patient is then instructed to "scrub" a plywood board using a back and forth motion beginning with three minute sessions of steady scrubbing three times per day. The program is increased to 7 minutes after 2 weeks; alternatively, a 10 minute session twice a day may be substituted if tolerated by the patient. *Carry*—The patient loads the extremity by carrying a weight with the affected arm in elbow and wrist extension. The amount of weight is determined at the first session, generally ranging from 1 to 5 pounds (a purse or briefcase). The weight should be carried throughout the day whenever the patient is standing or walking. The amount of weight carried is recorded daily on a record sheet. Increases in the amount of weight are incremental.[6]
- *Thermotherapy* is by way of hot packs or a paraffin bath to relax muscles and soften scar tissue to facilitate improved range of motion. *Fluidotherapy* is ideal for desensitization of the limb affected by RSD as well as for softening of scar tissue. Heat is often helpful if coupled with elevation.[3]
- Jobst *intermittent compression treatment* is most effective in patients demonstrating pitting edema. The treatment lasts 45 minutes to 1 hour with compression set at 60 to 90 mm Hg while the affected limb is elevated. If the Jobst unit is used to increase passive interphalangeal flexion, compression must be reduced to a range of 30 to 60 mm Hg, and the fingers should be positioned alternately in flexion and extension. After compression treatment, gentle *retrograde massage* for 10 minutes with lanolin-based cream as a lubricant to decrease edema, desensitize the extremity, soften scar tissue, and facilitate further gain in range of motion.
- Use a pressure wrap or a thermoelastic compression glove after Jobst treatment and massage.
- Use gentle joint mobilization to facilitate gain in range of motion and softening of tightened joint capsules.
- *Ice treatment* for 20 minutes in contrast baths may decrease edema, though this, similar to other edema-reducing modalities, is often not well tolerated in RSD patients because it may cause painful vasoconstriction.[3]
- Advise patients to stop smoking so as to avoid tissue ischemia from vasoconstriction.
- The use of a *hot* whirlpool bath is *contraindicated*[3] because heat applied with the extremity in a dependent position will cause stagnation of the lymphatic and venous system and result in increased swelling.

- *Splinting* to relieve pain on motion and relieve muscle spasm has been proposed. The goal of splinting is to, by means of exerting passive motion on the joint, return the hand to the "resting-hand" position of 45-degree wrist extension, slight ulnar wrist deviation, 70-degree metacarpophalangeal joint flexion, and 30-degree proximal interphalangeal joint flexion. The value of this position is that it is that range in which the least number of deforming forces act upon the joints of the hand. The key to splinting at the wrist is to understand that one cannot expect to reduce extensor contractures of the PIP joints without first getting the wrist into extension. This is accomplished by a volar thermoelastic splint with Velcro straps customized with as much wrist extension as the patient can comfortably tolerate. The splint is periodically reheated to accommodate increasing wrist extension. Vigorous contracture reduction of the flexed PIP joints and the extended MP joints may be attempted after reduction of the wrist flexion contracture. The former reductions are facilitated by use of dynamic splints in the form of a dorsal thermoplastic splint with an outrigger and rubber-band slings that produce a gentle extension force over the IP joints; this, however, may be achieved only if an equal or greater force is exerted on flexing of the MP joints. This is accomplished by use of a lumbrical bar that pushes down on the dorsum of the proximal segments of the fingers (so as to yield MP joint flexion) with the same or greater force than is used to extend the IP joints. This setup may also be achieved by the use of flexion rubber bands and slings affixed to a wristlet band, thus providing a respectable flexion force applied to the MP joints. The passive forces applied to the joints will be detrimental if the patient experiences pain from an ill-fitting or too tightly adjusted dynamic splint. Although the splints ought to be worn the majority of the time, they may be removed every 30 minutes for the duration of the exercise program.[3]
- Skateboard exercises for the shoulder and elbow (Fig. 6-4).
- Begin gentle exercises distally in the fingers and progress proximally with time. Initially, very gentle passive motion is administered as far as possible without coming to the point of pain, followed by active assistive movement to the limit of painless motion and maintenance of this position for 10 seconds. These exercises are performed in both flexion and extension, with selective isolation of each joint of each finger while providing proximal stability. Similar exercises are performed in finger adduction and abduction as well as for the wrist in all planes of motion. This entire regimen should be ideally repeated once every 30 minutes.[3]
- Active dowel or wand exercises to increase shoulder, elbow, and forearm range of motion and strength (Fig. 6-5). A Velcro cuff weight may eventually be added for resistance.[7]

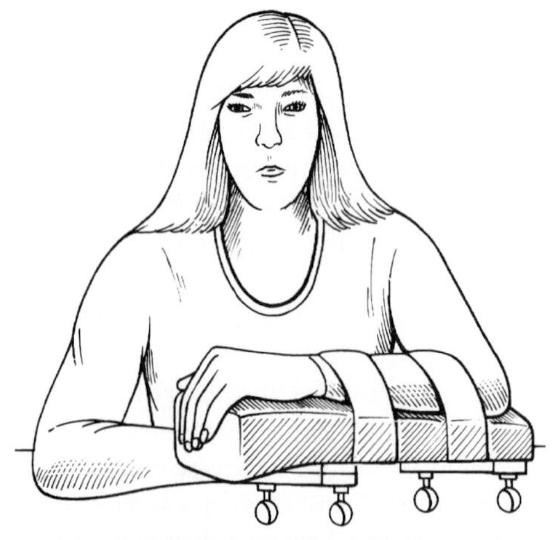

Fig. 6-4 Skateboard exercises for the shoulder and elbow.

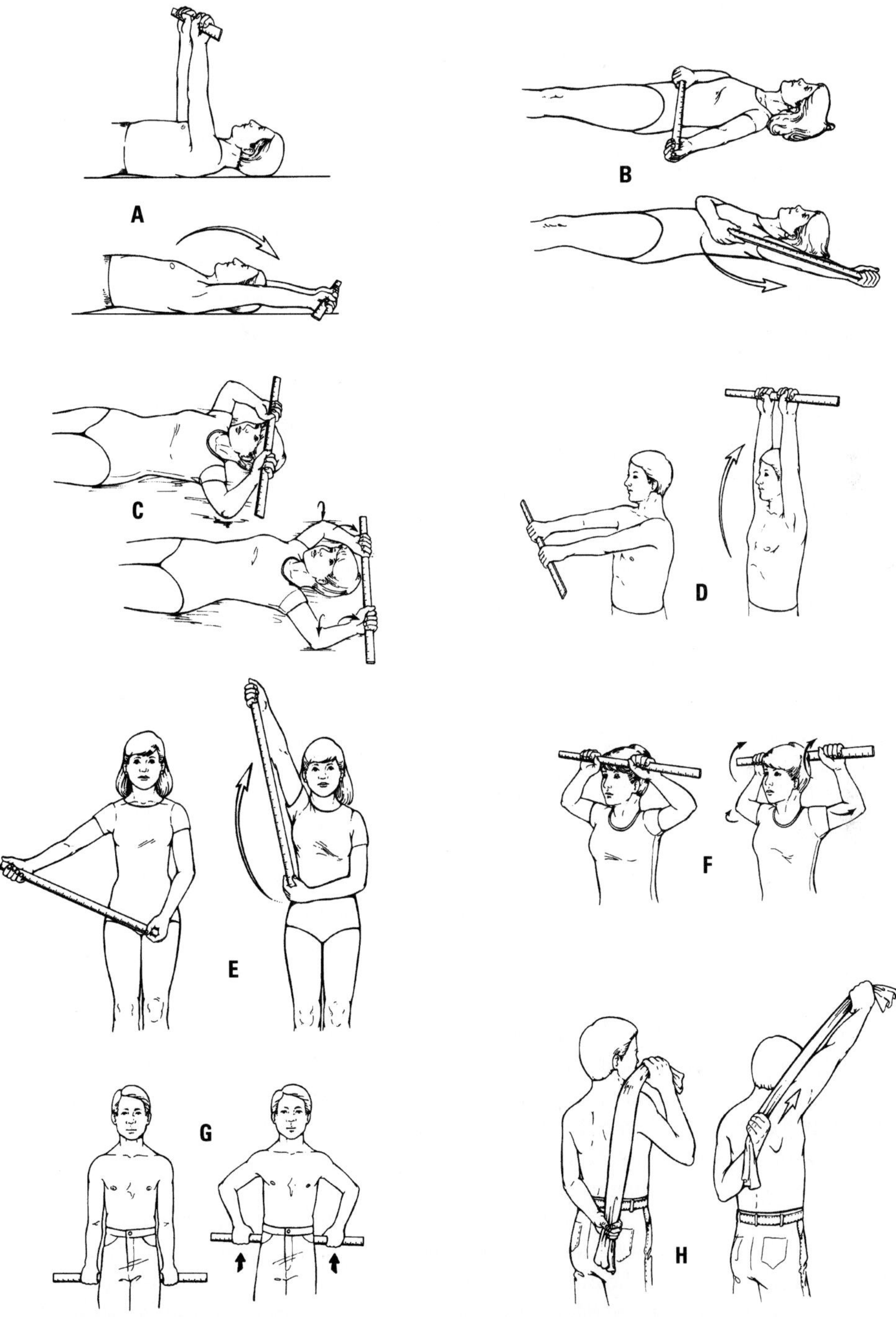

Fig. 6-5 Wand exercises to increase range of motion in the shoulder. **A,** Supine flexion. **B,** Supine abduction. **C,** Supine external rotation. **D,** Standing flexion. **E,** Standing abduction. **F,** Standing external rotation. **G,** Standing internal rotation. **H,** Standing internal rotation with towel. (From Saunders HD: *Evaluation treatment and prevention of musculoskeletal disorders,* Bloomington, Minn., 1985, Education Opportunities.)

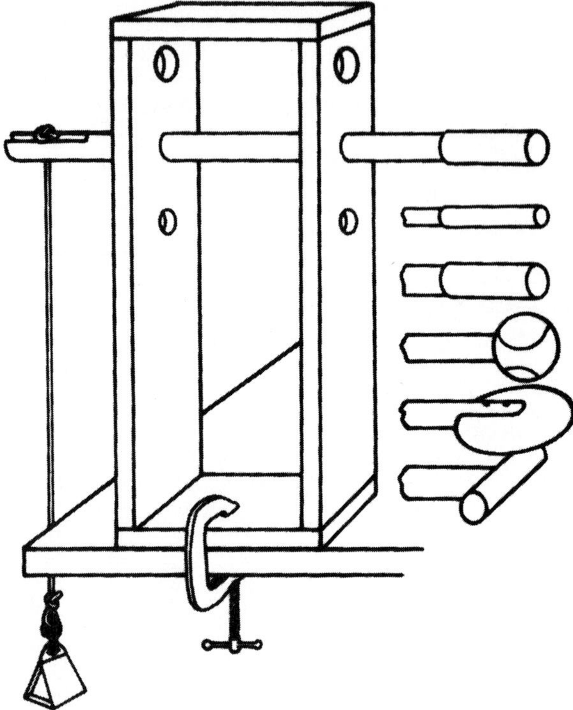

Fig. 6-6 Weight well exercise device with interchangeable handles for wrist and hand exercises. (From Hunter JM, Schneider LH, Mackin EJ, Callahan AD, editors: *Rehabilitation of the hand: surgery and therapy,* ed 3, St. Louis, 1990, Mosby.)

- Progressive resistive exercises by means of the *treppe* (German for "staircase") *method* gradually warming up the muscle for maximum exertion without risk of overstretching the muscle by increasing muscle contractions gradually against resistance. This system employs a series of 10 contractions against 100% of maximum weight.[7]
- *Weight well exercises,* (Fig. 6-6), in addition to active strengthening, elevate the hand to decrease edema and assist venous flow through the pumping action of the forearm and hand musculature.[7]
- Activities of daily living and craft activities are extremely important with patients suffering from RSD, since these patients typically avoid using the upper extremity. Through simple accomplishments in craft projects, the patient is made aware that his or her hand is functional and, as such, will begin to use it once again. Simple rote crafts such as linking a belt, stacking blocks, or placing wooden rings over round pegs reincorporate the spontaneous use of the injured hand into their lives. This is accomplished because the patient has no set expectations about a craft activity never before attempted but is often unwilling to accept substandard performance of self-feeding and other forms of activities of daily living. The therapist should try to be one step ahead of the patient in the setting of goals, with appropriate adulation expressed that will psychologically boost the patient and spur him or her on to new levels of accomplishment.[3] Eventually the therapist should guide the patient into performing the kind of functional activities that simulate the kind of work the patient will perform when he or she will return to employment.

References

1. Dawson DM, Hallet M, Millender LH: *Entrapment neuropathies,* ed 2, Boston, 1990, Little, Brown & Co.
2. Genant HK, Kozin F, Bekerman C, et al: The reflex sympathetic dystrophy syndrome, *Radiology* 117:28, 1975.
3. Lankford LL: Reflex sympathetic dystrophy. In Hunter JM, Schneider LH, Mackin EJ, Callahan AD, editors: *Rehabilitation of the hand: surgery and therapy,* ed 3, St. Louis, 1990, Mosby.
4. Mitchell SW, Morehouse GR, Keen WW: *Gunshot wounds and other injuries of nerves,* Philadelphia, 1864, Lippincott.
5. Schumacher HR, Bomalski JS: *Case studies in rheumatology for the house officer,* Baltimore, 1990, Williams & Wilkins.
6. Watson HK, Carlson L: Treatment of reflex sympathetic dystrophy of the hand with an active "stress loading program," *J Hand Surg* 12A(5)(part 1):779, 1987.
7. Waylett-Rendall J: Therapist's management of reflex sympathetic dystrophy. In Hunter JM, Schneider LH, Mackin EJ, Callahan AD, editors: *Rehabilitation of the hand: surgery and therapy,* ed 3, St. Louis, 1990, Mosby.

Recommended reading

Lankford LL: Reflex sympathetic dystrophy. In Hunter JM, Schneider LH, Mackin EJ, Callahan AD, editors: *Rehabilitation of the hand: surgery and therapy,* ed 3, St. Louis, 1990, Mosby.

Patt RB, Balter K: Posttraumatic reflex sympathetic dystropy: mechanisms and medical management, *J Occup Rehab,* vol 1, No. 1, 1991.

Waylett-Rendall J: Therapist's management of reflex sympathetic dystrophy. In Hunter JM, Schneider LH, Mackin EJ, Callahan AD, editors: *Rehabilitation of the hand: surgery and therapy,* ed 3, St. Louis, 1990, Mosby.

Bilateral Epicondylar Elbow Pain

7

A middle-aged man enters your office with complaints of both right and left elbow pain. The gentleman underwent his second divorce 2 months previously and spends most of his time away from the office avidly playing golf. The gentleman is right handed and leads his golf stroke with his left elbow. He does not play tennis. He reports that daily high doses of aspirin are helping him. There is no history of injury or injection to either elbow, nor is there any history of gout.

OBSERVATION Both elbows appear normal; there is neither swelling nor redness.

PALPATION Palpation yields point tenderness immediately anterior, medial, and distal to the left lateral epicondyle, directly over the extensor brevis, and distally 1 to 2 inches along the course of pronator teres and flexor carpi radialis, as well as the right medial epicondyle; there is no tenderness over the olecranon process. Both epicondyles feel slightly warm.

ACTIVE RANGE OF MOTION Full and painless with no evidence of contracture.

MUSCLE STRENGTH There is good minus strength in the extensor-supinator muscle group in the left arm, as well as in the flexor-pronator muscle group in the right arm as compared to the contralateral arm.

JOINT PLAY Movements are full and painless.

SPECIAL TESTS No pain to left elbow below outer epicondyle after a varus stress test, and no pain to right elbow below inner epicondyle after valgus stress test. Normal compression and distraction test results of the cervical spine.

CLUE *Selective tension* reveals the following patterns for the left and right elbows:

Left elbow. *Resisted* wrist extension (with elbow extended) and radial deviation, forced passive wrist flexion and ulnar deviation, and forearm pronation (with elbow extension) reproduce pain in the vicinity of the lateral epicondyle.

Right elbow. Pain elicited on *resisted* wrist flexion (with the elbow straight) and pronation, as well as extremes of passive wrist extension with forearm supination (and elbow extension) and ulnar deviation, all mimic pain at the medial epicondyle.

1. **What is the cause of this man's pain?**
2. **What is the sequential progression of this disorder?**
3. **Which vocations or avocations are commonly associated with lateral epicondylitis?**
4. **What are the three types of tennis elbow?**
5. **Why does lateral tennis elbow most commonly present as a chronic disorder?**
6. **What is the histologic basis for this disorder?**

7. **What are radiographic findings?**
8. **What is pitcher's elbow?**
9. **What may account for the lesser incidence of medial epicondylitis?**
10. **What adjacent ligamentous disorder may pitchers incur from excessive valgus stress at the elbow?**
11. **What is the epidemiology of tennis elbow?**
12. **What factors contribute to lateral epicondylitis in tennis players?**
13. **What is the significance of provocative testing with the elbow in extension?**
14. **What is the differential diagnosis for tennis elbow?**
15. **What is radial tunnel syndrome?**
16. **Why is lateral tennis elbow a persistent disorder that does not tend to resolve spontaneously?**
17. **What therapeutic management best serves the patient?**
18. **At what point does surgery become a treatment option?**

1. **What is the cause of this man's pain?**

This gentleman has lateral epicondylitis of the left elbow and medial epicondylitis of the right elbow (Fig. 7-1). The most common contractile lesions occurring in the elbow region involve the proximal attachments of the wrist extensors and flexors.[10] Both are an overuse syndrome involving strain and inflam-

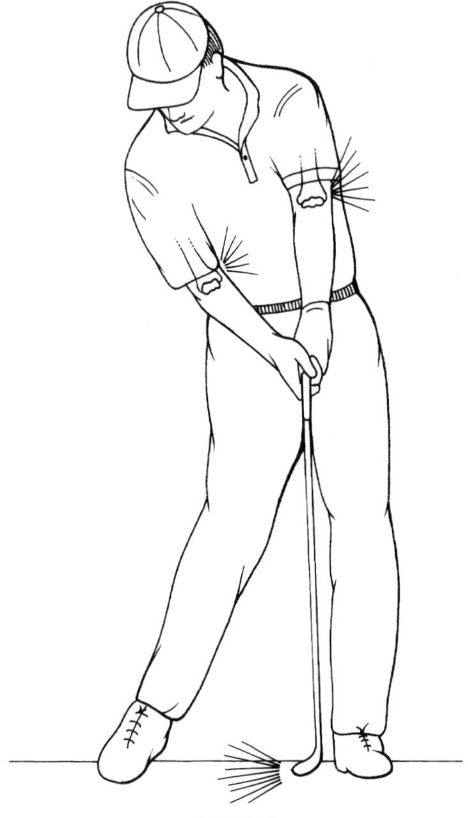

Fig. 7-1

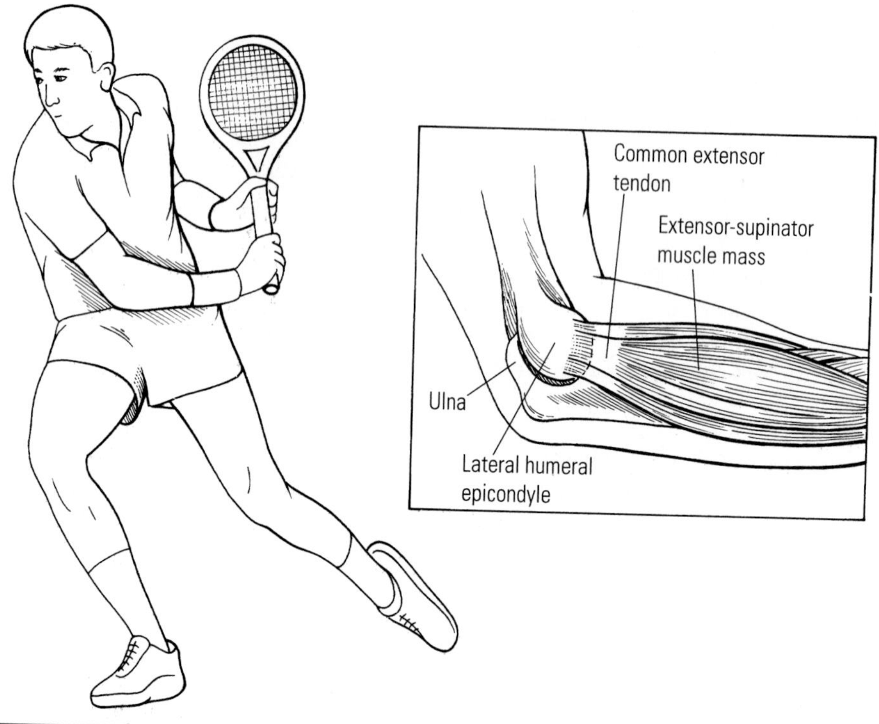

Fig. 7-2 A faulty backhand technique is implicated as the mechanism in classic tennis elbow disorder. Excessive stress is transmitted through the extensor-supinator muscle mass, particularly the extensor carpi radialis brevis, to the lateral epicondyle.

mation of a common tendon and share a common mechanism of disorder: the pull of many muscles on a small origin creates a high load per unit area.[20] However, both disorders are quite different in several ways. *Lateral epicondylitis,* or *(lateral) tennis elbow,* is a disorder deriving from a faulty backhand stroke (Fig. 7-2) and involves the lateral humeral epicondyle serving as the origin of the superficial layer of forearm wrist and finger extensors by way of a common extensor tendon. Provocation occurs by resistive wrist extension, radial deviation, and passive stretching of the wrist flexors, ulnar deviators, and forearm pronators. In contrast, *medial epicondylitis,* otherwise known as *golfer's elbow* (or *medial tennis elbow*), is a less common disorder that may result from a faulty forehand tennis stroke.[8] This involves a disorder of the medial humeral epicondyle, which serves as a proximal attachment for all the middle and superficial layer wrist flexors and extrinsic finger flexors by way of the common flexor tendon. Provocation of this disorder occurs by means of resisted wrist flexion and forearm pronation as well as wrist extension with passive supination and ulnar deviation. Tennis is by no means the only cause of tennis elbow; here, a right-handed golf player succumbed to left-sided tennis elbow. Both disorders affect those who play neither tennis nor golf.

2. What is the sequential progression of this disorder?

Grade I. Generalized elbow soreness with activity is an early warning signal that most players ignore.[17] A vicious cycle of irritation, inflammation, inadequate healing, pain, and weakness is initiated and gains full expression in subsequent grades of injury.

Grade II. Playing or working through the soreness may increase pain, which becomes localized at the lateral condyle or radial head[22] and persists after activity. The lateral aspect of the elbow becomes tender to touch and may become swollen and warm. Pain will interfere with his or her game and the player may find that he or she can no longer take a backhand stroke. As the condition persists, pain may radiate down the extensor surface of the forearm toward the wrist or it may extend into the upper arm and shoulder.[9]

Grade III. As the condition progresses, even simple activities of daily life such as shaking hands, turning a doorknob, holding a pen or pencil, or lifting a cup (positive *coffee-cup sign*) may become difficult or painful. There may occur sudden twinges that render the grip momentarily powerless so that the patient may even drop the teacup or racket he holds.[8] Continued playing can cause secondary problems such as rotator cuff tendinitis, biceps tendinitis, and low back pain as other joints attempt to compensate and help attenuate stresses. The result is the alteration of normal biomechanics of the upper extremity and trunk. If playing continues and pain is ignored, arthritic changes in the proximal radioulnar joint may eventually occur.

3. Which vocations or avocations are commonly associated with lateral epicondylitis?

Carpentry, gardening, dentistry, politicians (from handshaking), racquetball players, squash players, golfers, bowlers, baseball players, javelin throwers, needlework,[20] or scouring pots[8] all involve repetitive forearm use while gripping an object. The common denominator of the aforementioned repetitive tasks involve wrist ulnar deviation combined with wrist extension or forearm pronation contributing to excessive tensile stress on the extensor-supinator muscle mass, passed along the flattened common extensor tendon and delivered to the lateral epicondyle.

4. What are the three types of tennis elbow?

- *Lateral tennis elbow* commonly involves the origin of the extensor-supinator muscle mass in the following descending order: extensor carpi radialis brevis, extensor digitorum communis, extensor carpi radialis longus, extensor carpi ulnaris, and supinator. The extensor carpi radialis is most commonly involved probably because the positions of wrist flexion, elbow extension, and forearm pronation stretch the tendon over the prominence of the radial head. The most common cause of lateral epicondylitis in almost 90% of afflicted tennis players is technique related, particularly an incorrect backhand technique.[17] By incorrectly leading with the elbow on the backhand stroke, the racket head will lag behind the elbow only to accelerate faster than the elbow as it moves in to meet the ball. At impact the racket immediately decelerates, resulting in transmission of impact forces along the upper extremity to the lateral epicondyle.
- *Medial tennis elbow* (synonym: golfer's elbow) is medial epicondylitis[20] and involves the flexor-pronator muscle mass: the pronator teres, the flexor carpi radialis, and occasionally the palmaris longus, flexor carpi ulnaris, and flexor digitorum superficialis. Golfer's elbow may occur in recreational tennis players using a faulty forehand technique[20] or in top-level players who use a serving action during which the wrist is flexed and radially deviated at the same time the forearm is pronated. It may also occur in players who excessively pronate while hitting an exaggerated top spin, in swimmers after they make pullthrough strokes, or in baseball pitchers.
- *Posterior tennis elbow* involves a sudden severe strain to the triceps tendon as the arm is fully extended and can result from a twisted serve in competitive players.[20] This rare condition occurs from intrinsic overload of the triceps tendon in activities that require a sudden snapping of the elbow into extension, as in javelin throwing.[6] Pain is reproduced by fully resisting elbow extension while the patient stands with the elbow flexed and the forearm fully supinated.[12]

5. Why does lateral tennis elbow most commonly present as a chronic disorder?

Lateral tennis elbow is more commonly a chronic disorder related to a degenerative process. The majority of patients presenting with this disorder are 35 years of age or older. Except in sports clinics where the majority of patients present with the acute form of tennis elbow, the majority of patients do not relate the onset or aggravation of the disorder to playing tennis. In contradistinction to the acute presentation, most patients with lateral epicondylitis relate the onset of symptoms as being gradual and usually appearing after an activity.

With aging, the loss of mucopolysaccharide chondroitin sulfate results in decreased tendon extensibility. If activities are not modified or curtailed as senescence advances, the energy of tensile loading must be absorbed as internal strain of the collagen fibers rather than temporary deformation of the tendon. This decrease in the tensile modulus may result in fatigue and microfractures of the collagenous fibers composing the tendon. An inflammatory response occurs as an attempt at tissue healing by the laying down of immature collagen.[12]

6. What is the histologic basis for this disorder?

There seems to be controversy whether lateral epicondylitis and medial epicondylitis are primarily a disorder of the musculotendinous junction (MTJ)[4,13,24] or of the tenoperiosteal junction (TPJ).[8] In the former, scar tissue fills in the space between torn fibers that, over time, reduces the widened gap between the two edges. Eventually, enough scar tissue fills the gap so that the two edges lie in apposition and any tension on the scar ceases. Periosteum is a layer of connective tissue that invests most bone; tendons attach to bone by means of the periosteum. In the latter scenario, a periosteal avulsion, a cleft, forms between the cortical bone below and the periosteum above. The body treats this insult like a fracture and lays bone down in the cleft forming an *exostosis.* Without rest this bone spur will grow and result in more inflammation as soft tissues rub against it.

7. What are radiographic findings?

Radiographs of the elbow joint can be unremarkable[1] and are important to rule out other pathoses. However, there may be evidence of dystrophic calcific deposits[14] in the area of degeneration in the extensor muscle origin[23] as well as evidence of traumatic arthritis in the form of bone spurring.[14]

8. What is pitcher's elbow?

Pitcher's elbow is medial epicondylitis incurred when a curve ball is imparted a spin by rapid acceleration (that is, whipping) of the elbow into the extremes of extension, forearm supination, and ulnar deviation. This motion focuses considerable traction on the pronator-flexor muscle mass and their common origin by way of the common flexor tendon. It is essential to realize that the movement into this range occurs by concentric and eccentric contraction of the pronator-flexor muscle group. Baseball pitchers are better off using a tissue-sparing pitch such as a knuckle ball.

9. What may account for the lesser incidence of medial epicondylitis?

Because the medial epicondyle is somewhat larger than the outer epicondyle,[11] the pressure, defined as force per unit area, delivered through the common flexor tendon is more widely dissipated. In addition, pressure is further dissipated by virtue of the forearm flexor muscles having more bulk. Both factors may account for the statistic that medial epicondylitis is approximately 10 times less common than lateral epicondylitis.

10. What adjacent ligamentous disorder may pitchers incur from excessive valgus stress at the elbow?

Repetitive valgus stress to the medial epicondyle may result in a strain of the ulnar collateral ligament (Fig. 7-3). The pitcher most commonly presents with a vague medial elbow pain that worsens during activity. Upon evaluation, the patient presents with palpable tenderness just inferior to the medial epicondyle, along the anterosuperior portion of the ligament. Pain or instability provocation on valgus stress testing the elbow at 30° (Fig. 7-4) confirms the diagnosis. Radiographs may show traction spurs and loose bodies. Additionally there may also be heterotrophic ossification of the ulnar ligament. Ulnar

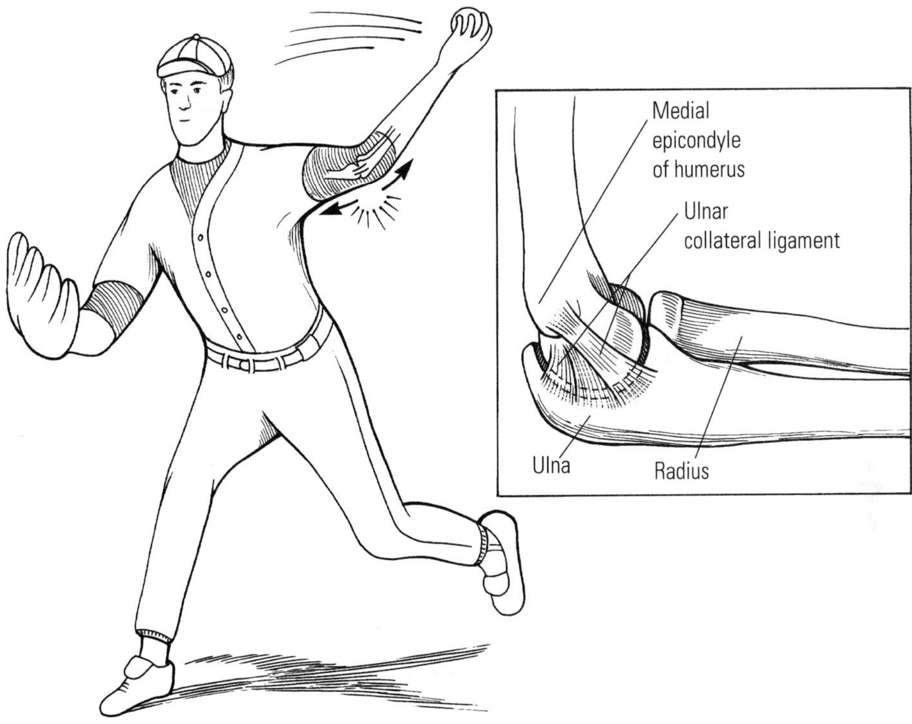

Fig. 7-3 Excessive valgus stress to the elbow during the acceleration phase of pitching or other throwing activities may sprain the ulnar collateral ligament.

collateral ligament strain generally responds to conservative treatment such as rest, ice, nonsteroidal anti-inflammatory medication, and modification of the sport technique.[14]

11. What is the epidemiology of tennis elbow?

Almost one third of today's 32 million regular tennis players suffer from lateral epicondylitis at some point in their game, and the risk is even greater among those who play tennis for more than 2 hours per week, with an estimated 45% developing tennis elbow.[5] Lateral epicondylitis is a form of nonarticular rheumatism, most commonly occurring in the dominant elbow, though it occurs in bilateral elbows some 60% of the time. Patient age averages between 40 and 50 years.[20] Because of this, age is implicated as a causative factor possibly related to tendon degeneration. Prevalence is equal for men and women.

12. What factors contribute to lateral epicondylitis in tennis players?

- *Improperly sized racket grip.* A grip that is too small can increase muscle fatigue and make it more difficult to stabilize the wrist at impact.
- *A hard court surface* such as concrete will cause the ball to travel faster, thereby increasing the impact force against the racket.
- *Heavy tennis balls*—wet or dead balls—require a greater force to stop as well as to propel forward than normal balls.
- *High string tension* increases the impact, which means that the racket can absorb less shock, which subsequently is transmitted to the arm.

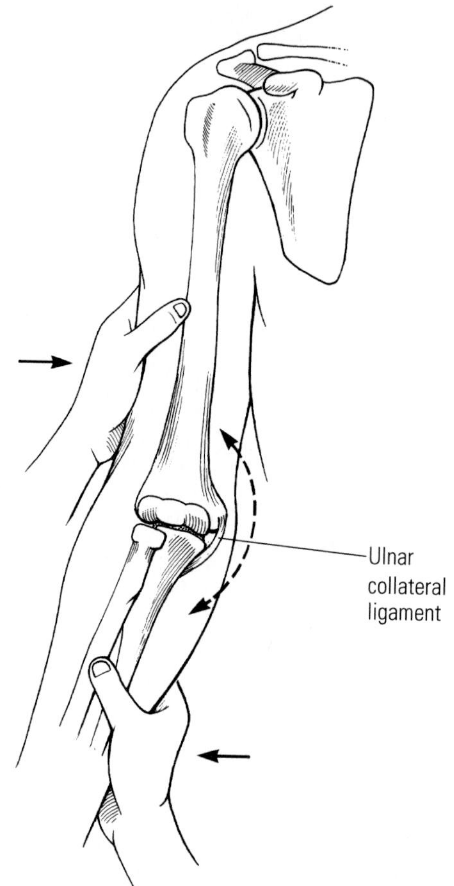

Fig. 7-4 Valgus stress test for assessment of stability of the integrity of the ulnar collateral ligament at the elbow.

- A *small racket size* reduces the sweet spot available for optimal force contact. A sweet spot is the mathematical center of percussion located in the racket face where minimal torsion occurs on impact. Striking the ball outside the perimeter of this spot produces a moment arm about which the force of the ball may create a high pronatory torque. If the player's wrist extensors are weak, the wrist may be forced into flexion. The combined effects of active and passive tension created in the extensor-supinator muscle mass result in high loading of the extensor tendons. These combined sources of tension are reproduced during provocative tennis elbow testing (Fig. 7-5).
- *Increased racket stiffness,* that is, using metal rackets, which vibrate at impact.
- *Wrong racket size.* A casual player should best use a light racket because a heavier one may cause greater load.[20]

13. What is the significance of provocative testing with the elbow in extension?

Because the soft tissues implicated span more than one joint, placing them on stretch will more clearly reveal presence of a disorder by provoking the inflamed portion of the tissue. Otherwise, a false-negative result may be obtained. In lateral tennis elbow pain is reproduced when one asks the patient to make a fist and extend the wrist. Sudden, severe pain is elicited at the lateral epicondyle when the examiner forcefully extends the patient's wrist (Fig. 7-5).

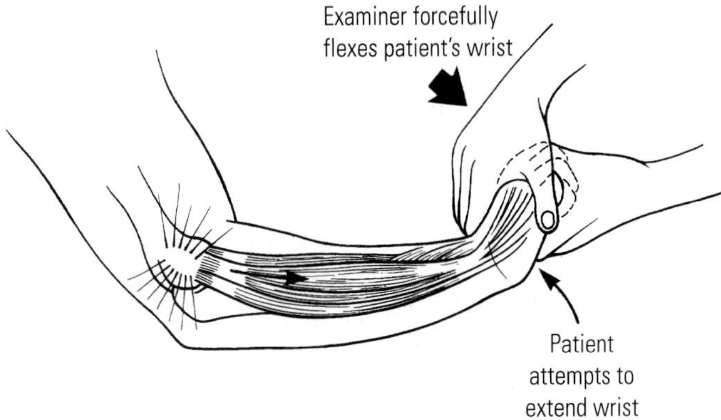

Fig. 7-5 Provocation test for lateral tennis elbow generates active and passive tension delivered to the lateral epicondyle. With the forearm in pronation the patient attempts to make a fist and to extend the wrist, as the therapist forcefully overcomes the patient by flexing the wrist.

14. What is the differential diagnosis for tennis elbow?

Radiographs of the radiohumeral joint are important when another pathologic condition is suspected. The radiograph may confirm suspicions by showing only soft-tissue swelling. Tennis elbow should not produce swelling at the elbow joint.

- *Cervical spine disease.* Pain from impingement of a cervical nerve may radiate to the elbow and be mistaken for tennis elbow.
- *Radiohumeral joint inflammation* and swelling may occur from rheumatoid arthritis, gout, or infectious arthritis, especially in the last if there has been a history of injections to this area, such as repeated steroid injections for recalcitrant tennis elbow; swelling, if present, will occur between the lateral epicondyle and the olecranon process below.[25] Fluid extraction with examination for crystals as well as fluid cultures for aerobic and anaerobic bacteria, mycobacteria, fungi, and other organisms are appropriate; if these studies have normal results, a synovial biopsy is performed with biopsy material cultured and examined histologically.[25]

15. What is radial tunnel syndrome?

Radial tunnel syndrome may occur concomitantly with lateral epicondylitis, is a common cause of treatment-resistant cases, and should be considered suspect when tennis elbow fails to respond to conservative treatment. The radial nerve runs down the medial posterior humeral wall en route to the forearm and is transmitted laterally through the musculospiral groove in the distal third of the humerus. The nerve does not cross the antecubital fossa but rather runs laterally to it in a cleft between the brachioradialis muscle and the biceps brachii. As soon as it leaves that cleft, it crosses directly over the supinator and splits into two major branches; a deep motor branch supplies the dorsal musculature whereas a sensory branch supplies the dorsal forearm and radial dorsum of the hand.

The radial nerve is susceptible to compression at four different sites (Fig. 7-6) listed here in proximal to distal order: (1) the fibrous bands surrounding the radial head and joint capsule; (2) the recurrent radial arteries; (3) the arcade of Frohse[15]—a fibrous arcade overlying the deep radial nerve as it enters the supinator; and finally (4) the most common site of compression the fibrous edge of the origin of the extensor carpi radialis brevis.[21] Although patients suffering from radial tunnel syndrome often present with complaints resembling that of lateral epicondylitis, the former contrasts the clinical presentation of the latter in the following manner: pain over the proximal dorsal forearm, maximal tenderness at the site of the radial tunnel (that is, 4 cm distal to the lateral epicondyle) over the posterior interosseous nerve, radial

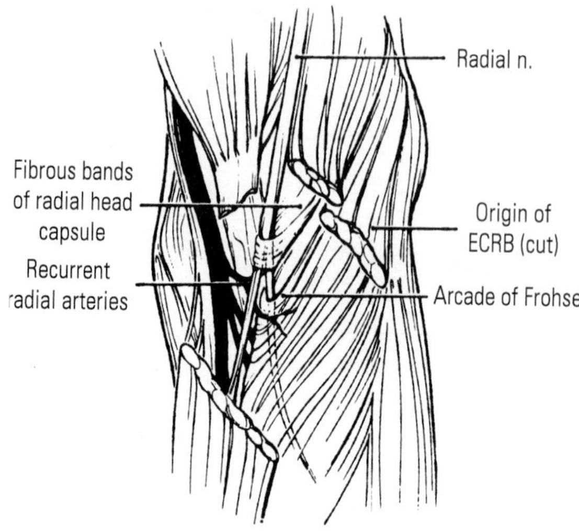

Fig. 7-6 Common sites of compression in radial tunnel syndrome. ECRB, Extensor carpi radialis brevis. (From Chabon SJ: Uncommon compressive neuropathies of the forearm. *Physician Assistant,* p 60, Sept 1990.)

nerve paresthesia heightened by direct compression over the radial tunnel, weakness of the extensor digitorum communis, and pain localized to the radial tunnel upon resisted supination, will all be characteristic of the radial tunnel syndrome and not of lateral epicondylitis.[3] The therapist may tension-test the radial nerve tract to further confirm a suspicion of involvement of that deep radial nerve known as the *posterior intersoseous nerve.* This may be performed by superimposition of the following sequence of limb postures upon the upper extremity: shoulder depression (that is, adducted close to the side), medial rotation, extension or abduction forearm pronation, elbow extension, wrist flexion, and ulnar deviation, together with lateral head flexion away from the involved side.[2] Several months of nonoperative treatment should be taken before surgical consideration.

16. Why is lateral tennis elbow a persistent disorder that does not tend to resolve spontaneously?

A dilemma arises when we consider an appropriate treatment strategy for lateral tennis elbow. If total rest is imposed upon the patient, there may not be adequate stress to the new collagen to stimulate maturation. In this case, the immature collagen composing the scar may break down after resumption of activities. On the other hand, if the patient continues to perform activities that aggravate the condition, the immature collagen produced by an attempted repair is broken down before it has a chance to mature and the chronic inflammatory process continues. Because of this, lateral epicondylitis tends to persist chronically in many individuals.[12]

17. What therapeutic management best serves the patient?

- *Selective rest.* Preferably avoid stressful activity until the pain has subsided; however pain-free movement is encouraged.[24] Excessive activity or early return to activity may direct excessive stress to healing scar tissue. Activities that involve strong, repetitive grasping, such as hammering or tennis playing, should be restricted until there is minimal pain on resisted isometric wrist extension and little or no pain when the tendon is passively stretched.
- *Ice massage* for 20 minutes, three times a day in the acute stage and the use of heat during acute or subacute stages. Elevation and compression are not necessary because appreciable swelling does not occur.

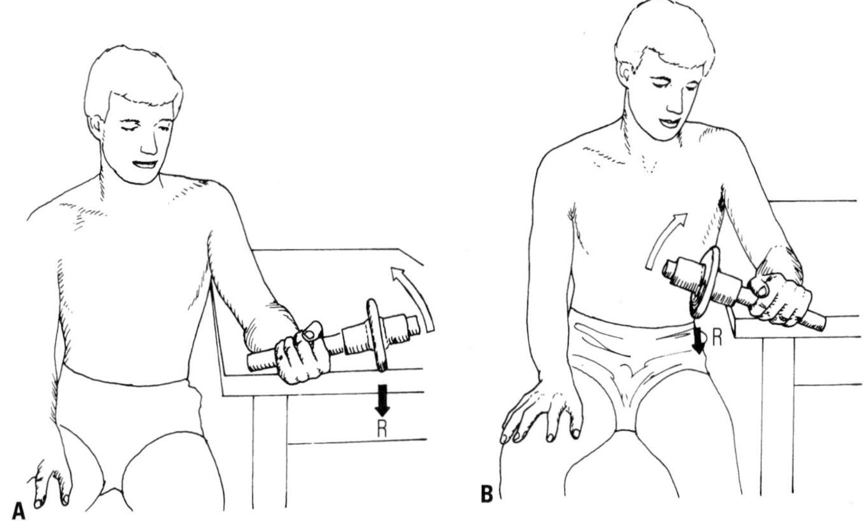

Fig. 7-7 Mechanical resistance exercise using a small bar with asymmetrically placed weight for strengthening forearm pronators, **A,** and supinators, **B.** (From Kisner, C, Colby LA: *Therapeutic exercise: foundations and techniques,* ed 2, Philadelphia, 1990, FA Davis Co.)

- In the acute state, total rest is achieved by immobilization of the wrist, hand, and fingers in a resting *splint.* The splint may be removed several times a day, so that the patient can gently and slowly actively move the wrist into flexion, the forearm into pronation, and the elbow into extension to maintain muscle and tendon extensibility.[12]
- *Gentle cross-fiber massage* within tolerance to the site of lesion to mechanically influence tissue maturation so that immature collagen becomes oriented along the lines of stress. Transverse friction massage is essentially intentional stress that is limited to helping toward maturation of new collagen and permits resolution of the healing process. In this fashion the defect heals with a maximum degree of tissue extensibility and is less likely to be overstressed as activity is resumed.
- *Ultrasound* provides a deep heating effect that may enhance increased blood flow and resolution of inflammatory exudates including lysosomal enzymes and other cellular "debris."[12]
- *Lateral counterforce brace.* A 4-inch strap[1] worn tightly around the forearm just distal to the elbow splints the area and alters the biomechanics such that the origin of the wrist extensors is transferred more proximally. This shift ensures that forces delivered to this area are absorbed by the bulk of muscle bellies, which presumably withstand greater forces than the tendon can.[26] This tennis elbow splint is applied when the arm is relaxed and should be worn until the rehabilitation period is completed[20] as well as during a graduated return to sports activity. The patient should be gradually weaned from brace use as strength, mobility, and painless function increase. This device may also be applied to the forearm flexors for medial tennis elbow. Cybex testing and biomechanical studies have confirmed the clinical validity of this treatment adjunct.[18,19]
- *Strengthening.* Gradual concentric as well as eccentric strengthening (Fig. 7-7) is important, as different authorities ascribe, since each of these modes of contraction is culpable in the development of a pathosis.[7,16] Since the common extensor tendons suffer a loss of tensile adaptation with age and the mechanism of injury involves tensile overloading of those tendons, a logical strategy would emphasize eccentric work, since this in large part is the nature of the force producing the injury. Increased muscle bulk

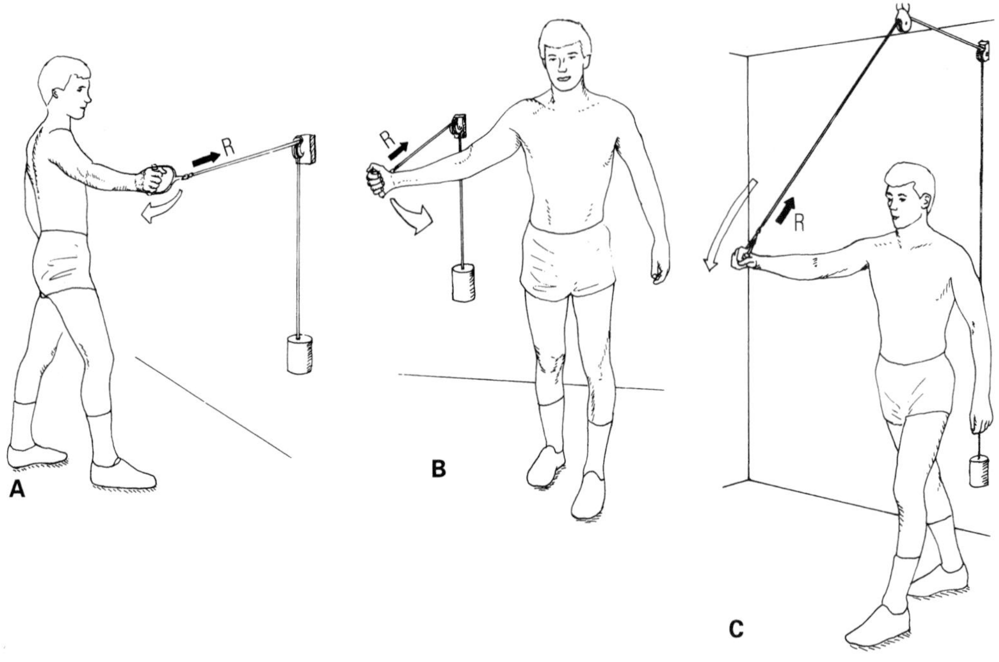

Fig. 7-8 Mechanical resistance exercise using wall pulleys to stimulate tennis swings; backhand stroke, **A;** forehand stroke, **B;** and serve, **C.** (From Kisner, C, Colby LA: *Therapeutic exercise: foundations and techniques,* ed 2, Philadelphia, 1990, FA Davis Co.)

by way of hypertrophy helps attenuate stress because there is more soft tissue to dissipate disruptive forces. Exercises should include strengthening of the ipsilateral shoulder. All exercises of the extensor-supinator group should be started with the elbow in flexion.[24] Wall pulleys may be used to simulate tennis swings (Fig. 7-8).

- *Stretching regimen.* Gaining length in the extensor-supinator muscle mass will take up some of the pull placed on the origin of those muscles. Stretching of the entire hand, forearm, and shoulder complex should be performed emphasizing normal muscle balance. This may be especially helpful after ultrasound and friction massage. Teaching the patient to self-stretch is very helpful as part of the home exercise program. Self-stretching exercises include the following three:
  - To stretch the *flexor palm muscles,* hold the hand flat on a table with the elbow extended and the wrist extended to 90°. Gently pull up on your fingers, stretching the flexor muscles of the palm. Hold for 10 seconds and repeat twice (Fig. 7-9).
  - To stretch the *wrist flexors,* keep your hand flat on the table and gently lean forward over your hand stretching the flexor muscles in your forearm. Hold for 10 seconds and repeat twice (Fig. 7-10).
  - To stretch the *wrist extensors,* place the back of your hand flat on the table while keeping your elbow straight. Gently lean back over your palm stretching the extensors in your forearm. Hold for 10 seconds and repeat twice (Fig. 7-11).
- *Proper equipment.* A fiberglass, graphite, or wood racket is more flexible than a metal one. A large sweet spot is preferable. Gut strings give more resilience and less vibration than nylon ones do. The strings should ideally be strung to a range of 52 to 55 pounds of tension. If nylon is used, 16-gauge strings are preferred. Increasing the racket handle diameter helps the player with relatively weak wrist extensors

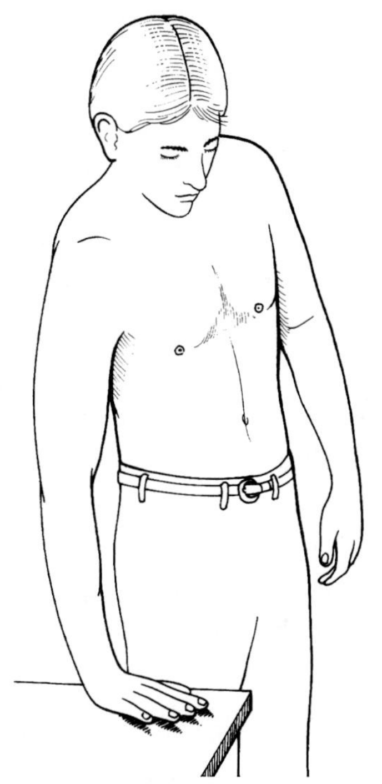

Fig. 7-9 Technique to stretch the flexor palm muscles.

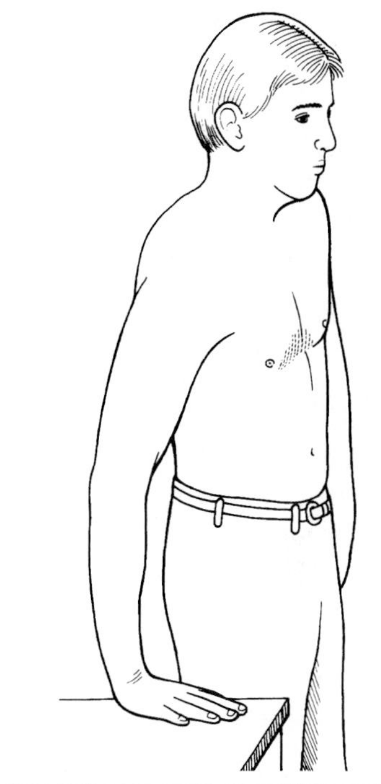

Fig. 7-10 Technique to stretch the wrist flexors.

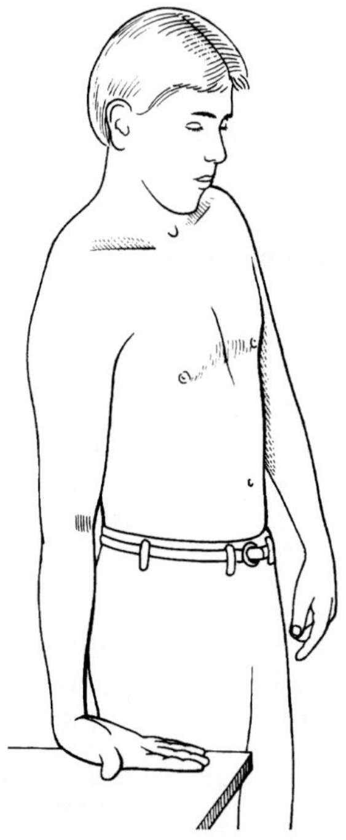

Fig. 7-11 Technique to stretch the wrist extensors.

from incurring a passive pronatory torque when the ball is struck outside the sweet spot. Modifying the playing surface is also helpful. The common denominator in all equipment modifications is a reduction of tensile force applied to the lateral epicondyle.

- *Proper technique.* An emphasis should be made on recruiting the whole of the shoulder and trunk in hitting the ball so as to dissipate forces as widely as possible. With a correct backhand stroke the elbow is held straight and the stress of the ball's impact is transmitted up along the arm and shoulder musculature. Additionally it is imperative to hit strokes with a firm wrist and not to return the ball by the use of wrist movements. The wearing of an elastic wrist splint may help. Use of a two-handed backhand may be helpful to some. Players with poor technique should consider obtaining a lesson to identify areas where technique can be improved upon. It is helpful to learn to strike the ball with the center point of the strings while avoiding the periphery.
- *High-voltage galvanic stimulation*[14] has been found helpful in relieving pain and inflammation.
- *Gradual return to activity* is predicated upon normal restoration of strength and return of normal range of motion without pain.
- *Anti-inflammatory medication* as prescribed by a physician may help relieve pain and inflammation.
- *Local anti-inflammatory treatment, although often resulting in dramatic relief of symptoms,* ***has no lasting benefit*** *because it does not influence the cause of the pathologic process.* ***Often, the patient misinterprets sudden relief as license to play tennis with all the vigor he or she can muster only to return soon to treatment because of relapse.*** *Local anti-inflammatory treatment, at best, is used as an adjunct management of the acute state.*
- *Iontophoresis or phonophoresis* with hydrocortisone cream and lidocaine (Zylocaine) or dexamethasone (Decadron).[24]
- *Steroid injections* are not to exceed two or three and are administered with the intent of providing pain relief only to allow progression of rehabilitation effort; healing occurs through rehabilitation not from steroid injection.[14]

18. At what point does surgery become a treatment option?

The prognosis for tennis elbow is generally good. On rare occasions operative treatment is warranted only after a trial of quality rehabilitation of some 3 to 4 months.[14] Surgery involves division and distal retraction of the fascial attachment of the extensor muscles to the lateral epicondyle.[23] After surgery, an interval of 8 to 11 weeks should elapse before tennis playing is resumed.[20]

References

1. Berkow R: *The Merck manual of diagnosis and therapy,* Rahway, N.J., 1987, Merck, Sharp & Dohme Research Laboratories.
2. Butler D: *Mobilisation of the nervous system,* Melbourne, 1991, Churchill Livingstone.
3. Chabon SJ: Uncommon compressive neuropathies of the forearm, *Physician Assistant,* p 65, Sept 1990.
4. Chusid J, McDonald J: *Correlative neuroanatomy and functional neurology,* ed 17, Los Altos, Calif., 1979, Lang Medical Publications.
5. Constable G, editor: *Restoring the body: treating aches and injuries,* Alexandria, Va., 1987, Time-Life Books.
6. Corrigan B, Maitland GD: *Practical orthopaedic medicine,* Stoneham, Mass., 1985, Bitterworth Pubs.
7. Curwin S, Standish WD: *Tendinitis: its etiology and treatment,* Lexington, Mass., 1984, Collamore Press.
8. Cyriax J: *Textbook of orthopaedic medicine,* vol 1: *Diagnosis of soft tissue lesions,* Philadelphia, 1982, Bailliere-Tindall.
9. Ellison MD et al, editors: *Athletic training and sports medicine,* Chicago, 1985, American Academy of Orthopedic Surgeons.
10. Gould JA: *Orthopaedic and sports physical surgery,* ed 2, St Louis, 1990, Mosby.
11. Gray H: *Anatomy, descriptive and surgical,* ed 15, New York, 1977, Bounty Books.
12. Hertling D, Kessler RM: *Management of musculoskeletal disorders,* ed 2, Philadelphia, 1990, Lippincott.

13. Kapjandi IA: *The physiology of the joints,* vol 1, Edinburgh, 1970, Churchill Livingstone.
14. Lillegard WA, Rucker KS: *Handbook of sports medicine—a symptom oriented approach,* Boston, 1993, Andover Medical Publishers.
15. Moss SH, Switzer H: Radial tunnel syndrome: a spectrum of clinical presentations, *J Hand Surg* 4:414-419, 1983.
16. Nirschl RP: Tennis elbow, *Orthop Clin North Am* 4:787-800, 1973.
17. Nirschl RP: The etiology and treatment of tennis elbow, *Am J Sports Med* 2:308-319, 1974.
18. Nirschl RP: *Medial tennis elbow: the surgical treatment.* Presented at the annual meeting of the American Academy of Orthopaedic Surgeons, Atlanta, March 1, 1980.
19. Nirschl RP: Muscle and tendon trauma: tennis elbow. In Morrey BF, editor: *The elbow and its disorders,* Philadelphia, 1985, Saunders.
20. Peterson L, Renström P: *Sports injuries: their prevention and treatment,* London, 1986, Martin Dunitz, Ltd (distributor in USA: Mosby, St Louis).
21. Ritts G, Wood M, Linshield R: Radial-tunnel syndrome: a ten-year surgical experience, *Clin Orthop* 219:201-205, 1987.
22. Rodman GP, Schumacher HR: *Primer on rheumatic diseases,* ed 8, Atlanta, 1983, Arthritis Foundation.
23. Salter RB: *Textbook of disorders and injuries of the musculoskeletal system,* ed 2, Baltimore, 1983, Williams & Wilkins.
24. Saunders HD: *Evaluation, treatment, and prevention of musculoskeletal disorders,* Bloomington, Minn., 1985, Educational Opportunities.
25. Schumacher HR, Bomalski JS: *Case studies in rheumatology for the house officer,* Baltimore, 1990, Williams & Wilkins.
26. Wadsworth PT et al: Effects of the counterforce armband on wrist extensor and grip strength and pain in subjects with tennis elbow, *Orthop Sports Phys Ther* 11:192-197, 1989.

Recommended reading

Hertling D, Kessler RM: *Management of commmon musculoskeletal disorders,* ed 2, Philadelphia, 1990, Lippincott.

Peterson L, Renström P: *Sports injuries: their prevention and treatment,* London, 1986, Martin Dunitz, Ltd (distributor in USA: Mosby, St Louis).

Part Three

Shoulder

8

Persistent Pinpoint Tenderness over Bicipital Groove Despite Shoulder Rotation and Painful Arc during Resistive Supination and Elevation

A 51-year-old electrician spends most of his professional time installing ceiling light fixtures for several lighting stores in his area. He complains of right anterior shoulder pain. There is full range of motion with painful arc present on elevation and depression at approximately 50° on both the upswing and the downswing. There is no observed muscle wasting. Palpation yields tenderness over the bicipital groove. There is no cuff wasting, and the patient admits to a history of cuff impingement and suspected tear of his right shoulder of several years' duration that was operated on last year. His history also includes generalized arthritis and occasional bouts of gout since age 28, though there is no exacerbation at present. Muscle strength is good throughout, except for right forearm supination, which is decreased to good minus; elbow flexion is graded as good. Shoulder abduction in either direction of glenohumeral rotation is painful. Resisted flexion with the forearm fully pronated is mildly uncomfortable, whereas resisted flexion and supination is most definitely painful. Placement of the biceps muscle in passive insufficiency caused by simultaneous passive shoulder depression, elbow extension, and forearm pronation yields pain in the vicinity of the anterior deltoid. Flexibility testing also reveals tightness in the latissimus and pectoral muscle groups. There is normal joint play present in all joints of both shoulder girdles except for tightness of the posterior glenohumeral joint capsules of both shoulders. The patient takes no medications for his pain.

SPECIAL TESTS Negative Yergason's test, negative drop-arm test, negative Ludington's test, positive impingement sign, positive sawing test, positive Speed's test, positive deAnquin's test, positive Hueter's sign, negative Lippman's test, negative axial compression/distraction.

1. **What most likely accounts for this individual's anterior shoulder pain?**
2. **What anatomy is relevant to understanding biceps brachii disorders?**
3. **What is the kinesiology of the biceps brachii?**
4. **What effect if any does the long biceps brachii tendon have in contributing to humeral head depression?**

5. What other function does the long head of the biceps brachii share with the rotator cuff?
6. What is the most important restraint of the long tendon of the biceps brachii as it courses down the arm?
7. What osseous anatomy is relevant to understanding biceps brachii tendon disorders?
8. What unique functional relationship exists between the long tendon of the biceps brachii and the proximal humerus?
9. What is the function of the bicipital aponeurosis?
10. What happens to the tendon of the long head of the biceps brachii during rotator cuff attrition and tear?
11. What is the most common form of proximal biceps brachii tendinitis?
12. What comparative anatomy studies may shed light on the origin of biceps brachii tendinitis and rotator cuff disorders?
13. What are the clinical signs of proximal bicipital tendinitis within the glenohumeral joint?
14. Describe five provocative tests implicating lesions of the biceps brachii tendon.
15. What accounts for painful nocturnal exacerbation in many painful shoulder conditions?
16. What is primary biceps brachii tendinitis?
17. Which sports are associated with proximal biceps brachii tendinitis and subluxation?
18. What happens to the long tendon of the biceps brachii during subluxation or dislocation?
19. How is the bicipital groove best palpated?
20. What forms of imaging are appropriate in detecting biceps brachii lesions?
21. What is the clinical sign of strain of the long head of the biceps brachii at its glenoid origin?
22. At which sites does the biceps brachii tendon most likely rupture, and who is most vulnerable?
23. What is the presentation of sudden proximal tendon rupture?
24. What is the mechanism for distal tendon avulsion?
25. What is bicipital tenosynovitis at the lower arm?
26. What is bicipital tendinitis of the lower arm?
27. How is a brachialis muscle disorder differentiated from a lesion of the biceps brachialis?
28. What is the differential diagnosis?
29. What rehabilitative treatment is most appropriate for proximal biceps brachii tendinitis, and when is surgery appropriate?
30. What postoperative care is appropriate to patients having undergone surgery for a proximal biceps brachii lesion?

---

1. What most likely accounts for this individual's anterior shoulder pain?

Bicipital tendinitis within the glenohumeral joint.

2. What anatomy is relevant to understanding biceps brachii disorders?

The biceps brachii, a long fusiform muscle that arises by two heads, has no direct connection with the humerus as it originates above the shoulder and inserts below the elbow joint. As such it can be moved about, when grasped, more easily than muscles that take their origin on the humerus. The tensile strength of the biceps tendon has been measured at between 150 and 200 lb.[6,12]

The tendon of the long head of the biceps arises from the supraglenoid tubercle and arches obliquely across the top of the humeral head within the capsule of the shoulder joint. This biceps tendon is intra-articular but extrasynovial. Imperative to understanding the pathology of the long tendon is that the

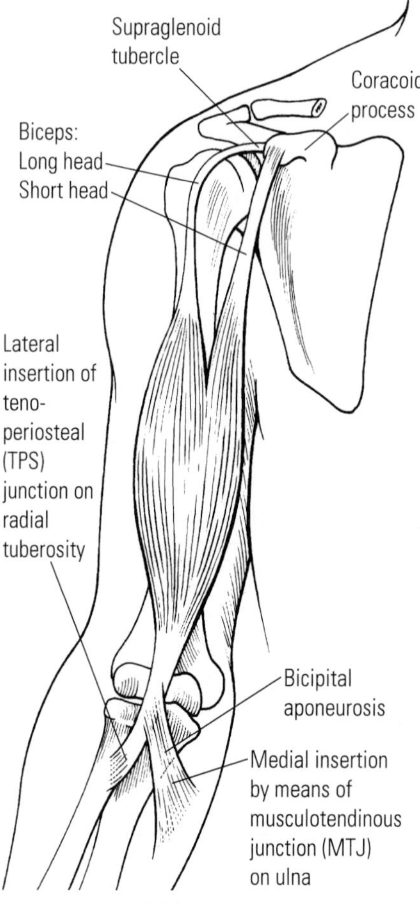

Fig. 8-1 Biceps brachii.

tendon penetrates the rotator cuff between the subscapularis and the supraspinatus tendons. The tendon then begins its descent superficially along the anterior humeral shaft via the bicipital groove (intertubercular sulcus) located in the anterior proximal humerus.

The short head of the biceps arises with the coracobrachialis from the scapula's coracoid process and runs down the medial side of the long head of the biceps. The two bellies join as a common distal tendon shortly above the elbow joint as a flattened tendon, only to separate into two distal insertions. Although the lateral insertion on the radial tuberosity is a *tenoperiosteal junction,* the main medial insertion attaches to the ulna as a *musculotendinous junction* by means of the bicipital aponeurosis, a triangular flat sheet running medially from the main tendon through the arm's deep fascia into the ulna (Fig. 8-1).

3. What is the kinesiology of the biceps brachii?

The significance of the two different origins and insertions of the biceps muscle as well as the humeral length that it traverses make the biceps a jack of all trades but master of none in relation to the shoulder joint, the elbow joint, and even the distal wrist joint.

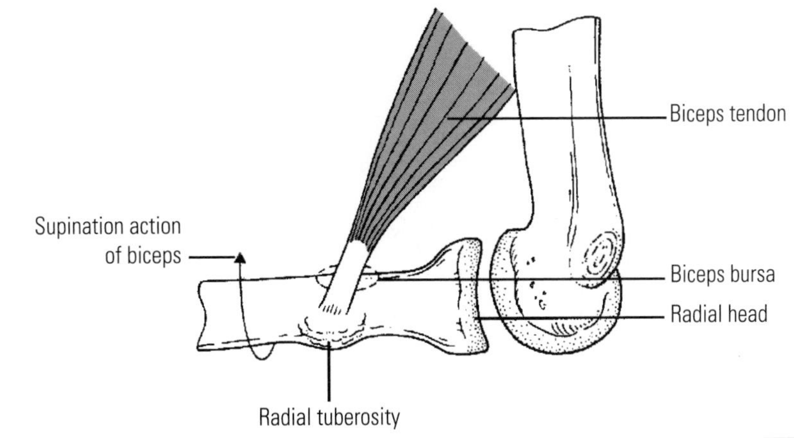

Fig. 8-2 When the biceps supinates the forearm, the radius is uncrossed relative to the ulna and lies parallel with that bone. Supination is most powerful when the elbow is flexed at the right angle. (From Ellis H: *Clinical anatomy*, ed 7, Oxford, 1983, Blackwell Scientific Publications.)

Aside from being a major forearm flexor by means of its ulnar insertion, the biceps is also a powerful supinator when the forearm is flexed by its radial insertion. During contraction, in addition to forearm flexion, there is concomitant radial unwinding as the tuberosity is rotated anteriorly (Fig. 8-2).

This second function, performed routinely when one opens a corkscrew or turns a screw into hardwood, is best performed in flexion (Fig. 8-3) because this position places the biceps muscle at its ideal length and optimum mechanical advantage.

4. What effect if any does the long biceps brachii tendon have in contributing to humeral head depression?

Electromyographic studies show that the biceps tendon does have a weak active head depressor effect. Based on its anatomic saddling of the humeral head it, at the very least, serves as a static checkrein preventing cephalad humeral excursion (Fig. 8-4). In the event of medial subluxation of the biceps tendon, this checkrein effect is lost.[2]

5. What other function does the long head of the biceps brachii share with the rotator cuff?

Another function that the long head of the biceps shares with the adjacent supraspinatus tendon is shoulder *abduction.* In the absence of deltoid strength, for example, from posterior joint dislocation with resultant axillary nerve injury, the biceps may be recruited to abduct the shoulder 50° in the context of the following substitution pattern: by externally rotating the shoulder, the biceps has a line of pull that is placed parallel with the coronal plane, making the biceps an abductor. Elevation above 50° is not possible as a function of a fixed lever arm secondary to a tethering of the tendon by the bicipital retinaculum. The biceps is also a shoulder flexor to 50° but only when the shoulder is in neutral with respect to rotation.

6. What is the most important restraint of the long tendon of the biceps brachii as it courses down the arm?

The gliding of the long tendon of the biceps is guided by the *coracohumeral ligament* (Fig. 8-5). This ligament runs through the interval between the subscapularis and supraspinatus tendons known as the

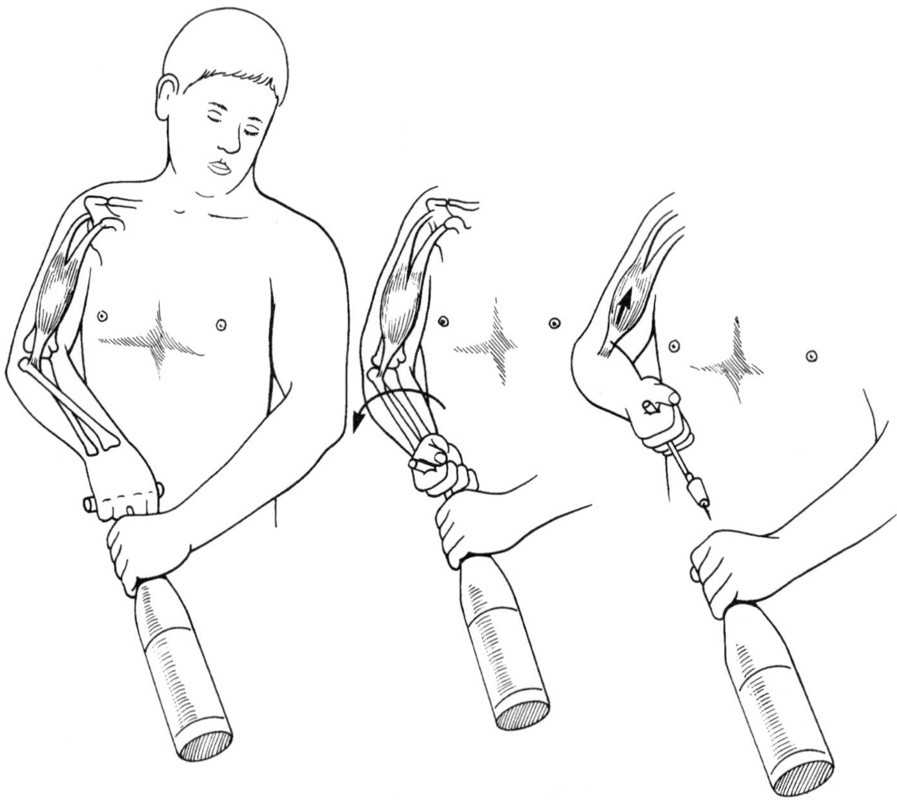

Fig. 8-3 The elbow flexion and forearm supination function of the biceps brachii illustrated by uncorking a bottle.

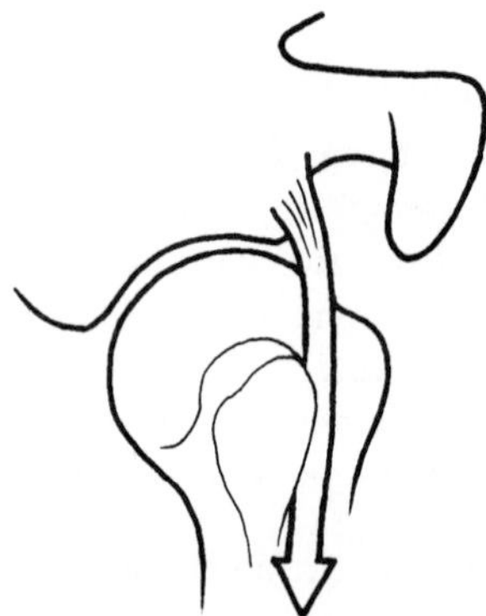

Fig. 8-4 Electromyographic analysis shows the long biceps tendon to be an active head depressor, albeit a weak one. Given its line of pull and the resultant vector, the biceps tendon is certainly at very least a static head depressor. (From Habermeyer P, Kaiser E, Knappe M et al: *Unfallchirurg* 90[7]:319-329, 1987.)

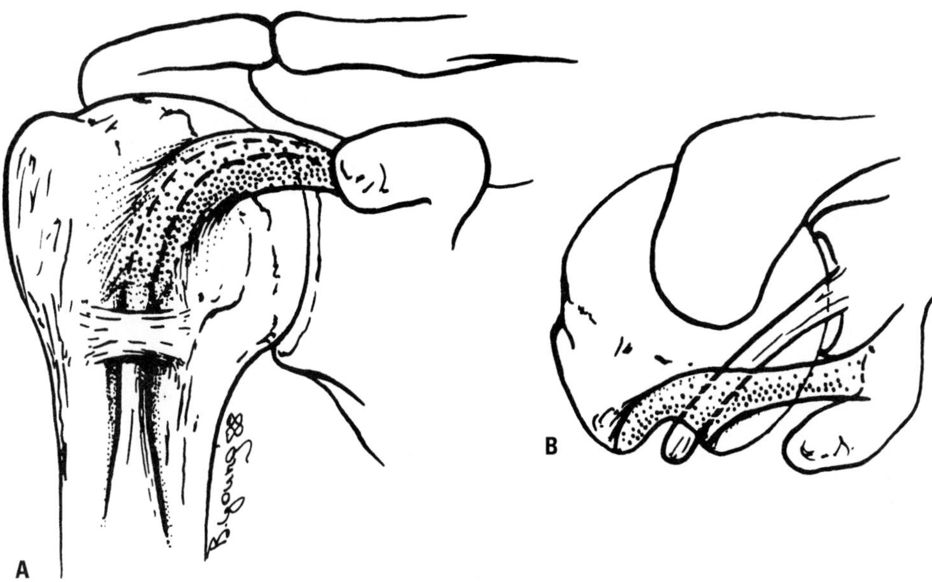

Fig. 8-5 The coracohumeral ligament thickens the rotator interval, inserts on either side of the bicipital groove, and is an important stabilizer of the biceps tendon. **A,** anterior view, **B,** superior view. (Modified from Paavolainen P, Slatis P, Aalto K: Surgical pathology in chronic shoulder pain. In Bateman JE, Welsh RP, editors: *Surgery of the shoulder*, St. Louis, 1984, Mosby.)

rotator interval and serves to reinforce the glenohumeral joint capsule at that locale. Additionally, this ligament together with the edges of the subscapularis and supraspinatus tendons thicken and reinforce that portion of the capsule so as to stabilize the tendon within the intertubercular groove. This portion of reinforced capsule serves as the principle obstacle to medial tendon dislocation. In cases of dislocation this ligament may become torn or stretched.

7. What osseous anatomy is relevant to understanding biceps brachii tendon disorders?

The bicipital groove is located between the lesser and greater tuberosities. Although the medial wall of this sulcus is formed by the lesser tuberosity, the lateral wall is formed by the edge of the greater tuberosity. The intertubercular sulcus is measured according to its width, depth, and medial wall angle (Fig. 8-6); medial wall angles in humans are unique among primates in that they vary widely between 15° and 90° but with the majority of the population falling between 60° and 75° (Fig. 8-7). Groove variations, whether too wide and shallow or excessively deep, may lead to problems. A positive correlation exists between lower medial wall angles (that is, shallower grooves) and subluxation or dislocation of the biceps tendon. Excessively deep grooves tend to be too narrow and may compress the tendon.[4,5] Furthermore, a bony anomaly, known as the *supratubercular ridge* (Fig. 8-8), extending from the lesser tuberosity is present in some people; when it is, the ridge decreases sulcus depth and diminishes the effectiveness of the tuberosity as a pulley. Medial wall spurs are much more common in individuals with supratubercular ridges.[13]

8. What unique functional relationship exists between the long tendon of the biceps brachii and the proximal humerus?

It is important to understand that, unlike most tendons, the long head of the biceps moves on a fixed area of bone (that is, the superior glenoid rim during shoulder motion). From vertical adduction and depression to

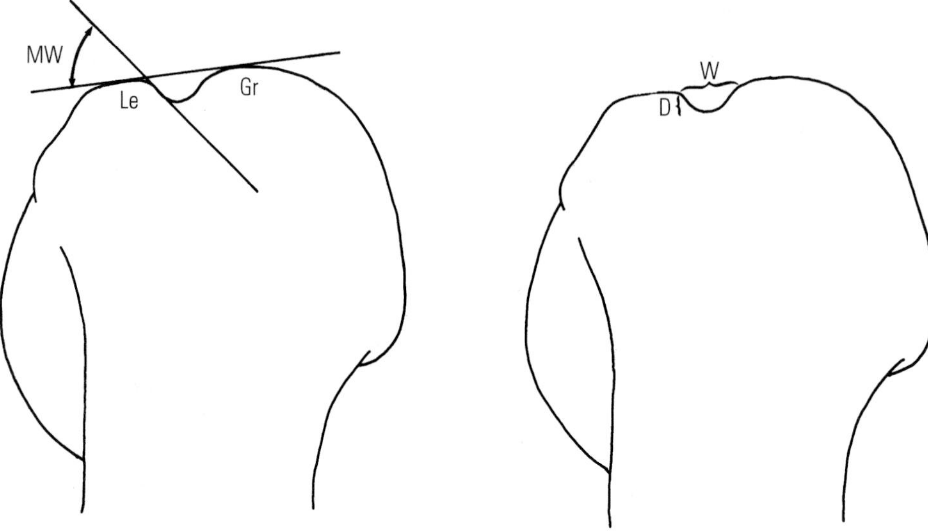

Fig. 8-6 Measurements taken by Cone and associates, including the medial wall angle as well as the width and depth of the bicipital groove. *D*, depth of groove; *Gr*, greater tuberosity; *Le*, lesser tuberosity; *MW*, medial wall angle; *W*, width of groove. (From Cone RO, Danzig L, Resnick D, Goldman AB: *Am J Roentgenol* 41:781-788, 1983.)

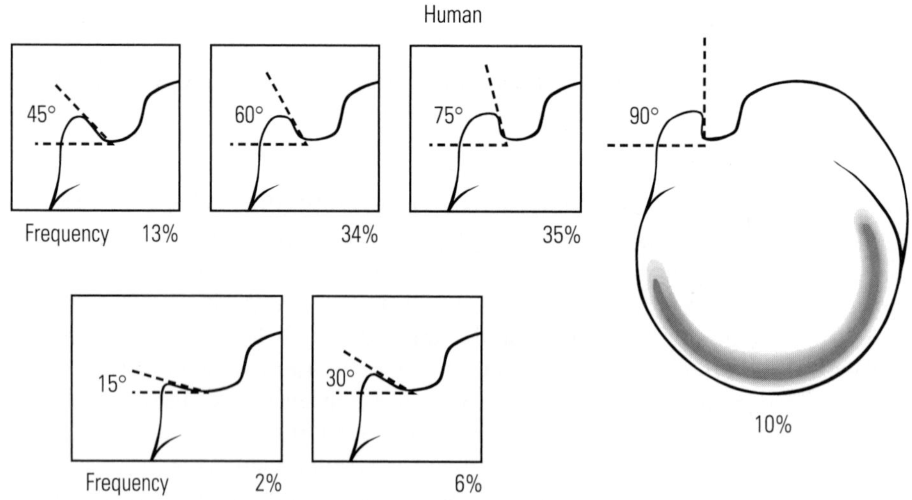

Fig. 8-7 Humans are unique among primates in exhibiting variations in bicipital groove characteristics, including depth, width, and hence medial wall angle. The average medial wall angle varies between 60°-75° throughout in the majority of people. Groove characteristics in all other primates are constant within the species. (Modified from Hitchcock HH, Bechtol CO: Painful shoulder: Observations in the role of the tendon of the long head of the biceps brachii in its causation. *J Bone Joint Surg.* 30 A:263-273, 1948.)

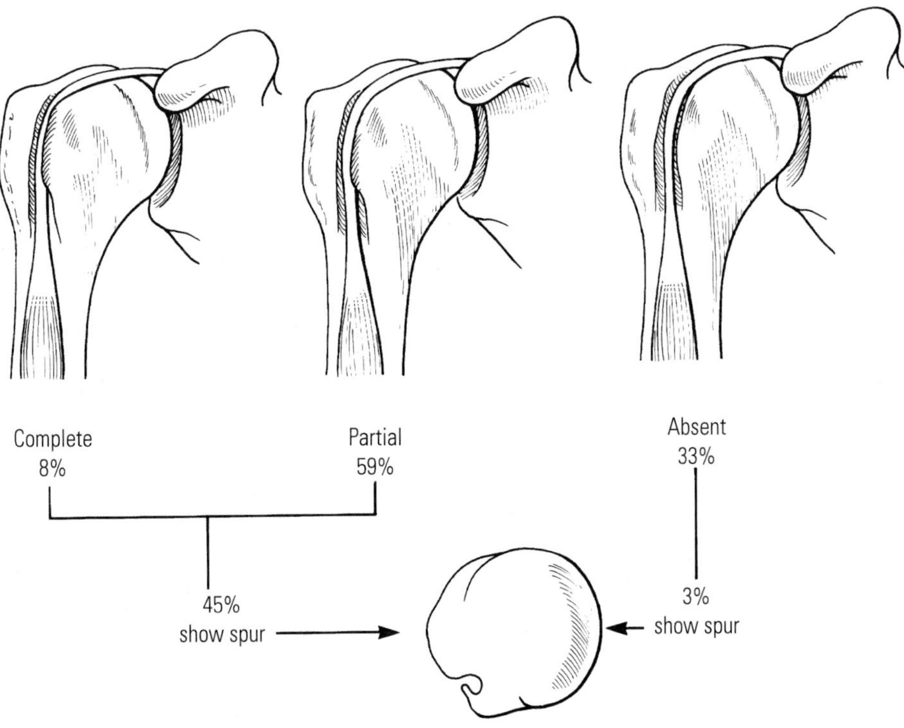

Fig. 8-8 Medial wall spurs are more common in individuals with supratubercular ridges.

complete shoulder elevation the bicipital groove moves along the tethered long tendon of the biceps for a distance of as much as 6-8 cm. Motion of the long tendon in its groove occurs with motion of the shoulder joint. At any given point, a different amount of biceps tendon is found within the joint (Fig. 8-9). For example, on abduction and flexion, the intra-articular portion of this tendon is only a few centimeters long, whereas on adduction or extension this length increases to 4 cm. To facilitate ease of motion, the synovial pouch of the glenohumeral joint extends distally to line the greater extent of the bicipital groove.

9. What is the function of the bicipital aponeurosis?

The bicipital retinaculum (Fig. 8-10) serves to hold the tendon of the long head of biceps against the proximal humerus within the bicipital groove. The functional significance of this becomes apparent during shoulder elevation, which limits biceps contribution to either flexion or abduction by tethering of the long tendon within the bicipital groove. By way of analogy, the humerus travels on the biceps tendon like a monorail on its track.[2] The retinaculum prevents the biceps from deflecting away from the humerus during contraction by keeping it straddled between the two tuberosities, thus limiting its leverage as a significant elevator.

10. What happens to the tendon of the long head of the biceps brachii during rotator cuff attrition and tear?

The triad of proximal bicipital impingement, tendinitis, and tearing must be viewed against the backdrop of that tendon's intimate association with the rotator cuff. The biceps tendon is well situated to produce

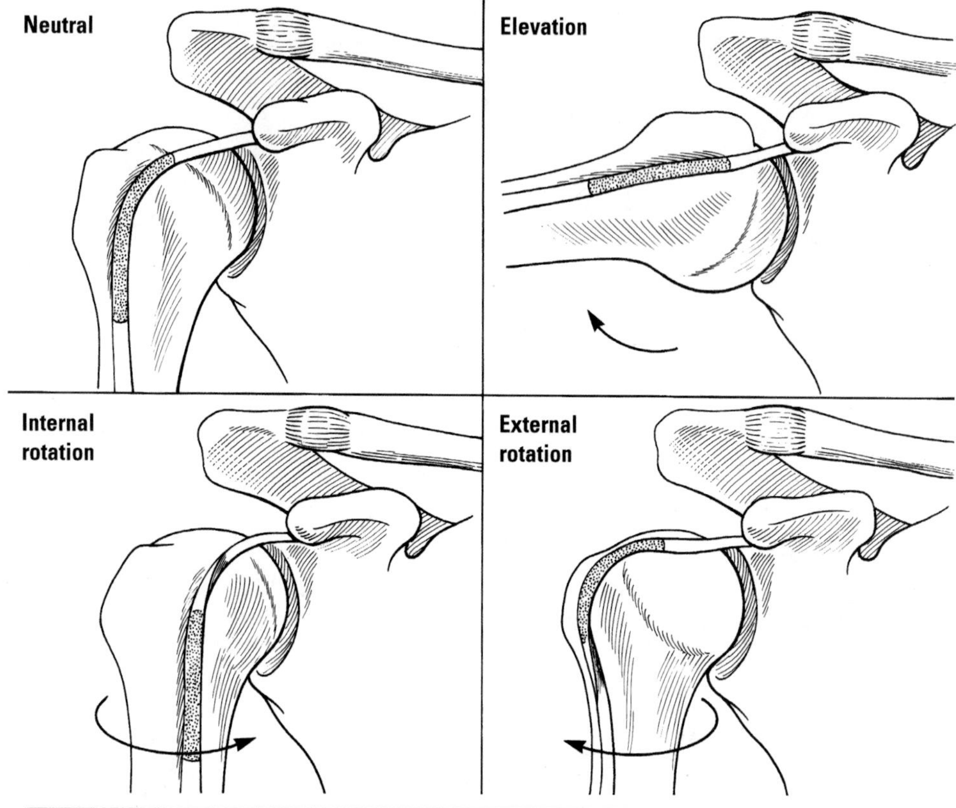

Fig. 8-9 A different amount and portion of biceps tendon is located with the glenohumeral joint, depending on the plane of shoulder movement. Tendon excursion occurs because the biceps tendon is tethered against the bone. Movement occurs when the humerus moves on the tendon. Tendon excursion is greatest during shoulder elevation, particularly in abduction.

humeral head depression in partnership with the cuff and thus bears additional load when the rotator cuff ruptures. In many cases of surgical exposure the biceps is revealed to be hypertrophied and flattened to the contour of the humeral head almost as if it were trying to become a substitute cuff. The missing downward force by the cuff results in upward displacement of the humeral head causing greater impingement of the coracoacromial arch on the biceps tendon. *Because of the intimate relationship of the biceps tendon with the rotator cuff, whenever one considers the diagnosis of a biceps long tendon disorder, one should also consider impingement of the rotator cuff.* A complete tear of the biceps tendon will usually produce no shoulder pain; thus, the patient with a rupture of the long tendon of the biceps may also be suspected of having a cuff tear.[2] Rotator cuff rupture increases exposure of the long biceps tendon to compression from the acromion above and the humeral head below. As with the rotator cuff, impingement may progress to tendinitis.

11. What is the most common form of proximal biceps brachii tendinitis?

The most common cause (95% to 98%) of bicipital tendinitis actually results as a secondary involvement of the biceps after primary impingement or tearing of the rotator cuff (Fig. 8-11). This is more easily imagined when we appreciate that the biceps tendon passes directly under the critical zone of the supraspinatus

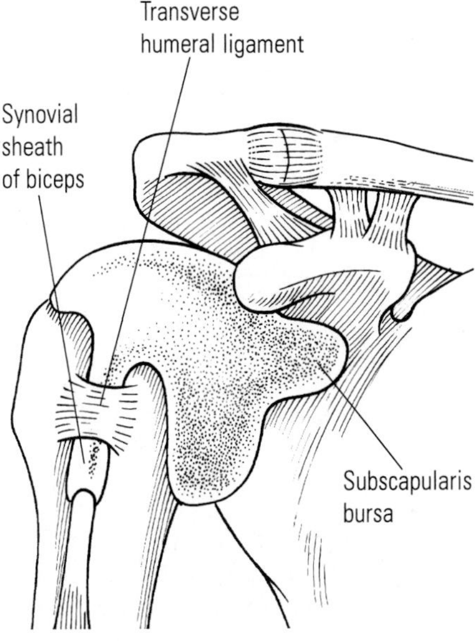

Fig. 8-10 Transverse humeral ligament.

tendon. In fact, the intracapsular portion of the biceps tendon has its own *critical zone* of avascularity caused by a "wringing-out" phenomenon when the arm is abducted.[18] In fact, the close functional relationship between the rotator cuff and the biceps long tendon is emphasized by the frequency with which tears of these two structures coincide.

Bicipital tendinitis may also occur secondary to an intra-articular problem such as rheumatoid or osteoarthritis.

12. What comparative anatomy studies may shed light on the origin of biceps brachii tendinitis and rotator cuff disorders?

When we look comparatively at the progressive changes in the relationship between the scapula and the bicipital groove, we notice a pronounced shift in the transition from quadruped mammals such as the opossum to that of biped primates. The human arm is essentially derived from the foreleg of a quadruped with a principal function of weight bearing. Subsequently, when locomotion evolved from quadruped to biped, the upper limb, no longer operating in a closed kinetic chain, moved away from the body to enable the arm to operate in a wide range of circumduction.

This modification was accomplished by (1) a progressive anteroposterior flattening of the thorax (Fig. 8-12) resulting in an increased angle formed between the scapula and the thorax as well as a relative lateral scapular displacement; (2) a shortened forearm that, along with changes in scapular position, necessitates a greater medial humeral rotation for the hand to reach midline. These two changes were incompletely compensated for by torsion of the humerus.

In the opossum, for example, the biceps tendon runs a *straight* course through the bicipital groove and is therefore an effective shoulder elevator. In humans, however, by virtue of an approximately 35° retroversion, the biceps tendon is left behind on the anterior aspect of the shoulder joint straddled by the tuberosities as the distal tendon courses *obliquely* over the glenohumeral joint.[2]

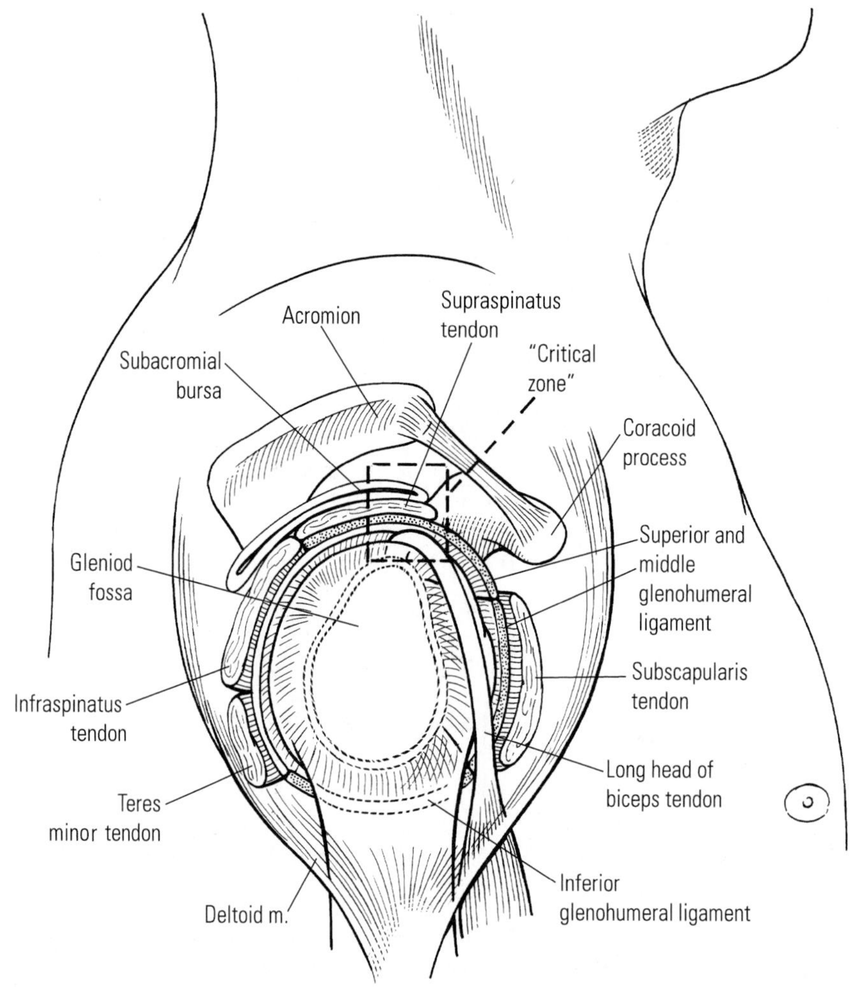

Fig. 8-11 Right shoulder. Orientation of tendinous origins of supraspinatus and the long tendon of the biceps brachii in relation to the "critical zone" vis-à-vis the subacromial arch.

The idea has been advanced[1] that the human embryo, during the course of its growth, metamorphoses through many stages of its evolutionary advancement; thus, the genetic code that guides the growing human neonate is expressed as an evolutionary metamorphisication of the various stages of man's vertebral ancestory that includes fish, amphibians, reptiles, and mammals.[15a] An example of ontogeny recapitulating phylogeny is how gill slits actually develop early on, only to mature into lungs as the neonate grows; similarly, the tail bud is resorbed into the coccyx, which is hidden by no more than a pronounced skin dimple. In the same vein upper limb rotation occurs at the elbow and is reflected at the elbow as humeral retroversion during the ninth week of gestation.

Thus, with the advent of *Homo erectus,* the biceps tendon became lodged against the lesser tuberosity (see Fig. 8-7), where the presence of either a medial supratubercular ridge or a shallow groove created a milieu for increased likelihood of a pathologic condition. This was further disadvantaged by the shortened forearms (and hence power arms) that no longer needed to be of equidistant height with the hind legs and most often worked resistively against the weight of held objects in an open kinetic chain. In this unfavorable mechanical situation the short lever arm is forced to work against a longer lever arm[2] (that is, the

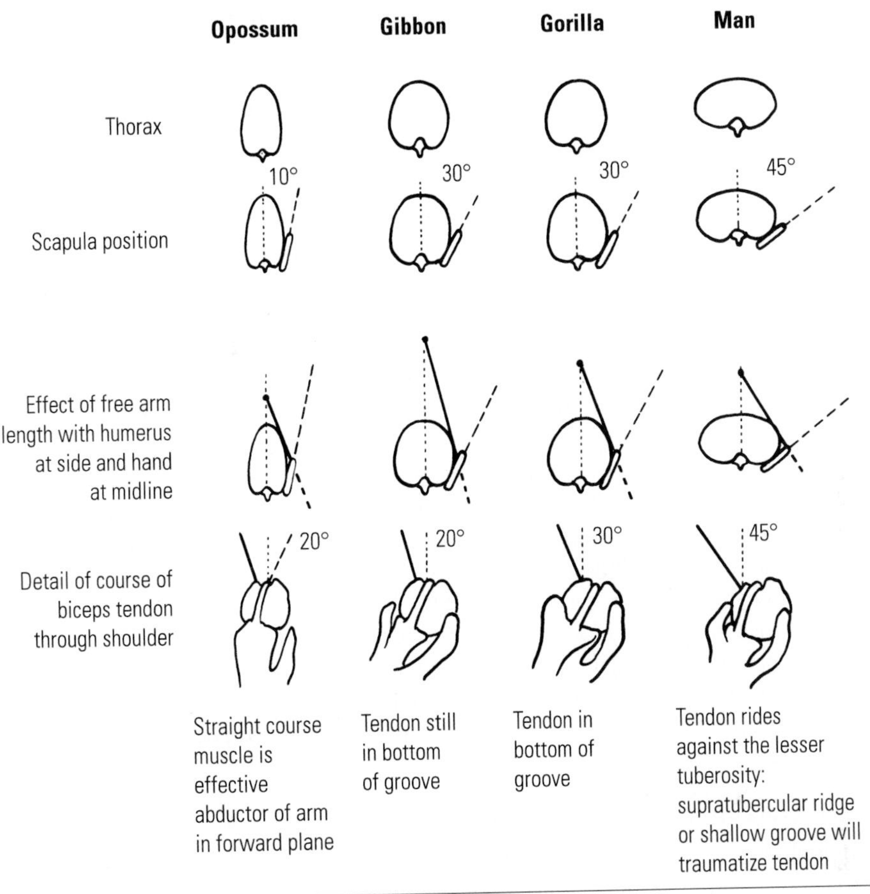

Fig. 8-12 Progressive changes in anteroposterior flattening of the thorax scapular position and migration of the biceps tendon from the quadruped to the biped. (Modified from Hitchcock HH, and Bechtol CO: Painful shoulder: Observations on the role of the tendon of the long head of the biceps brachii in its causation. *J Bone Joint Surg.* 30 A:263-273, 1948.)

object held), and this situation focuses undue excessive disruptive force, which may lead to tendinitis of the biceps or the rotator cuff. As such, bicipital tendinitis is yet another one of those disorders that are heir to the legacy of mankind's evolutionary advancement.

13. What are the clinical signs of proximal bicipital tendinitis within the glenohumeral joint?

Proximal biceps tendinitis is evidenced by proximal anterior shoulder pain and possibly a painful arc[16,20] during shoulder flexion and extension while the biceps is tensed *(sawing test)* and by tenderness in the bicipital groove on palpation. Pain may radiate distally to the muscle belly or proximally, like pain from cuff impingement, radiate to the deltoid insertion. There is no radiation into the neck or distally beyond the biceps muscle belly. The patient is typically young or middle aged with a history of overhead repetitive arm use. Pain is less intense during rest and worse with use. Nighttime exacerbation is common. Active or passive internal rotation with abduction is often painful because the long tendon works against the medial wall of the groove and thereby tenses that tendon. Similarly, abduction with external rotation is also painful when the long tendon occupies the floor of the groove and is again made taut when that tendon pulls downward on the humeral head. Resisted forward flexion may be painful.

14. Describe five provocative tests implicating lesions of the biceps brachii tendon.

See the provocative tests implicating lesions of the biceps tendon (Fig. 8-13).

15. What accounts for painful nocturnal exacerbation in many painful shoulder conditions?

Painful conditions of the shoulder are made worse at night for the following reasons:

- The supine position places the shoulder at or below the level of the heart.
- Rolling over the involved shoulder further increases the problem by decreasing the venous return from the upper extremity.
- Compression loading.[2]

16. What is primary biceps brachii tendinitis?

Primary bicipital tendinitis is uncommon as an isolated entity. However, this condition often accompanies cuff impingement and contributes to anterior shoulder pain. It involves changes in the tendon and enveloping synovial membrane within the bicipital groove; as such, it may be referred to as *bicipital tenosynovitis* of the upper arm. Tendinitis also goes by the name of *palm-up pain syndrome,* since symptoms are elicited during the supination portion of Yergason's maneuver. Pathologic changes are akin to other disease entities involving the passage of tendons through a fibro-osseous tunnel, such as de Quervain's tenosynovitis in the wrist region. Synovial reaction includes edema, intense erythema, thickening of the transverse humeral ligament, as well as tendon narrowing and attrition beneath the sheath. A bony spur may develop, causing stenosis and attrition of the long tendon of the biceps. This type of bicipital tendinitis (attrition tendinitis, see fig. 8-19) may be very painful and contributes to complete tendon rupture.[2] Treatment is by local rest with an arm sling, and one or more steroid injections may be required. Occasionally symptoms are so severe as to warrant operative treatment in which the degenerated tendon is divided and the distal stump is sutured to the bicipital groove.

17. Which sports are associated with proximal biceps brachii tendinitis and subluxation?

Degenerative processes are common in football quarterbacks because of the weight of the ball and the need for additional pushing action in softball pitchers because of forceful supinator strain with the arm and forearm in flexion.[11,17] Bicipital tendinitis is frequently seen in patients who participate in golf, tennis, swimming, pitching, or other throwing sports. The common denominator here is that humeral rotation at or above the level of the horizontal approximates the tuberosities, the intervening groove, the biceps tendon, and rotator cuff in direct contact with the anterior acromion or coracoacromial ligament.[2]

18. What happens to the long tendon of the biceps brachii during subluxation or dislocation?

Subluxation of the tendon of the long head may be isolated and result from attrition but is often concomitant with moderate to massive tears extending into the anterior portion of the cuff. A fully displaced bicipital tendon lies in the sling of the ruptured cuff and may, in the early phase of this lesion, slip in and out of the groove. As the sulcus gradually fills with scar tissue, the groove becomes shallower, and so finally the tendon remains in a medially dislocated position[2] (Fig. 8-14).

When an excessive load is applied to the arm in the position of abduction and external rotation, the line of pull of the long bicipital tendon is placed in the coronal plane and presses against the medial wall of the groove but is restrained from bowstringing by the lesser tuberosity acting as a simple pulley. In the event of a shallow groove or excessive force the tendon is restrained by the coracohumeral ligament as well as the restraining aponeurosis but may nonetheless luxate medially out of the groove and over the lesser medial tuberosity in one of two patterns: (1) rupture of the transverse ligament and subluxation of the biceps tendon out of the groove, with the tendon lying anterior to the subscapularis muscle, or (2) tendon

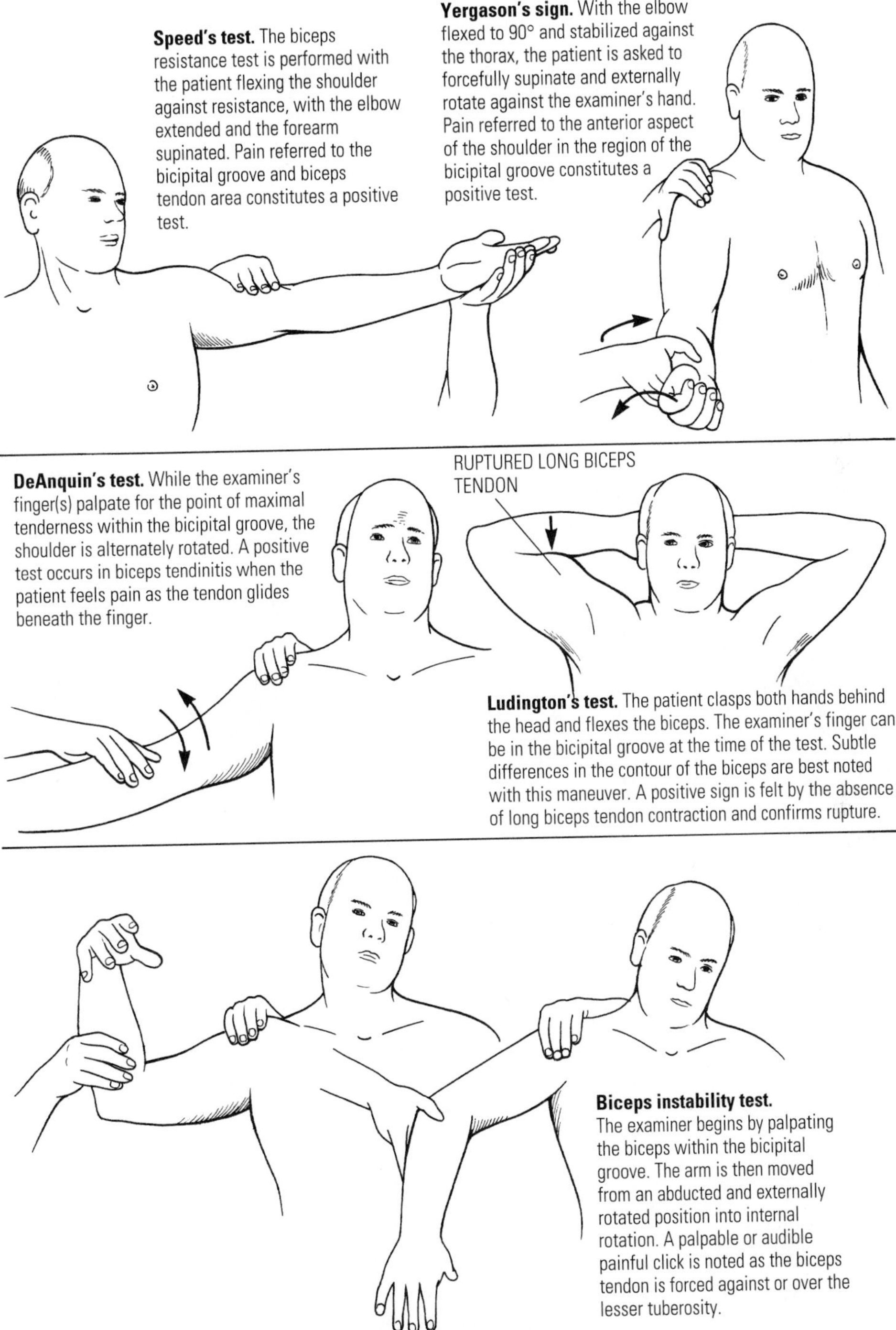

Speed's test. The biceps resistance test is performed with the patient flexing the shoulder against resistance, with the elbow extended and the forearm supinated. Pain referred to the bicipital groove and biceps tendon area constitutes a positive test.
Yergason's sign. With the elbow flexed to 90° and stabilized against the thorax, the patient is asked to forcefully supinate and externally rotate against the examiner's hand. Pain referred to the anterior aspect of the shoulder in the region of the bicipital groove constitutes a positive test.
DeAnquin's test. While the examiner's finger(s) palpate for the point of maximal tenderness within the bicipital groove, the shoulder is alternately rotated. A positive test occurs in biceps tendinitis when the patient feels pain as the tendon glides beneath the finger.
RUPTURED LONG BICEPS TENDON
Ludington's test. The patient clasps both hands behind the head and flexes the biceps. The examiner's finger can be in the bicipital groove at the time of the test. Subtle differences in the contour of the biceps are best noted with this maneuver. A positive sign is felt by the absence of long biceps tendon contraction and confirms rupture.
Biceps instability test. The examiner begins by palpating the biceps within the bicipital groove. The arm is then moved from an abducted and externally rotated position into internal rotation. A palpable or audible painful click is noted as the biceps tendon is forced against or over the lesser tuberosity.

Fig. 8-13 Provative tests implicating long bicipital tendinitis, rupture, and instability.

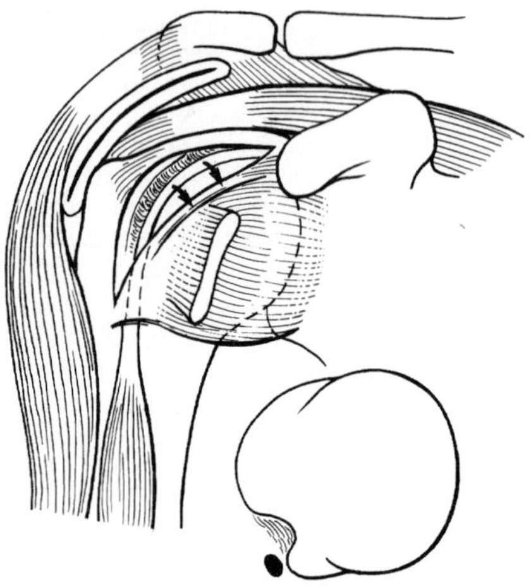

Fig. 8-14 Subluxation of the biceps. A tear in the medial portion of the coracohumeral ligament causes subluxation and medial displacement of the tendon out of the bicipital groove. (Redrawn from Paavolainen P, Slatis P, Aalto K: Surgical pathology in chronic shoulder pain. In Bateman JE, Welsh RP, editors: *Surgery of the shoulder,* St. Louis, 1984, Mosby.)

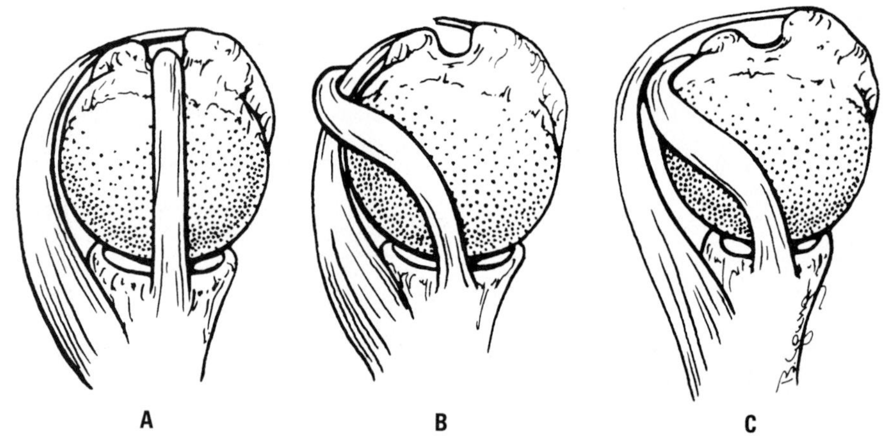

Fig. 8-15 **A,** The normal relationship of the biceps tendon in the groove corerel by the transverse humeral ligament. **B,** Rupture of the transverse ligament and subluxation of the biceps tendon out of the groove with the tendon lying anterior to the subscapularis muscle. **C,** Interatendinous disruption of the subscapularis commonly occurs in which the subscapularis insertion degenerates and the tendon subluxates beneath the muscle-tendon belly. The subscapularis tendon may be attached to the greater tuberosity through the coracohumeral and transverse ligaments. (Modified from Petersson CJ: *Aeta Orthop Scand* 54: 277-283, 1983.)

subluxation beneath the subscapularis muscle belly (Fig. 8-15). The long tendon will then return of its own accord back into the groove once the upper arm is rotated medially and then laterally while the forearm is flexed at the elbow[14] as in the provocative test of Yergason (Fig. 8-16). A positive test reproduces pain, and the examiner may feel the tendon snapping in and out of the groove. Motion is often accompanied by a palpable snap or pop. This may be attributable to actual subluxation of the biceps tendon but is more likely caused by the roughened edges of the cuff tendons catching against the anterior edge of the

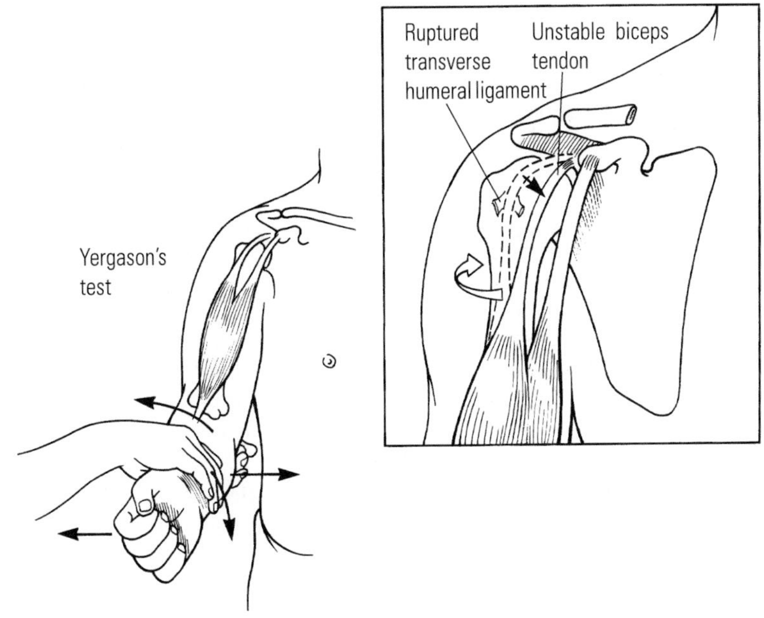

Fig. 8-16 Yergason's test for long biceps tendon stability. The examiner resists supination as the patient simultaneously externally rotates the shoulder against resistance.

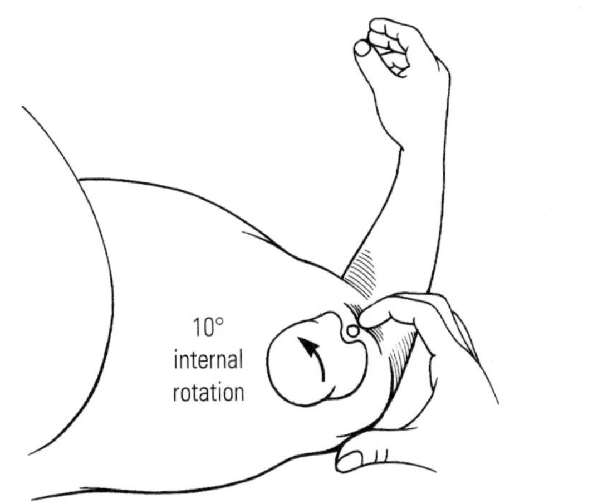

Fig. 8-17 The biceps tendon may be palpated directly anteriorly with the arm in 10° of internal rotation.

acromion and coracoacromial ligament. Pain is felt at the front of the shoulder, and one may reproduce it by simply raising the upper arm to 90°.

19. How is the bicipital groove best palpated?

Pinpoint tenderness in the biceps groove is best localized with the humerus in about a 10° of internal rotation, placing the long tendon to face directly anteriorly and located 6 cm below the acromion (Fig. 8-17). This point tenderness should move with rotation of the arm and often disappears as the lesser tuberosity and groove rotate internally under the short head of the biceps and the coracoid. This "tenderness in motion" is likely the most specific sign implicating bicipital lesions. It does not, however, differentiate biceps tendinitis from long biceps tendon instability. Although some authorities claim that the long tendon can actually be felt subluxating in and out of the groove, it is in reality difficult to discern whether what one is feeling is actually a subluxating tendon or deltoid muscle bundles rolling up against the humerus by the examiner's hand pressed against the humerus; this is especially so in a well-muscled individual.[2]

20. What forms of imaging are appropriate in detecting biceps brachii lesions?

Because routine plain radiographs of the shoulder appear normal with proximal biceps tendinitis, special views are indicated when biceps involvement is suspected. The bicipital groove view determines medial wall angle; the width, presence, or absence of bicipital groove spurs; coexisting degenerative changes in the greater or lesser tuberosity; and the presence or absence of a supratubercular ridge. In addition, a caudal tilt view may reveal the degree of anterior acromial prominence or spurring, which would implicate a commonly missed source of proximal biceps tendon lesions: coracoacromial arch impingement syndrome.[2]

Shoulder arthrography may also provide information on the state of the biceps tendon; for example, whether a shallow groove appearing on a plain radiograph is associated with a dislocation of the long tendon. Arthrography in patients with biceps tendinitis shows an intact rotator cuff but with the biceps poorly outlined, having a thickened sheath, or elevated at its origin.

The long tendon as well as the bicipital groove can also be assessed with computerized tomographic arthrography.

21. What is the clinical sign of strain of the long head of the biceps brachii at its glenoid origin?

Localized pain is felt at the acromioclavicular joint. All passive and resistive movements of the shoulder and elbow, including pronation and supination, are painless. Only resisted adduction is painful, and only when the elbow is kept extended. This characteristic is suggestive of the constant-length phenomenon and implicates the long tendon of biceps.[4] Treatment is by steriod injection.[3]

22. At which sites does the biceps brachii tendon most likely rupture, and who is most vulnerable?

Rupture of the biceps most commonly occurs in the long head at one of three locations: (1) in the shoulder joint, (2) at the bicipital groove, or (3) distally at the musculotendinous junction on the ulna. A fourth location, the origin of the long tendon on the supraglenoid tubercle, may also occur.[15]

Ruptures most commonly affect middle-aged individuals, most likely as a result of attritional and degenerative changes in the tendon. Rupture may occur spontaneously or as the result of muscular strain as from lifting a heavy load.

23. What is the presentation of sudden proximal tendon rupture?

During sudden tendon rupture the patient experiences immediate sharp pain[15] at the time of rupture, a feeling that something has snapped[5] or "given way."[9] There is sometimes an audible pop in the shoulder. Mild swelling and ecchymosis of the upper anterior arm[15] as well as a change of contour of the biceps muscle occurs over the next several days because of subcutaneous bleeding.[5] Weakness of the forearm supinators and elbow flexors also develop. With time, swelling and bruising will subside and the muscle fibers comprising the long head may still contract, albeit unrestrained proximally. This takes the appearance of a firm ball of muscle[5] that is more distal than normally expected and is palpable as a soft hump when the elbow is flexed or the forearm is supinated,[15] especially against resistance. This deformity will persist and is sometimes called the *Popeye sign* after the well-known cartoon sailorman (Fig. 8-18). The short head of the biceps continues to function and may even hypertrophy. There is little loss of power because of the contractile[5] contributions of the short biceps head and brachialis and brachioradialis muscles.[15] Movement of the shoulder is little affected.[15] Surgical repair

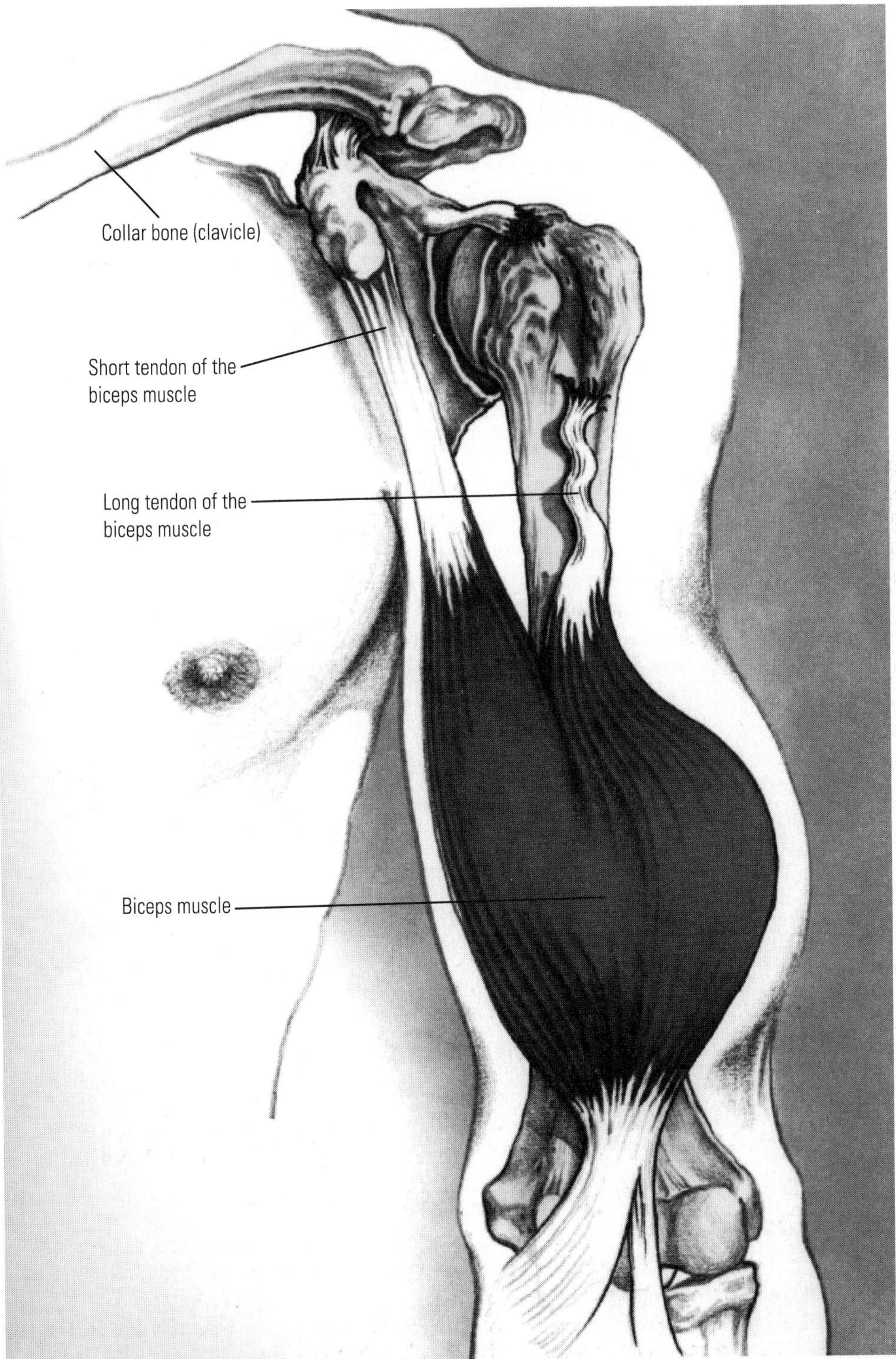

Fig. 8-18 Proximal long tendon biceps rupture with retraction of torn tendon ends. (From Peterson L, Renström P: *Sport injuries: their prevention and treatment*, London, 1986, Martin Dunitz, Ltd.)

is not necessary, since the resulting disability is mild and is indicated only for individuals involved in strong physical work that requires strong elbow flexion, as well as for cosmesis. Surgery is therefore appropriate in young or athletic patients and in those individuals performing heavy physical labor.[15]

24. What is the mechanism for distal tendon avulsion?

Avulsion or rupture of the distal tendon off the ulna is uncommon and is caused by sudden forceful flexion of the elbow against resistance.[15] There may be a history of heavy exertion against a major resistance[7] that may have, in times past, initiated degenerative changes in the tendon or at its insertion at the radial tuberosity.[15] Pain is sudden and profound[5] and is accompanied by pronounced swelling. Forearm supination is considerably weakened, whereas elbow flexion strength has a good muscle grade because of substitution of other muscles. Unlike with proximal tendon rupture, there is minimal upward retraction deformity because of the yet-intact second distal attachment at the radial tuberosity. Long-term symptoms of moderate aching and supination weakness are sometimes permanent and lead to moderate disability of the arm. Surgical repair consists of reattaching the tendon to the radial tuberosity is usually indicated but not mandatory unless the bicipital aponeurosis is also ruptured. Results of surgery are generally good.[15]

25. What is bicipital tenosynovitis at the lower arm?

This disorder usually occurs in athletes who engage in repetitive activities such as weight lifting, bowling, and gymnastics. Symptoms include elbow pain and weakness, with the former exacerbated by direct palpation of the distal end of the tendon and provoked by resisted flexion and supination,[7] just as full passive pronation does at the elbow joint. This exacerbation is especially noted when the elbow is held flexed because this position presses the radial tuberosity against the ulna.[3] Pain may radiate down the anterior forearm as far distally as the wrist. X-ray findings are unremarkable. Treatment includes rest, ice, elevation, compression, NSAID, modalities, deep friction massage, iontophoresis, and modification of training errors.[7] Deep transverse friction massage is performed by application of the tip of the thumb to the top of the radial tuberosity anteriorly while the therapist's other hand alternately pronates and supinates the forearm while grasping the patient's hand.[4] Therapeutic exercises should focus on increasing flexibility of the flexor mechanism as well as muscle strength.[7] Steroid injection may be performed but is best avoided because of the risk of tendon rupture.

26. What is bicipital tendinitis of the lower arm?

With bicipital tendinitis of the lower arm, pain is confirmed by palpation over the distal musculotendinous junction into the ulna and is confirmed by local anesthesia. Treatment includes deep friction massage,[4] modalities, stretching, strengthening, and NSAID.

27. How is a brachialis muscle disorder differentiated from a lesion of the biceps brachialis?

Pain elicited on resisted flexion with the forearm fully pronated is produced only by the brachioradialis, whereas pain on flexion with supination implicates the biceps as well as the brachialis. The position of the forearm does not affect brachialis function, since this muscle is recruited under all conditions of flexion. The biceps is recruited to assist the brachialis if heavy resistance is required in supination or to move very quickly.

28. What is the differential diagnosis?

Differential diagnosis includes the following:

- *Anterior shoulder instability* caused by glenohumeral joint dislocation has several features in common with dislocation of the long biceps tendon. Pain is present in the anterior shoulder, is episodic in nature, and is, like the biceps lesion, associated with a palpable and audible clunk. Indeed the mechanism of injury described for both of these conditions is very similar in that they most commonly occur with forced abduction and external rotation. The differential diagnosis can be even more confusing in the event that anterior shoulder instability and impingement syndrome coexist. The differences between these two pathologic conditions are quite noticeable, and so the examiner need not confuse one with the other. In anterior shoulder instability, aside from there often being an obvious swelling within the patient's armpit, the maximum point of apprehension and clicking should be at 90° abduction and maximum external rotation (that is, a positive apprehension sign). Whereas in the patient with a medially subluxating biceps tendon, pain is not maximal until the arm is brought down from the position of maximum abduction and external rotation and the click occurs as the examiner begins to internally rotate the arm *(biceps instability test)*. Yergason's and Speed's signs should not be present in patients with anterior shoulder instability. In addition to provocative testing, roentgenographic shoulder views clarify the diagnosis. Computerized tomography (CT) is helpful in demonstrating both the biceps tendon within the groove as well as lesions of the anterior cartilaginous labrum in patients with instability. If, after the above studies, the diagnosis still remains unclear, glenohumeral arthroscopy may be performed and allows direct visualization of the anterior labrum as well as the intra-articular portion of the biceps tendon, the aperture of the sulcus, and the surrounding cuff tissue.[2]

- *Glenoid labrum tears without instability,* such as those that occur in the superior one third of the labrum adjacent to the biceps origin, may demonstrate symptoms similar to those of biceps tendon subluxation and rotator cuff tear. Superior labrum tears occur in athletes who throw, such as baseball players, and result in an audible or palpable clunk occurring as the tear flips in and out of the joint, impinging on normal humeral head excursion during rotation above the horizontal plane. When encountering a throwing athlete with shoulder pain, one finds that patients may report more pain on ball release because of the deceleration effect of the biceps pulling on the torn labrum. Computerized tomography may occasionally not reveal this lesion, and the best way to differentiate this disorder from that of a subluxating biceps tendon may be by glenohumeral arthroscopy.[2]
- The *coracoid impingement syndrome* shares similar symptoms to biceps tendinitis and instability. The normal coracoid-to-humeral distance is calculated at 8.6 mm and is noted to be decreased to some 6.7 mm in patients with coracoid impingement syndrome. Thus this condition is associated with patients who have excessively long or laterally placed coracoid processes, or in those individuals who have undergone bone block or osteotomy procedures for instability. Symptoms of coracoid impingement include dull pain in the front of the shoulder with referral to the front and upper arm and occasionally extending into the forearm. Symptoms are consistently provoked by forward flexion and internal rotation or abduction and internal rotation, and it differs from the more common type of impingement syndrome by being most painful on forward flexion between the unusual ranges of 120° to 130°. Suspicion of this condition is confirmed by obliteration of the patient's pain by a subcoracoid injection.[2]
- The tenderness of *cuff impingement* is often diffuse, is located more proximally, and is accompanied by tenderness in the arm, anterior acromion, coracoacromial ligament, coracoid process, and supraspinatus insertion. Additionally, pain does not move with rotation of the arm. Primary biceps tendinitis rarely exists as an isolated entity and occurs secondarily to cuff impingement syndrome. If one is in doubt, selective injection with a local anesthetic is an indispensable part of the physician's evaluation. Patients suffering from either primary or secondary bicipital tendinitis, unlike those with rotator cuff tendinitis, find no relief from lidocaine injection into the subacromial space. Injection is performed at the lateral or posterolateral corner of the acromion into the subacromial space so as to avoid inadvertent injection into the groove. It is important to remember that the subdeltoid bursa, which extends to the groove, is continuous with the subacromial bursa, and so inadvertent injection into the groove area will anesthetize the

subacromial bursa. If an isolated biceps injection relieves all pain and restores 100% of motion, a diagnosis of primary biceps tendinitis is justified.[2]

- Tenderness of *subdeltoid bursitis* is generally more diffuse and should not change with arm rotation.[2]
- Early *glenohumeral joint arthritis* frequently presents as anterior shoulder pain with limited range of motion. Because the long biceps tendon is an intra-articular structure, it may become involved with any process within the joint. Thus inflammatory changes occur in the synovia of the biceps recess just as they do in the subscapular and axillary recess. Plain radiographs may show bone spurring of the proximal humerus with a ring osteophyte and flattening of the glenoid. Double-contrast arthrography may reveal thinning of the articular cartilage before the development of obvious osseous spur formation.[2]
- *Brachial neuritis* (syndrome of Parsonage and Turner) is an extremely painful condition that frequently presents as anterior shoulder pain. The early course of this condition, usually preceded by viral illness, manifests as pain exceeding neurologic findings, and the examiner may be fooled into thinking that he or she is dealing with an acute calcific tendinitis. Later, numbness and weakness with obvious atrophy become prominent. This condition occurs mainly in young men and produces supraclavicular pain, weakness, and diminished reflexes in the distribution of the brachial plexus as well as minor sensory abnormalities. The rostral plexus and thus proximal musculature become involved in two thirds of all cases. Profound weakness may occur within a day to a week of onset, only to regress over the subsequent 3 months. The cause is unknown, though viral or immunologic inflammatory processes are suspected. The course is variable.[2]
- *Thoracic outlet syndrome* (see Chapter 18) is ruled out when provocative tests such as Wright's maneuver, Adson's test, or Roo's overhead grip test score positive with negative or equivocal findings in Yergason's, Speed's, and impingement tests. Subacromial and bicipital injections should not completely alleviate pain.[2]
- *Frozen shoulder* (see Chapter 13) is differentiated from biceps lesions by the presence of severely diminished joint play in the former. Additionally, when the physician injects and infiltrates the biceps tendon sheath with 2 to 3 ml of lidocaine and the patient's pain is obliterated but there is no appreciable change in motion, adhesive capsulitis is suspected.[2]
- *Cervical radiculopathy*, especially at the level of C5-C6, may also mimic primary shoulder lesions. Similarly, *peripheral nerve entrapment* caused by carpal tunnel syndrome (see Chapter 4) ulnar neuritis, or posterior interosseous nerve entrapment may refer pain proximally to the shoulder. These pathologic conditions may be a source of differential confusion in the patient with proximal bicipital tendinitis. These entities however are distinguished from biceps disorders by careful neurologic examination, provocative testing, and electromyograph and nerve conduction velocity testing when in doubt.[2]
- In patients with persistent anterior shoulder pain in whom a work-up for a primary shoulder disorder shows normal results and neurologic examination is unrevealing, a tumor may be suspected.[2]

29. What rehabilitative treatment is most appropriate for proximal biceps brachii tendinitis, and when is surgery appropriate?

The treatment of the varied lesions of the biceps tendon, except for acute traumatic rupture in the young patient or in association with massive cuff tear in an active patient, is best managed with conservative care and repeated evaluation. The guiding criterion is that, as long as the patient is making gradual improvement, surgical intervention is not recommended. Surgery is indicated only after a minimum of 6 consecutive months of conservative care. This is especially so in patients over 65 years of age.[2]

In the case of proximal biceps *impingement tendinitis*, treatment initially closely follows that of rotator cuff impingement and tendinitis (see pp. 113-118, and 133-135). In the event of a failed conservative treatment outcome, surgical treatment primarily focuses on repair of the rotator cuff and decompression

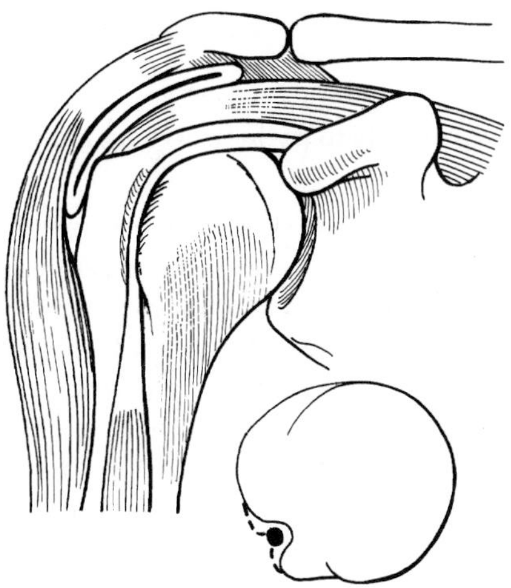

Fig. 8-19 The cuff is exposed to show the constriction of the biceps tendon within the groove. Local formation of new bone and connective tissue causes stenosis of the bicipital groove, leading to attrition of the tendon of the long head of the biceps. (Modified from Paavolainen P, Slatis P, Aalto K: Surgical pathology in chronic shoulder pain. In Bateman JE, Welsh RP, editors: *Surgery of the shoulder*, St. Louis, 1984, Mosby.)

of the subacromial arch (acromioplasty procedure). Biceps tenodesis is appropriate only in the event that the tendon is extremely frayed as from severe attrition wear, such that rupture appears to be imminent, or in the event that reconstruction of the fibrous roof of the arch is impossible.

No attempt is usually made to repair chronic ruptures (greater than 6 weeks) of the long biceps tendon; here, surgery involves only removal of the intra-articular portion of the tendon. The patient is informed preoperatively that he or she will continue to have a bulge in the lower portion of the arm.

Surgical treatment of *biceps instability* is often recommend in patients under 50 years of age, especially if the injury is acute. *Once dislocation of the biceps tendon is clinically suspect and then confirmed by sonography, one may also assume concomitant rupture of a portion of the rotator cuff. This concomitance depends on the intimate relationship the biceps tendon shares with the rotator cuff tendons just proximal to the groove, where the latter serve as a significant medial restraint to the long tendon of the biceps. The idea here is that if the long tendon restraint is compromised the probability of medial subluxation is greatly increased because of loss of the cuff's dynamic checkrein preventing subluxation and dislocation.* Indeed, surgically proved biceps instability is virtually always related to a degenerative process in the cuff, restraining capsule, and coracohumeral ligament in the proximal portion of the groove. As such, confirmed instability warrants open tendon reduction and reconstruction of the rotator cuff and subacromial decompression.[2]

Patients who suffer from *attrition tendinitis* (Fig. 8-19) best respond to judicious use of rest, NSAID, moist heat, and gentle exercises. Judicious use or corticosteroid injection may also be helpful; however, it is absolutely imperative that injection be into the bicipital sheath and not into the tendon so as not to cause collagen necrosis. There may be as much as a 35% loss of tendon strength immediately after injection, and such a loss reverses after approximately 2 weeks. However, ultrastructural changes within the tendon do not completely revert for 6 weeks. Because of this, patients should avoid any strenuous activity for 3 weeks. These injections frequently make the patient more comfortable quickly and shorten the course of the illness. Although injection has been shown to be equally efficacious to the use of indomethacin (Indocin), some patients unfortunately cannot tolerate a nonsteroidal anti-inflammatory agent in the doses required. Surgery is recommended only if the patient fails to respond to conservative care over a 6 to 12-month period.[2]

30. What postoperative care is appropriate to patients having undergone surgery for a proximal biceps brachii lesion?

During the first 3 postoperative weeks a Velcro elastic immobilizer is often utilized, and the patient is encouraged to take his or her elbow out of the immobilizer and gently flex and extend it passively with the opposite hand. Gentle pendulum exercises are initiated on the first postoperative day, and passive elbow flexion is initiated on the second postoperative day. Pulley exercises should be avoided during the immediate postoperative period, since holding onto a pulley handle requires some active contraction of biceps; instead, passive shoulder flexion and external rotation are appropriate. At 1 month, a pulley may safely be introduced and gentle, active elbow flexion started. Strengthening of the repaired cuff, deltoid, and biceps generally begins at 2 months and becomes more vigorous at 3 months. Jobs that require lifting should be avoided until approximately 6 months postoperatively.[2]

References

1. Asimov I: The human body, New York, 1992, NAL-Dutton.
2. Burkhead WZ: The biceps tendon. In Rockwood CA, Matsen FA, editors: *The shoulder,* vol 2, Philadelphia, 1990, Saunders.
3. Cyriax J: *Textbook of orthopaedic medicine,* vol 1: *Diagnosis of soft tissue lesions,* ed 8, London, 1982, Bailliere-Tindall.
4. Cyriax J: *Textbook of orthopaedic medicine,* vol 2, ed 11, London, 1984, Bailliere-Tindall.
5. Dandy DJ: *Essential orthopaedics and trauma,* Edinburgh, 1989, Churchill Livingstone.
6. Gilcreest EL: Rupture of muscles and tendons, particularly subcutaneous rupture of the biceps flexor cubiti, *JAMA* 84:1819-1822, 1925.
7. Lillegard WA, Rucker KS: *Handbook of sports medicine: a symptom-oriented approach,* Andover, Mass., 1993, Butterworth-Heinemann.
8. Lippman RK: Frozen shoulder, periarthritis, bicipital tenosynovitis, *Arch Surg* 47:283-296, 1943.
9. Lippman RK: Bicipital tenosynovitis, *NY State J Med* 44:2235-2240, 1944.
10. Magee DJ: *Orthopaedic physical assessment,* Philadelphia, 1989, Saunders.
11. McCue FC III, Zarins B, Andrews JR, Carson WG: Throwing injuries to the shoulder. In Zarins B, Andrews JR, Carson WG, editors: *Injuries to the throwing arm,* Philadelphia, 1985, Saunders.
12. Mercer A: Partial dislocations: consecutive and muscular affectations of the shoulder joint, *Buffalo Med Surg J* 4:645-652, 1959.
13. Meyer AW: Spolia anatomica: absence of the tendon of the long head of the biceps, *J Anat* 48:133-135, 1913-1914.
14. Moore KL: *Clinically oriented anatomy,* ed 2, Baltimore, 1985, Williams & Wilkins.
15. Netter FH: *The CIBA collection of medical illustrations,* vol 8: *Musculoskeletal system,* Part II, Summit, N.J., 1990, CIBA-Geigy Corp.

15a. Netter, F: *The CIBA collection of medical illustrations,* vol 8, part I.

16. Neviaser RJ: Painful conditions affecting the shoulder, *Clin Orthop* 173:63-69, 1983.
17. O'Donohue D: Subluxating biceps tendon in the athlete, *Clin Orthop* 164:26, 1982.
18. Rathbun JB, McNab I: The microvascular pattern of the rotator cuff, *J Bone Joint Surg* 52B:540-553, 1970.
19. Salter RB: *Textbook of disorders and injuries of the musculoskeletal system,* ed 2, Baltimore, 1983, Williams & Wilkins.
20. Simon WH: Soft tissue disorders of the shoulder: frozen shoulder, calcific tendinitis, and bicipital tendinitis, *Orthop Clin North Am* 6:521-539, 1975.

Recommended reading

Burkhead WZ: The biceps tendon. In Rockwood CA, Matsen FA, editors: *The shoulder,* vol 2, Philadelphia, 1990, Saunders.

Lillegard WA, Rucker KS: *Handbook of sports medicine: a symptom-oriented approach,* Andover, 1993, Butterworth-Heinemann.

Peterson L, Renström P: *Sport injuries: their prevention and treatment,* London, 1986, Martin Dunitz, Ltd.

Loss of Active Right Shoulder Elevation after Injury without Painful Arc

9

A 43-year-old male house painter spent the past 21 years of his working life engaged in the vocation of ceiling painting as his specialty. He reports having a history of bilateral shoulder tendinitis with "clicking" while raising his arms overhead. About 2 weeks ago he reports how half a can of paint fell onto his right shoulder. Since that time he complains of not quite being able to use his shoulder the same as before and feels stiff and weak when attempting to elevate his right arm overhead. When asked to elevate actively, he does so with the following bizarre substitution: by placing his hand on the outer side of his ipsilateral thigh and then twitching his hip outwardly while bending his trunk over to the opposite side. There is no report of pain anywhere along the active range; nor is there any painful arc of passive range, though passive movement seems guarded after 110° of elevation. When asked to elevate without substitution, he attempts what appears to be an overexaggerated right shoulder shrug that manages to elevate to some 40° momentarily before flopping down to his side (positive Mosely test).

OBSERVATION There is no ecchymosis observed at the shoulder.

PALPATION Mild tenderness is elicited over the right proximal humeral tuberosities and bicipital groove.

RANGE OF MOTION There is full active as well as passive medial and lateral rotation of the right shoulder joint, though some pain is reported through these ranges.

MUSCLE STRENGTH The muscle strength was not clearly tested with secondary guarding in various ranges; nevertheless, external right shoulder rotation appears to show decreased strength by at least one entire muscle grade. Otherwise normal.

SELECTIVE TENSION Symptoms of pain and guarding as well as apprehension are elicited on passive right shoulder internal rotation. Resistive external rotation yields similar results. Otherwise normal.

SPECIAL TESTS Negative Ludington's test, negative Yergason's test, negative Allen test, negative impingement sign, positive drop arm test, negative Speed's test, negative Adson's maneuver.

SENSATION Normal.

DEEP TENDON REFLEXES Normal.

After referring the patient for a radiographic series of both shoulders, the radiologist confirms your suspicion.

Clue:

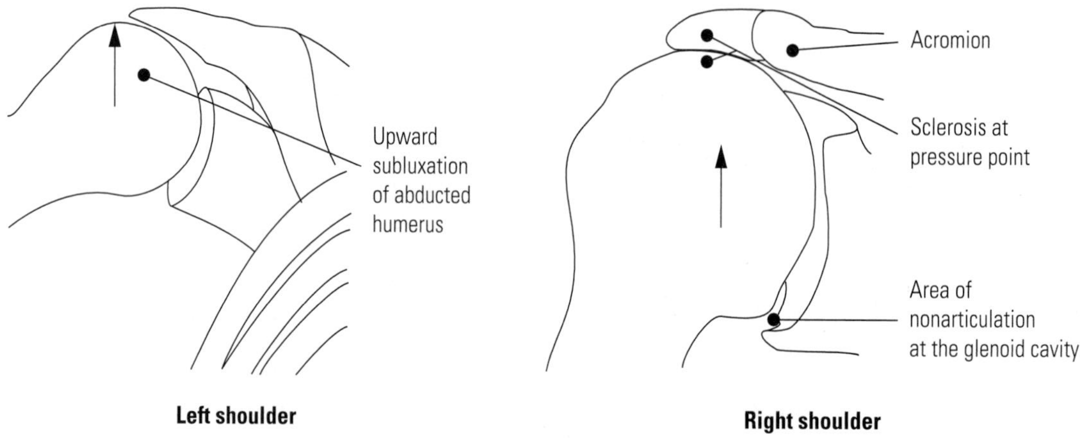

Xeroradiograph schematic of right and left shoulder. (From Dieppe PA, Bamji AN, Watt I: *Atlas of clinical rheumatology*, Baltimore, 1980, Lea & Febiger.)

1. **What is most likely wrong with this painter's shoulder?**
2. **What is the mechanism of injury?**
3. **What four stages successively occur during the evolution of rotator cuff disorders?**
4. **What area of the cuff tendon or tendons is most susceptible to involvement of rotator cuff injury?**
5. **What occurs during fiber failure, and what are the adverse effects, if any?**
6. **What is the likelihood for self-repair after cuff tear?**
7. **How do the cuff tendons contribute to humeral head elevation after cuff tear?**
8. **Is there an age-related epidemiologic correlation associated with rotator cuff tears?**
9. **What is the classification of injury in rotator cuff tendon disorders?**
10. **What is the differential diagnosis?**
11. **Is the presence of painful arc on passive or active elevation clinically revealing?**
12. **Can diagnosis of cuff tears be reliably made from the patient's history and physical examination alone?**
13. **What imaging techniques are best suited for confirmation of cuff tear?**
14. **What conservative treatment is appropriate in the stage I lesion?**
15. **What rehabilitative therapy is appropriate for the stage II and chronic stage III shoulders?**
16. **When is surgery appropriate?**
17. **What is the most commonly used surgical technique?**
18. **What factors account for decreased likelihood of success after surgical attempt at cuff repair?**
19. **What rehabilitation is appropriate after surgery?**
20. **How are partial- and full-thickness cuff tears managed in the elderly?**

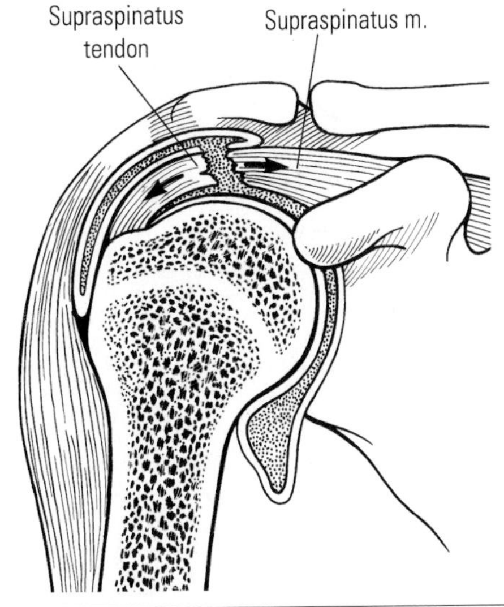

Fig. 9-1 Full-thickness tear of the rotator cuff tendons.

1. What is most likely wrong with this painter's shoulder?

Full-thickness tear of the right rotator cuff (Fig. 9-1), and partial-thickness tear of the left rotator cuff tendons. The former is obviated when viewing radiographs of the right shoulder showing cephalic humeral head subluxation and compression leasion at the head of the acromion.[8a]

2. What is the mechanism of injury?

The proposed causes of cuff tendon failure have included trauma,[4] attrition,[8] ischemia,[18] impingement,[23] and steroid injection.[19] Age-related changes in the rotator cuff include diminution of tendon vascularity, diminution of fibrocartilage at the cuff insertion, fragmentation of the tendon with loss of cellularity, disruption of the attachment to bone via Sharpey's fibers,[2] and eventually tendon infarct.[26] Let us assume that the normal cuff starts life out well vascularized and with a full complement of fibers; throughout its active life the cuff is subjected to repeated adverse exposure the likes of which include traction, contusion, impingement, inflammation, injections, and age-related degeneration, each of which place the cuff tendons at jeopardy for increased risk of injury[19] (Fig. 9-2). It is perhaps a wonder then that pathologic states do not occur more commonly than they do.

3. What four stages successively occur during the evolution of rotator cuff disorders?

Stage I *Edema and hemorrhage*[11] initiated by repeated microtrauma and presenting as a toothache-like discomfort felt after activity that is aggravated by provocative movements such as forced flexion at end range (impingement sign), forced internal rotation with the arm horizontally adducted and the shoulder at a 90° elevation, and a painful arc at around a 90° abduction. The supraspinatus tendon will be painful to palpation because of[11] impingement in this stage I disorder. Similarly the adjacent biceps tendon may also be tender at its bicipital groove exit in the event that it impinged under the subacromial arch. This *subacute stage*[11] is most often present in patients under 25 years of age,[24] but onset may occur at virtually any age. Stage I is *reversible* and may be viewed as a setting stage for the next level of disorder along the continuum of rotator cuff pathosis: tendinitis.

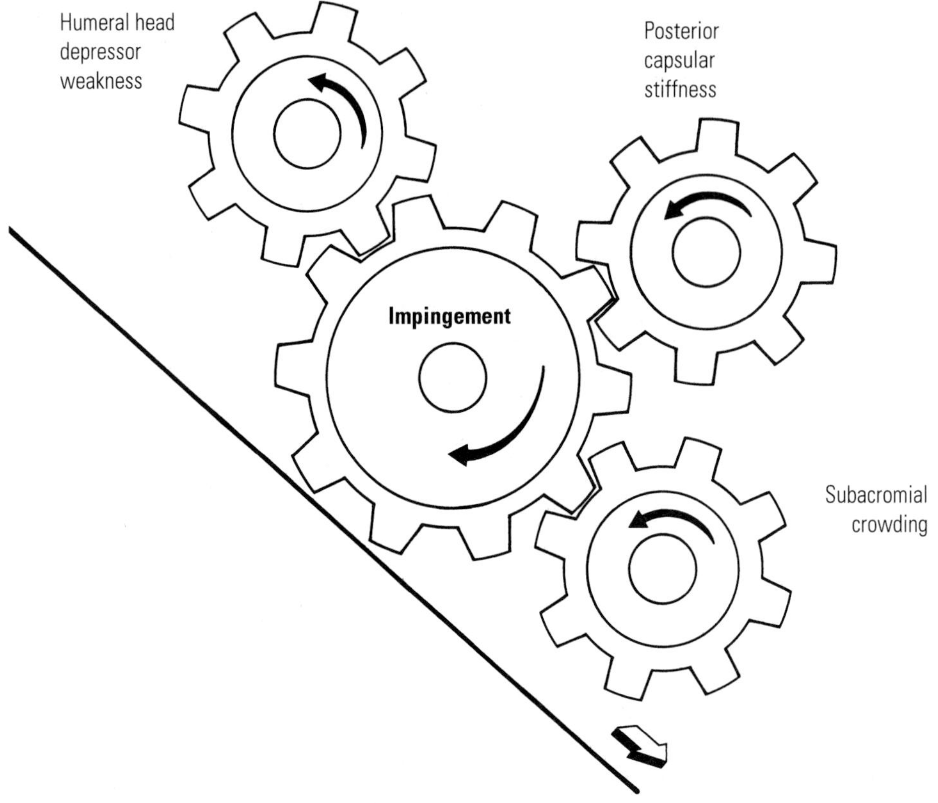

Fig. 9-2 Normal shoulder function is dependent on normal function of the humeral head depressors, normal capsular laxity, and adequate subacromial space. Some of the effects of impingement (weakness of the humeral head depressors, stiffness of the posterior capsule, and crowding of the subacromial space with thickened bursa) may further intensify impingement, producing a self-perpetuating process. (From Rockwood CA, Matsen FA, editors: *The shoulder,* ed 2, vol 1, Philadelphia, 1990, Saunders.)

Stage II *Tendinitis* is characterized by thickening and fibrosis of the tendons and bursae because of a vicious cyclic reinforcement of impingement vis-à-vis inflammation-edema–increased tendon volume with decreased suprahumeral space whose end result is further aggravation and impingement that eventually results in tendon infarct[11] and scarring. This stage most commonly occurs in the 25 to 40 year age group[23] and presents as a toothache-like pain most frequently experienced at night or after athletic activity.[23] The range of motion begins to decrease because of fibrosis and thickening of soft tissue. Rest, though important, is of limited value in that it can no longer reverse the pathologic process. Some stiffness may be reported.[11] All the previously mentioned signs applicable to the preceding impingement stage also apply here, including the presence of an impingement sign.

Stage III *Partial-thickness tear* caused by further tendon degeneration with toothache-like pain usually severe enough to cause a limitation of activity and loss of sleep occurs, and there may also be weakness reported and greater stiffness than before.[11] There is usually a history of tendinitis.[11] The patient can begin abduction but experiences pain or a painful arc during the attempt. Active abduction becomes more comfortable after injection of a local anesthetic, and this feature helps differentiate tendinitis or partial tear from a complete tear of the rotator cuff, since the patient with a large tear does not regain strength

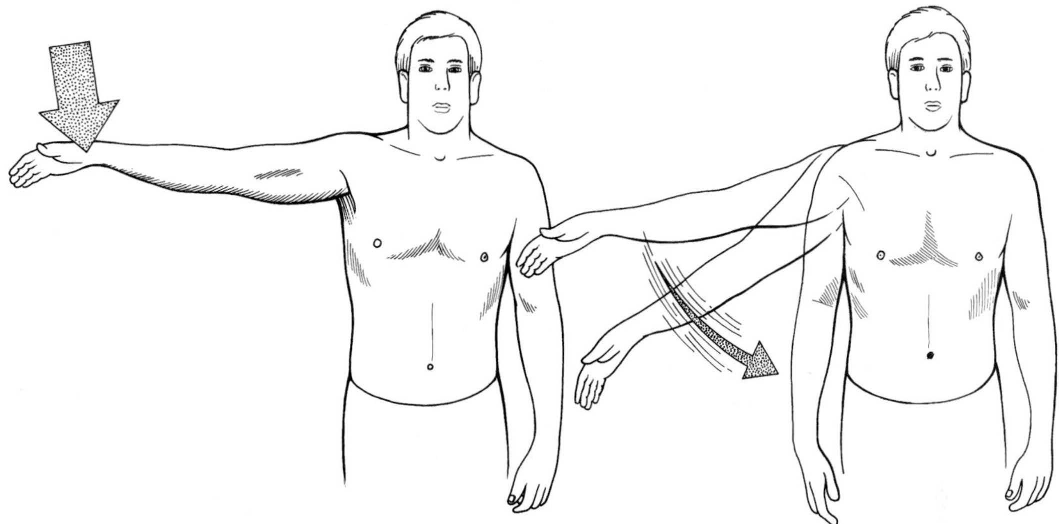

Fig. 9-3 A full-thickness tear of the rotator cuff is verified by a positive *drop-arm test.* The patient is unable to lower his arm slowly to the side in the presence of a torn cuff.

(i.e., active range of motion) after the subacromial space is anesthetized. If ignored, cuff tears, like a rip in nylon, tend to propagate themselves.[19]

Stage IV *Full-thickness tear* of the rotator cuff occurs as the final stage of a degenerative process in which the provoked tendon succumbs to something as trivial as opening up a stuck window or more seriously after sustaining a fall on the shoulder[28] or on an outstretched adducted arm.[11] A complete tear may also occur after greater humeral tuberosity fractures, or from shoulder dislocations. The patient, usually a man over 60 years of age, cannot initiate abduction and merely shrugs the shoulder on attempting to do so;[28] there is also weakness on flexion and external rotation.[19] Thus, while he exhibits a lack of active range, his passive range is not severely limited unless chronic or painful.[11] The synchronized force couple between deltoid and the rotator cuff muscle is lost, and the deltoid, acting unopposed, causes upward humeral migration that is visible on a radiograph and an observed altered glenohumeral rhythm. Altered biomechanics adversely influence the length-tension relationships of the remaining intact cuff musculature by placing them at a mechanical disadvantage, thus predisposing atrophy and wasting of these muscles. In long-standing cases, muscle wasting may be observed. If the arm is passively abducted to 90°, the patient is capable of maintaining this position by means of the deltoid muscle;[28] the drop-arm test scores as positive[11] (Fig. 9-3).

Many patients with full-thickness cuff tears have palpable cuff defects, as well as mild tenderness over the proximal humeral tuberosities, bicipital groove,[19] and anterior acromion and usually over the acromioclavicular joint.[13] Muscle wasting in the suprascapular and infrascapular fossae may occur, especially when the condition is long standing.[13] A large tear will preclude active shoulder abduction even when local anesthesia is administered to block pain perception.[20] After complete tear the proximal portion of the tendon will retract, allowing the glenohumeral joint to freely communicate with the subacromial bursa. Thus arthrography provides confirmation of the suspected full-thickness tear when injected radiopaque dye into the glenohumeral joint spreads into the bursae.

4. What area of the cuff tendon or tendons is most susceptible to involvement of rotator cuff injury?

Tears of the rotator cuff are usually *longitudinal* but may be transverse and occur in a *critical zone* (see Fig. 8-10) situated at the anterior portion of the cuff located within the subacromial space between the supraspinatus tendon and the coracohumeral ligament.

5. What occurs during fiber failure, and what are the adverse effects, if any?

Cuff tendon ruptures clinically present as soft-tissue disruption both at the tendon insertion as well as at its midsubstance. Fibers fail when the applied load (whether repetitive or abrupt, compressive or tensile) exceed tendon strength and may fail a few at a time or en masse (known as an acute tear or acute extension). Because fibers are under a load even with the arm at rest, they will retract after rupturing. Each instance of fiber failure has, at the very least, three adverse effects: (1) it increases the load on the neighboring soft tissue because there are now fewer fibers to share the load; (2) it detaches muscle fibers from bone and therefore diminishes the force the cuff can deliver; (3) it risks the anastomotic vascular elements in proximity by distorting their anatomic features.[19]

6. What is the likelihood for self-repair after cuff tear?

Although some tendons such as the Achilles tendon have a remarkable propensity to heal after rupture, rotator cuff tendons lack a similar resiliency since the intra-articular environment does not favor the rebuilding of new fibers. The reason is that cuff ruptures communicate with joint and bursal fluid, which removes any hematoma that might contribute to cuff healing.[19] Additionally the tear itself compromises the cuff tendon blood supply,[19] and even if the tendon could heal with a scar, scar tissue lacks the normal resilience of tendon and is therefore under increased risk for failure with subsequent loading.[19] Finally, rupture itself is accompanied by retraction of the torn ends of the tendon. The cumulative effect of these factors considerably diminish the cuff's ability to repair itself effectively.

7. How do the cuff tendons contribute to humeral head elevation after cuff tear?

One of the major functions of the rotator cuff is humeral head depression though this function is progressively compromised during the evolution of rotator cuff disorder. With progressive loss of the depressor mechanism the humeral head rises higher and higher because of the unrelenting upward pull of the deltoid. In the event of a major defect in the rotator cuff after rupture, the humeral head can now migrate even further proximally by protruding through the defect. Eventually, the relationship of the cuff tendons to the humeral head is such that the tendons slip below the equator of the humeral head. The biomechanics are changed to such an extent that the action of the intact tendons are converted from depression to that of humeral head elevation. This *boutonniere deformity,* just like that in the finger, victimizes the buttonholed cuff by changing its line of pull so as to convert balancing forces into unbalancing forces[19] (Fig. 9-4).

8. Is there an age-related epidemiologic correlation associated with rotator cuff tears?

Yes. Patients with rotator cuff tears are almost always over 40 years of age.[25] The supraspinatus does not often rupture in young people because their tendons are so strong that they rather will avulse the tip of the greater tubercle of the humerus than rupture the tendon.[22]

9. What is the classification of injury in rotator cuff tendon disorders?

Many terms have been used to classify cuff tendon failure, such as partial- and full-thickness tears, acute and chronic tears, and traumatic and degenerative tears.

Full-thickness tear refers to when the tendon deficit extends all the way through the articular surface to the bursal surface of the rotator cuff. *Partial-thickness tear* refers to when the tendon defect involves only the deep surface, midsubstance, or superficial surface of the tendon; these tears occur twice as common as full-thickness tears.

Chronic tears are those that have existed 3 months or more; they may be insidious in onset and are degenerative in nature. *Acute tears* occur suddenly, usually the result of a definitive injury such as a fall. An

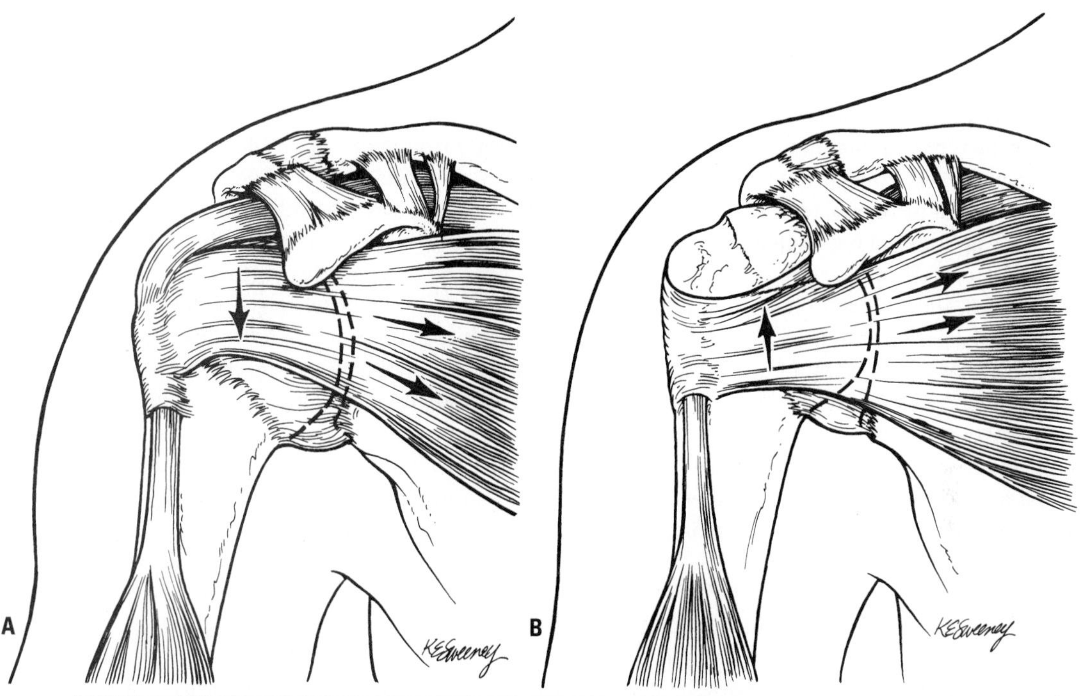

Fig. 9-4 **A,** In addition to the supraspinatus, the anterior and posterior rotator cuff muscles and the long head of the biceps tendon depress the humeral head and balance the upward-directed forces applied by the deltoid muscle. **B,** Major cuff fiber failure and retraction allow the humeral head to protrude upward through the cuff defect, creating *boutonniere lesion.* When the remaining cuff tendons slip below the equator of the head, their action is converted from humeral head depression to humeral head elevation. (From Rockwood CA, Matsen FA, editors: *The shoulder*, vol 1, ed 2, Philadelphia, 1990, Saunders.)

already chronic tear is at risk for an *acute extension*—the sudden failure of additional fibers with the production of acute symptoms superimposed on those of a chronic tear.

Cuff tears are also characterized according to the length of detachment from the humerus, the specific tendons involved, and the state of the detached tendon or tendons, such as retracted, atrophic, or absent. It is important to realize that cuff failure is always almost peripheral, near the tenoperiosteal junctions on the tuberosities, and nearly always on the supraspinatus tendon because that tendon runs adjacent to the biceps tendon.[19]

10. What is the differential diagnosis?

Differential diagnosis includes the following:

- *Cuff tendinitis* and *bursitis* are differentiated from cuff tears through arthrography or ultrasonography.
- Whereas partial-thickness cuff defects may demonstrate motion restriction, patients with full-thickness defects usually have a good range of passive motion but may be limited in strength or active range of motion.
- Although *cervical spondylosis* at C5 or C6 may produce pain and weakness in a pattern similar to rotator cuff involvement, radiculopathy is also inclusive of sensory, motor, and reflex abnormalities as additional diagnostic findings and furthermore as abnormal electromyographic findings, as well as pain often elicited on neck extension or when the chin is turned to the affected side.[19]

- *Suprascapular neuropathy* is characterized by dull pain over the shoulder exacerbated by shoulder movement, weakness in overhead activities, weakness of external rotators, spinal wasting, and normal radiographic evaluation, ultrasonography, and arthrography. Suprascapular neuropathy may arise from one of three causes: (1) *traction* injury to the suprascapular nerve as in an Erb's palsy type of injury, (2) *stenosis* at the suprascapular notch causing suprascapular nerve entrapment and resulting in chronic recurrent pain and weakness aggravated by shoulder use, (3) *brachial neuritis*, such as acute brachial neuropathy of unknown causes characterized by spontaneous onset of rather intense shoulder pain lasting several weeks with onset of weakness noted as pain subsides; atrophy and weakness occur chiefly in the rotator cuff, deltoid, and triceps as well as in muscles not supplied by the brachial plexus (that is, serratus anterior, trapezius, and the diaphragm); additionally there is occasionally minor sensory deficiency mainly affecting the axillary nerve distribution. The diagnosis of brachial neuritis is based on this observed pattern, recorded by electromyography, and occurring only in those individuals with no history of trauma.[32]
- A *snapping scapula* may produce shoulder pain on elevation and a catching sensation reminiscent of a rotator cuff tear. However, whereas the latter is usually elicited regardless of whether the scapula is stabilized or is allowed to rotate freely, scapular snaps arise from the superomedial scapular corner with just mere shoulder shrugging and without the presence of glenohumeral joint motion.[19]
- A superior sulcus *(Pancoast's) tumor*[19] (see p. 226).

11. Is the presence of painful arc on passive or active elevation clinically revealing?

Most probably yes. Cyriax maintained that active elevation yielding painful arc is indicative of tendinitis only, whereas a positive test for painful arc on passive elevation indicates rupture of supraspinatus.[7] Other authorities do not differentiate between active or passive pain-provoking movement possibly because of clinical evidence of full active range of motion in many cases of supraspinatus rupture.

12. Can diagnosis of cuff tears be reliably made from the patient's history and physical examination alone?

No. Imaging evaluation is necessary because cuff tears are not always symptomatic.[19] Patients with full-thickness and certainly partial-thickness tears have been known to exhibit strong active shoulder elevation, possibly attributable to substitution by other intact shoulder elevators.

13. What imaging techniques are best suited for confirmation of cuff tear?

Plain radiographs are usually normal in small cuff tears, except for some sclerosis on the acromial undersurface, but demonstrate upward humeral head displacement (that is, *subluxation*) with respect to both glenoid and acromion in partial tears because of loss of the tendons interposed between the humerus and acromion; this feature is better viewed by external rotation of the arm as the patient attempts isometric abduction. Plain radiographs of full-thickness tears are additionally characterized by several outstanding features: (1) appearance of a narrowed interval or even articulation between the humeral head and the acromion; this *acromiohumeral interval* normally measures between 7 and 14 mm; (2) concomitant widening or even nonarticulation of the inferior aspect of the humeral head with the inferior glenoid fossa; and (3) frequent sclerosis and osteophyte formation on the anteroinferior acromion and possibly on the greater tuberosity[13] as well.

Diagnostic ultrasonography reliably demonstrates the location and extent of cuff tears greater than 1 cm,[19] has the advantage of speed and safety, and is usually half the cost of an arthrogram and one eighth the cost of a magnetic resonance imaging (MRI) scan, all this despite the fact that ultrasonography does not detect small full-thickness tears and partial-thickness defects.[19] Arthrography shows intravasation of dye into the subacromial space (bursa) after injection and vigorous exercise that extends beyond the normal cuff attachment at the greater tuberosity, as well as a *geyser sign*, that is, dye leakage into the acromioclavicular joint. Arthrography is particularly effective in revealing suspected partial-thickness tears as well as larger tears but cannot reveal midsubstance or superior-surface tears. Shoulder MRI suffers from problems of image resolution.[19]

14. What conservative treatment is appropriate in the stage I lesion?

(See pp. 133-135 for a hypothetical treatment strategy of supraspinatus impingement syndrome.)

Stage I treatment: Because stage I is reversible, the primary thrust of treatment must be prevention of the underlying process causing injury. This is accomplished by vocational or athletic activity modification so as to permit noninjurious and biomechanically efficient motion. By educating the patient, coach, and trainer to understand how, for example, internal shoulder rotation during elevation may cause impingement vis-à-vis the subacromial arch, the patient may learn to substitute his or her motions with noninjurious movement patterns. This aspect of treatment cannot be overemphasized because treating the inflammation will do little good if the precipitating source of injury is still operative.

- Pain-limited *stretching* into external rotation in several positions of abduction is initiated because external rotation provides clearance, allowing the greater humeral tuberosity to swing back freely under the anterior acromion during active shoulder abduction; otherwise impingement will serve only to further exacerbate the injury.[11]
- Isolated *strengthening* of the supraspinatus, infraspinatus, and teres minor muscles while deemphasizing the deltoid muscle group serves to centralize the humeral head within the glenoid fossa and works to counter the tendency toward superior humeral invasion of the suprahumeral space.[11] The rotator cuff muscles are isolated for strengthening by the positions of (1) internal and external rotation in the neutral position, (2) external rotation at 90° of abduction,[16] and (3) shoulder abducted to 90° only, with the arm in slight forward flexed 30° to 45° and in full internal rotation[1] (Fig. 9-5). Electromyographic output of the supraspinatus is greatest in this last exercise.[16]

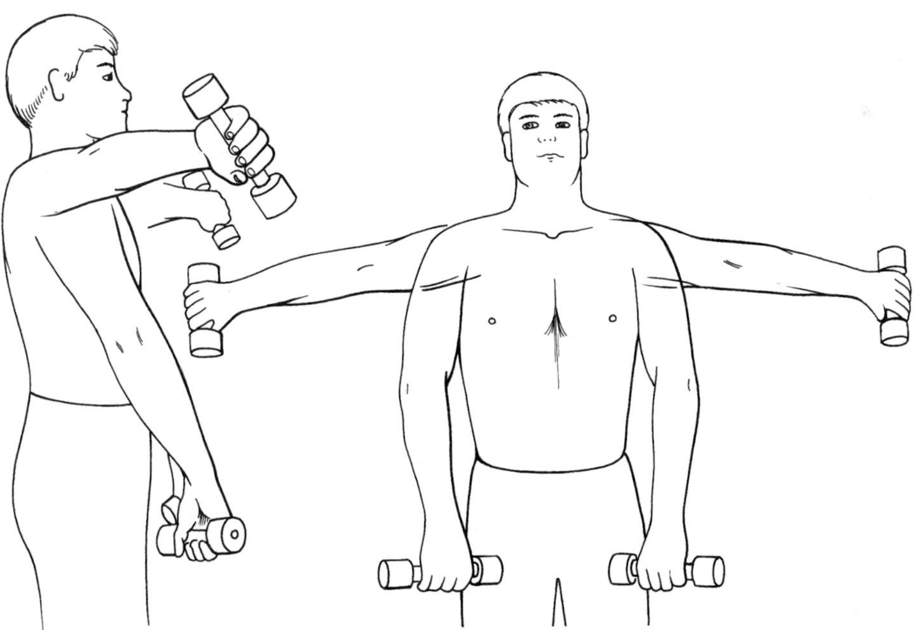

Fig. 9-5 Selective strengthening of the supraspinatus muscle. The patient should stand with the arm at the side and internally rotate the shoulder so as to pronate the forearm. The patient then starts elevation by moving diagonally toward abduction and arrives at 90° of abduction at 30° to 45° in front of the coronal position.

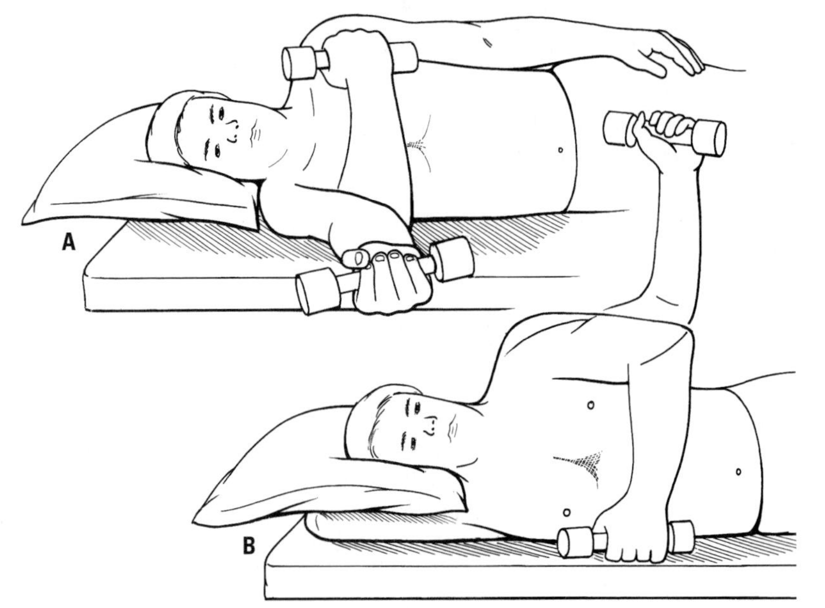

Fig. 9-6 Internal and external rotator-strengthening exercises using free weights. **A,** Internal rotator strengthening. **B,** External rotator strengthening.

Shoulder elevation above 90° should be initiated with a D1F (flexion–adduction–external rotation) proprioceptive neuromuscular (PNF) pattern before one advances to a D2F (flexion–abduction–external rotation) pattern.[29]

A light weight ought to be used (up to 5 lb), and the patient must remain in the pain-free range. Shoulder rotation exercises may initially be performed with the patient in side-lying position because the supraspinatus and subacromial bursae are unlikely to become irritated in this position. Also, this position is more likely to prevent reflex inhibition of muscles (Fig. 9-6).

The use of rubber tubing (Fig. 9-7) is especially helpful because the slow return of the limb to the rest position delivers an eccentric contraction to the muscles antagonistic to the desired direction of strengthening. Concentric and eccentric exercises may also be performed using wall weights (Fig. 9-8).

- *Selective strengthening* of the serratus anterior and other scapular rotators is essential. The scapula functions as a floating origin for the rotator cuff muscles, and its movement must be in synchrony with the demands of glenohumeral joint motion. By ensuring that the scapular muscles work in time with the demands of shoulder elevation, one can also ensure that the muscles and tendons of the rotator cuff will operate close to an ideal length and tension and are less likely to suffer fatigue and undergo attrition. Furthermore, kinesiologically sound scapular protraction permits timely elevation of the coracoid process allowing it to rotate clear of the abducting humerus.[17] Two exercises that help strengthen the upper trapezius and the serratus anterior are shoulder shrugs and push-ups with the arm abducted to 90°.[3]
- *Selective flexibility* of tightened shoulder girdle muscles. The affected muscles are slowly stretched while antagonistic isometric contraction is performed. After isometric contraction, the muscles relax, and further stretching may be applied (contract-relax technique). Contraction of the antagonist produces reciprocal relaxation of the agonist, permitting more effective stretching.[34] Stretching activities are recommended after a hot bath, as well as before and after aerobic exercise.[36]

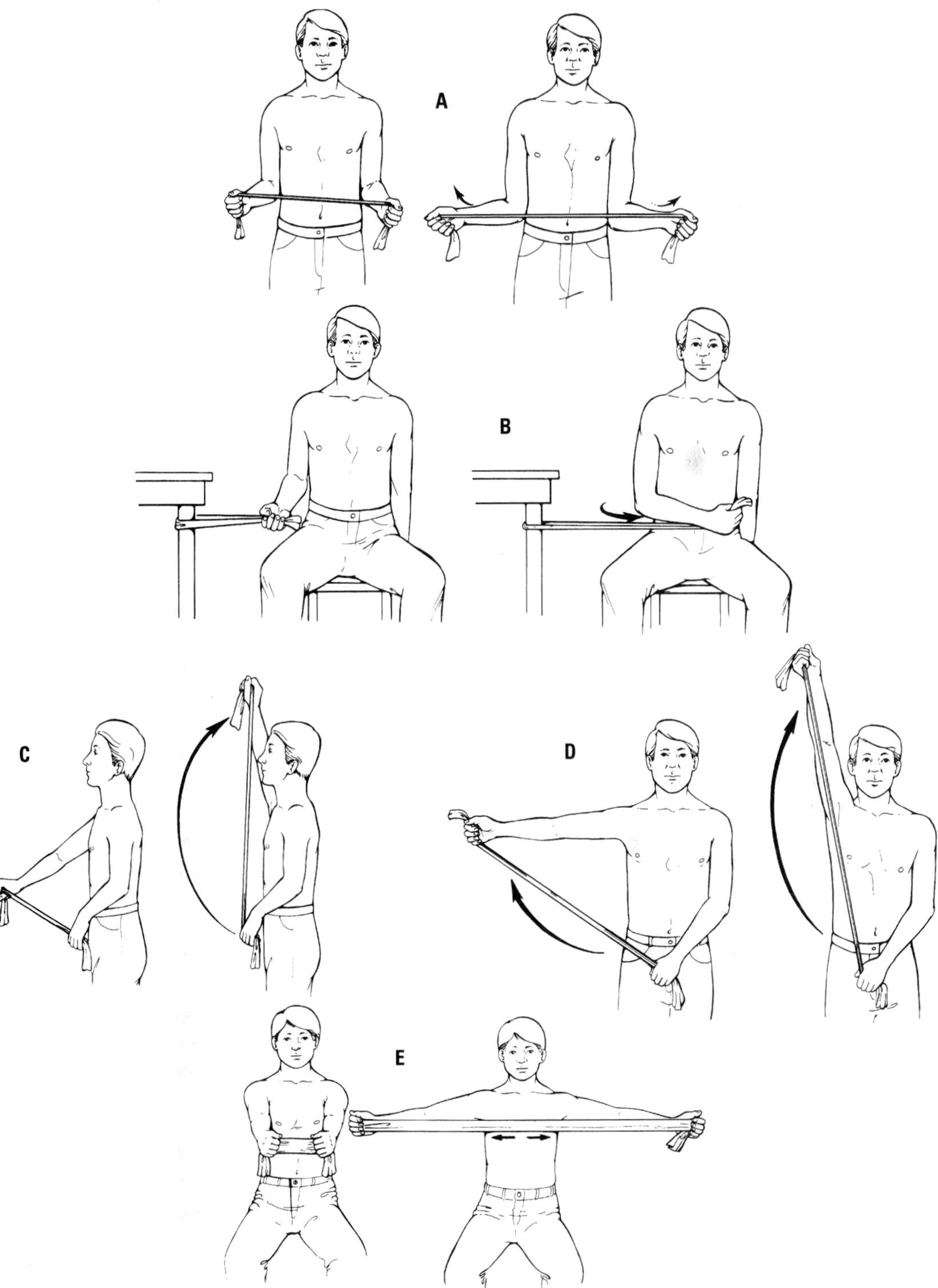

Fig. 9-7 Exercises to strengthen the shoulder muscles. **A,** External rotation. **B,** Internal rotation. **C,** Flexion. **D,** Abduction. **E,** Horizontal abduction. (From Saunders HD: *Evaluation, treatment and prevention of musculoskeletal disorders*, Bloomington, Minn., 1985, Educational Opportunities.)

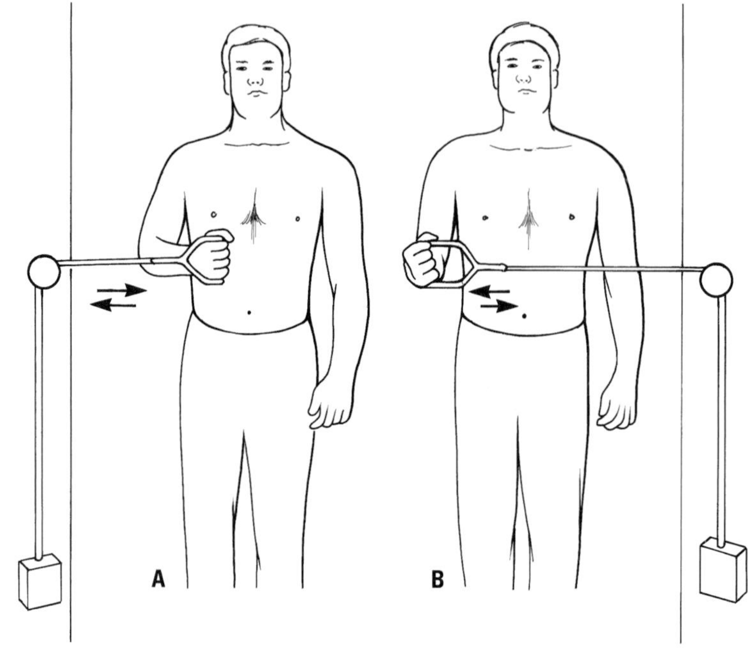

Fig. 9-8 External and internal rotator concentric and eccentric strengthening using wall weights.

Stretching activities may be performed in supine with a two to five pound cuff weight wrapped around the waist. Three important stretches are: (1) 90° of shoulder abduction and elbow flexion, with as much external rotation as possible will stretch the anterior shoulder capsule and soft tissues; (2) 135° of shoulder flexion with external rotation to stretch the anteroinferior capsule and soft tissues; and (3) reaching as far overhead as possible, with the palm toward the ceiling and the elbow extended will stretch the most inferior portion of the shoulder capsule[44] (Fig. 9-9).

- A valuable treatment in the management of a stage I lesion is the application of light to deep *transverse friction massage* to the supraspinatus tendon. Pressure is applied just proximal to the tendon insertion on the greater tubercle. Friction is applied in a direction perpendicular to the normal orientation of the tendon.[14]
- Selective total *rest.* Selective rest does not mean complete inactivity but rather an alternative motion that will permit the shoulder to achieve the movement objective. For example, a pitcher may resort to the use of a different pitching style while time is allowed for healing of the rotator cuff. However, some authorities maintain that pain sufficient to affect performance is an indication for total rest from the aggravating activity.

  Rest should extend beyond the activity, whether vocational or avocational, that precipitated impingement. It is important to emphasize to the patient the responsibility of elevating the arm in ways that avoid impingement in all his or her activities of daily living. This is very important during this potentially reversible stage.
- *Cryotherapy* for approximately 10 minutes after workouts[10] using an ice cup, slush bag, ice pack, or refreezable gel pack.
- *Therapeutic ultrasound* increases blood flow and increases permeability of cell membranes, resulting in improved exchange of metabolic products.[12] The ultrasound dosage to the treatment of the supraspinatus and bicep tendons vary according to the amount of interposing tissue. The more superficial biceps tendon requires between 0.8 and 1.2 watts/cm for 5 minutes daily for 10 days, whereas the supraspinatus

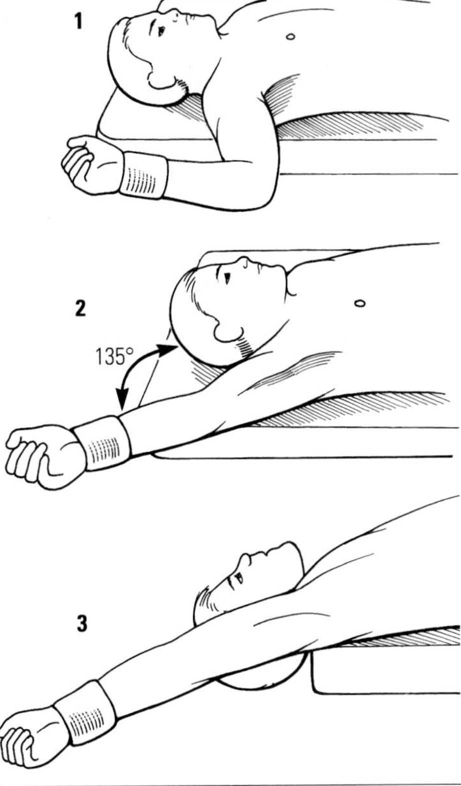

Fig. 9-9 Stretching of the rotator cuff muscles and glenohumeral shoulder capsule. Position 1 stretches the medial rotators and anterior shoulder capsule. Position 2 stretches the anterioinferior capsule. Position 3 stretches the inferior capsule.

tendon requires 1.2 watts/cm for 5 minutes daily for 10 days.[13] The use of ultrasound is controversial because being a deep-heat modality it may occasionally exacerbate symptoms.

- *Transcutaneous electrical nerve stimulation*[30] helps decrease pain. Electrotherapy may promote organization of collagen alignment because of a piezoelectric effect within the tendon during the healing phase.[6]
- An upper-arm *counterforce brace* may be placed high on the arm directly over the biceps tendon. It is theorized that the strap has a tenodesis effect on the biceps, making it a more effective humeral head depressor.[17]
- Emphasis on *prevention* cannot be stated enough at this still-reversible stage. Time therefore is an important ally in treatment. Warm-up routines should involve flexibility exercises and isometric contractions or light isotonic activities. The purpose of warm-up activities is to increase body temperature, particularly for muscles. As such, it is important to avoid fatiguing the shoulder with these preliminary exercises. Cooldowns after exercise are also important.
- *Massage* of shoulder muscles promotes increased circulation and relaxation and may be helpful before workouts.[13]
- Steroid injection into the adjacent subacromial bursa[11] is losing popularity because of catabolic effects to local metabolism. A less-invasive and more-benign form of relief provided by delivery corticosteroids is by *phonophoresis* or *iontophoresis*.[27]
- Pendulum exercises with[5] or without[9] weights may be performed during the acute phase.
- Orally administered *nonsteroidal anti-inflammatory medications*.

The advanced phase of rehabilitation concentrates on the progressive return to normal function. The patient may progress from the use of free weights to resistive activities performed on an exercise machine.

15. What rehabilitative therapy is appropriate for the stage II and chronic stage III shoulders?

A nonoperative trial of conservative therapy is attempted. The patient is forewarned that it may take up to 6 weeks to yield improvement and is admonished not to abandon therapy just because the shoulder is not better in a few days! Treatment includes all exercises of the previous stage except for the use of surgical tubing, which is contraindicated because it tends to overload the rotator cuff.[31]

- Rest.
- Nonsteroidal anti-inflammatory medication.
- Avoidance of precipitating activities.
- Steroid injections.[24]
- Gentle stretching activities to the rotator cuff muscles in all areas of tightness.
- Gentle internal and external rotation-strengthening exercises beginning with isometrics and progressing to rotation against resistance using rubber bands or light weights with instruction to the patient not to overdo exercise lest the cuff becomes further aggravated. A useful guide to the patient is that any soreness from exercises must subside within a few minutes after finishing the workout. Strengthening with the shoulder above 60° of elevation is avoided so as to prevent excessive tendon loading as well as tendon wear under the coracoacromial arch.
- Greater emphasis should be placed on range-of-motion activities to prevent adhesive capsulitis.

16. When is surgery appropriate?

If at the end of a 6-week conservative treatment regimen cuff imaging indicates an intact rotator cuff, patients are advised to continue working on their program for an additional 6 weeks. Patients with persistent symptoms are examined frequently and should not be lost to follow-up study; otherwise they may come back a year or so later with an irreparable cuff tear.[19] Criteria for operative treatment includes (1) a patient is younger than 60 years of age, (2) failure to improve after a nonoperative treatment regimen of not less than 6 weeks, (3) presence of a full-thickness tear, either clinically or by imaging techniques, (4) the patient's need to use the involved shoulder in a vocation or an avocation, (5) full passive range of motion that must be present to warrant operative treatment, (6) the patient's own willingness to forego loss of some active abduction in exchange for decreased pain and increased strength of external rotation, and (7) the ability and willingness of the patient to cooperate.[19] In addition, acute tears are best repaired within 3 weeks of initial injury before retraction, scarring, tendon-edge degeneration, and muscle atrophy occur to a substantial degree.

17. What is the most commonly used surgical technique?

Open acromioplasty (partial acromionectomy) accompanied by connective tissue reconstruction and surgical reattachment of the torn tendon complex into a bony trough created on the greater tuberosity.[11] However, when major amounts of cuff tissue have been lost, repair is not possible.[13]

18. What factors account for decreased likelihood of success after surgical attempt at cuff repair?

- An insidious, atraumatic onset of rotator cuff disorder
- Grade 3 or less of external shoulder rotation strength
- Age greater than 60 years
- Upward humeral head displacement relative to the glenoid and acromion
- History of multiple steroid injections

The surgeon may, in fact, find that the cuff tendons have all the strength of wet Kleenex.[19] This is the situation in which a neglected rotator cuff tear remains untreated and the lesion progresses to what is known as *rotator cuff arthropathy,* a term that denotes destruction of the humeral articulating surface occurring after a neglected massive cuff tear that is distinctly different from changes such as osteoarthritis, rheumatoid arthritis, and avascular necrosis of the humeral head. Whatever remains of these severely weakened cuff tendons are prone to failure after any attempted cuff repairs.

19. What rehabilitation is appropriate after surgery?

Postoperatively the patient's shoulder is immobilized in a position of abduction for 3 weeks[28] by an abduction bolster to protect against early tension on the repaired tendon from the adducted position. Horizontal adduction and internal rotation are also to be avoided. As early as the second postoperative day passive range of motion exercises with the splint in place are performed within the limits of comfort in the direction of forward flexion and external rotation so as to avoid adhesions and disuse atrophy.[13] Abduction with the shoulder in external rotation is also permitted this early but only if the patient is relaxed in a supine position because the sitting position increases the risk that the patient will assist in an antigravity movement,[11] which is not yet permitted.

The repair is likely to be weakest at 3 weeks when the healing process is underway but no enhancement of tensile strength has yet occurred.[19] During the first 3 postoperative months the cuff repair will not be stronger than it was immediately after surgery.[13]

Active range of motion, including active abduction, may begin at 6 weeks after operation, progressing from gravity-eliminated to gravity-resisted positions. Resistance training is begun at 7 to 8 weeks after operation beginning with 1 lb and focusing on isolated strengthening to each of the cuff muscles.[11] Challenging the repair with large loads should be avoided 6 months to a year.[19]

20. How are partial- and full-thickness cuff tears managed in the elderly?

In the elderly, the best treatment after injury is with simple active exercises as soon as possible with the strategy of preventing shoulder stiffness and palliative measures as well to reduce pain. Once the possibility of adhesive capsulitis is reduced, rest may eventually permit regain of some active range of motion as the small tear scars over.

Another school of thought advocates placement of the shoulder in a position that most closely approximates the ends of torn fibers while eliminating any movement that may elongate the cuff. This immobilization strategy continues for anywhere between 3 to 8 weeks and promotes the smallest span of scar tissue between the frayed tendon ends while avoiding abduction, forward flexion, and external rotation. Joint mobilization of those shoulder girdle joints not immobilized is imperative to minimize onset of adhesive capsulitis.[21]

References

1. Anderson TE: Rehabilitation of common shoulder injuries in athletes, *J Musculoskeletal Med,* p 17, Dec 1988.
2. Brewer BJ: Aging of the rotator cuff, *Am J Sports Med* 7(2):102-110, 1979.
3. Brewster CE, Shields CL, Seto JL, Morrissey MC: Rehabilitation of the upper extremity. In Shields CL, editor: *Manual of sports surgery,* New York, 1987, Springer-Verlag.
4. Codman EA: Complete rupture of the supraspinatus tendon: operative treatment with report of two successful cases, *Boston Med Surg J* 164:708-710, 1911.
5. Cuillo J: Swimmer's shoulder, *Clin Sports Med* 5: 115-136, 1984.
6. Curwin S, Stanish W: *Tendinitis: its etiology and treatment,* Lexington, Mass., 1984, Collamore Press.

7. Cyriax J: *Textbook of orthopaedic medicine*, vol 1: Diagnosis of soft tissue lesions, ed 8, London, 1982, Bailliere-Tindall.
8. DePalma AF, Gallery G, Bennet CA: Variational anatomy and degenerative lesions of the shoulder joint, *Instr Course Lect* 6:255-281, 1949.
8a. From Dieppe PA, Banjami AN, Watt I: *Atlas of clinical rheumatology,* Baltimore, 1980, Lea & Febiger.
9. Flicker P: The painful shoulder, *Prim Care* 7:271-285, 1990.
10. Gordon EJ: Diagnosis and treatment of common shoulder disorders, *Med Trial Tech Q* 28:25-73, 1981.
11. Gould JA III: *Orthopaedic and sports physical therapy*, ed 2, St. Louis, 1990, Mosby.
12. Hawkins RJ, Kennedy JC: Impingement syndrome in athletes, *Am J Sports Med* 8:57, 1980.
13. Hawkins RJ, Hobeika PE: Impingement syndrome in the athletic shoulder, *Clin Sports Med* 2(2):390, July 1983.
14. Hertling D, Kessler RM: *Management of common musculoskeletal disorders,* ed 2, Philadelphia, 1990, Lippincott.
15. Holt LE: *Scientific stretching for sports*, Halifax, Nova Scotia, 1973, Dalhousie University.
16. Jobe F, Moynes D: Delineation of diagnostic criteria and rehabilitation program for rotator cuff injuries, *Am J Sport Med* 10:336-339, 1982.
17. Johnson J, Sim F, Scott S: Musculoskeletal injuries in competitive swimmers, *Mayo Clin Proc* 62:289-304, 1987.
18. Lindblom K: Arthrography and roentgenography in ruptures of the tendon of the shoulder joint, *Acta Radiol* 20: 548, 1939.
19. Matsen FA, Arntz CT: Rotator cuff failure. In Rockwood CA, Matsen FA, editors: *The shoulder*, vol 1, Philadelphia, 1990, Saunders.
20. Meals RA: *One hundred orthopaedic conditions every doctor should understand*, St. Louis, 1992, Quality Medical Publishing.
21. Moffat M: *Musculoskeletal therapeutic exercise*, New York University Department of Physical Therapy Lecture, Nov. 1990.
22. Moore KL: *Clinically oriented anatomy*, ed 2, Baltimore, 1985, Williams & Wilkins.
23. Neer CS II: Anterior acromioplasty for the chronic impingement syndrome in the shoulder: a preliminary report, *J Bone Joint Surg* 54A:41-50, 1972.
24. Neer CS II: Impingement lesions, *Clin Orthop* 173:70-77, 1983.
25. Neer CS II, Flatow EL, Lech O: Tears of the rotator cuff: long term results of anterior acromioplasty and repair. Paper presented at the American Shoulder and Elbow Surgeons, fourth meeting, Atlanta, Ga., Feb 1988.
26. Nirsche RP, Pettrone F: Tennis elbow: the surgical treatment of lateral epicondylitis, *J Bone Joint Surg* 61A:8332, 1979.
27. Richardson A: Overuse syndromes in baseball, tennis, gymnastics and swimming, *Clin Sports Med* 2:379-389, 1983.
28. Salter RB: *Textbook of disorders and injuries of the musculoskeletal system*, ed 2, Baltimore, 1983, Williams & Wilkins.
29. Sullivan PE, Markos PD, Minor MA: *An integrated approach to therapeutic exercise: theory and clinical application*, Reston, Va., 1982, Reston Publication.
30. Sunderstrom WR: Painful shoulders: diagnosis and management, *Geriatrics* 38:77-92, 1983.
31. Thein LA: Impingement syndrome and its conservative management, *J Orthop Sports Phys Ther* 11:189, 1989.
32. Weaver HL: Isolated suprascapular nerve lesions, *Br J Accident Surg* 15:117-126, 1983.

Recommended reading

Blackburn TA: The off-season program for the throwing arm. In Zarins B, Andrews JR, Carson WG, editors: *Injuries to the throwing arm*, Philadelphia, 1985, Saunders.

Cofield RH: Current concepts review: rotator cuff disease of the shoulder, *J Bone Joint Surg* 67A:974-979, 1985.

Hawkins RJ, Hobeika PE: Impingement syndrome in the athletic shoulder, *Clin Sports Med* 2:394, 1983.

Moynes DR: Prevention of injury to the shoulder through exercises and therapy, *Clin Sports Med* 2(2):413-422, 1983.

Chronic Right Shoulder Pain and Crepitus during Elevation, Swimming, or Carrying a Briefcase

10

A 23-year-old female complains of pain when elevating her right shoulder and when carrying her briefcase in either hand to and from work. She has worked as a lifeguard specializing in swim instruction of the crawl and butterfly strokes for the past four summers at an all-girls summer camp. She appears to be in excellent physical condition and, when questioned, admits to swimming 200 laps a day during the three summer months for several years. She also complains of a slight "grinding" or "crunching" sensation when actively elevating her right shoulder. She admits that her left shoulder bothers her as well, though not as much as her right shoulder. There is no history of injury.

OBSERVATION There is no apparent muscle wasting of the suprascapular or infrascapular fossae. She has prominent pectoralis and anterior deltoid muscles because of hypertrophy.

PALPATION There is mild pinpoint tenderness slightly inferior to the anterior border of the acromion while the shoulder is passively extended. In addition, there is a slight sensation of crepitus felt upon active elevation.

RANGE OF MOTION Within functional limits but with a positive upward painful arc at 80° to 120°.

STRENGTH Normal.

FLEXIBILITY Normal.

JOINT PLAY There is mild posterior capsular tightness of the right glenohumeral joint.

SELECTIVE TENSION Presence of painful resisted external rotation and abduction as well as during passive internal rotation while the shoulder is elevated to 80°.

SPECIAL TESTS Negative drop-arm test, positive impingement sign, negative Speed's test, negative Adson maneuver.

1. **What is the most likely cause of this woman's pain?**

2. **What is "impingement syndrome"?**
3. **What is the subacromial arch and its components?**
4. **What osseous variations in acromial architecture predispose to a rotator cuff disorder?**
5. **What synergic relationship exists between deltoid and supraspinatus that is imperative to successful shoulder elevation?**
6. **Can elevation occur if either supraspinatus or deltoid is weak or paralyzed?**
7. **What is the pathokinesiology accounting for painful arc symptoms?**
8. **What accounts for the painful arc experienced at elevation end range in patients whose impingement has progressed to tendinitis?**
9. **What is the clinical presentation?**
10. **What provocative tests serve as important clinical confirmation?**
11. **Which pattern of capsular tightness of the glenohumeral joint is commonly found with the impingement syndrome?**
12. **What effect does an immobilized scapula have on the impingement syndrome?**
13. **What is the proposed mechanism of the pathologic condition in the young athletic population?**
14. **What accounts for the greater percentage of impingement syndrome in butterfly swimmers?**
15. **How do weight lifters become prone to supraspinatus tendinitis?**
16. **How do tennis players become vulnerable to supraspinatus tendinitis?**
17. **What is the proposed degenerative mechanism of the pathologic condition in the older population?**
18. **Are the subacromial arch disorders clinically differentiable?**
19. **Is there any single model that explains the mechanism of impingement?**
20. **Which occupations are particularly prone to development of impingement syndrome?**
21. **What cuff-imaging techniques are available to help diagnose this condition?**
22. **What therapeutic management is most appropriate to patients suffering from impingement syndrome?**
23. **Describe a hypothetical treatment sequence for this patient.**
24. **When is surgery appropriate?**
25. **What are the three surgical options?**
26. **What is the postoperative surgical program?**
27. **What is the success rate for returning athletes to competition after surgery?**

---

1. What is the most likely cause of this woman's pain?

Impingement of the right supraspinatus tendon (Fig. 10-1).

2. What is "impingement syndrome"?

The term "impingement syndrome" was popularized by Charles Neer in 1972.[18,20] Neer ascribed a unity to the range of pathologic conditions plaguing the shoulder by introducing the concept of a continuum of shoulder disorders that may begin with supraspinatus impingement and may eventually progress to partial or even complete tears of the rotator cuff. He also pointed out that physical as well as plain radiographic findings are often inadequate and unreliable in differentiating between chronic bursitis and partial-thickness tears versus full-thickness cuff tears.[19] Presumably the structures involved are quite small (as when compared to the larger soft-tissue structures of the lower extremity) and are packaged together so tightly that provocative movement of one structure, whether by active, passive, or resistive movement, may elicit pain in an adjacent structure by virtue of being in tight proximity.

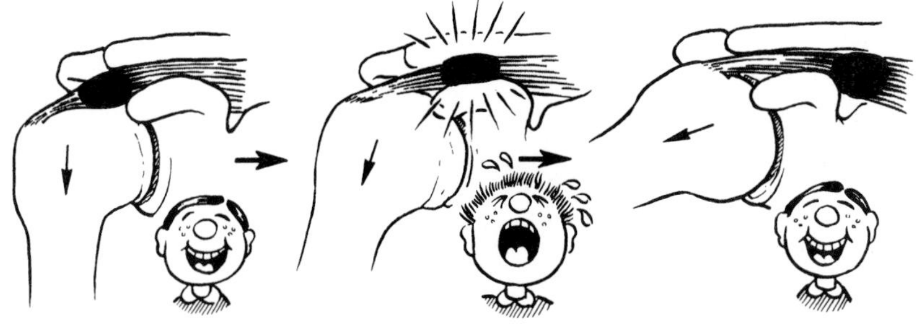

Fig. 10-1 Painful impingement of the right supraspinatus tendon. (From Dandy DJ: *Essential orthopaedics and trauma*, New York, 1989, Churchill Livingstone.)

"Impingement" of the supraspinatus or other cuff tendons within the narrow confines of the subacromial arch is not simply another way of saying rotator cuff tendinitis. Rather, impingement may be thought of as the predecessor of that next and worsened level of injury along the continuum of rotator cuff disorders known as *supraspinatus tendinitis* (see pp. 107-108).

3. What is the subacromial arch and its components?

The coracoacromial (synonym: subacromial) arch is a tunnel whose walls are formed by two scapular processes—the acromion located posteriorly and laterally and the coracoid processes located anteriorly and medially. The coracoacromial ligament connects these two processes and does so perforce by means of an oblique orientation of span. Finally the superior rim of the glenoid fossa (scapula) serves as the floor of the arch (Fig. 10-2).

The arch transmits the supraspinatus tendon, the tendon of the long head of the biceps, the subacromial (subdeltoid) bursa, and the coracohumeral ligament. These encased structures are subject to a potential lesion as a function of the arch's fixed volume because of increased pressure secondary to overactivity of the tendons, inflammation, bleeding, or edema.

4. What osseous variations in acromial architecture predispose to a rotator cuff disorder?

Variations in acromial shape are commonly observed in patients with impingement and rotator cuff tears[2] (Fig. 10-3). Three types of acromion are identified: type I (flat), type II (curved), and type III (hooked). The acromion, defining the posterolateral aspect of the subacromial arch, projects anteriorly from the lateral scapular spine. With type III acromia the anteriormost acromial projection is angled inferiorly. There appears to be a strong association between cuff tears and type III acromia.[17] Additionally, degenerative spurs on the anterior surface of the anterior acromial process[18] may further decrease the volume of the subacromial arch and predispose impingement.

5. What synergic relationship exists between deltoid and supraspinatus that is imperative to successful shoulder elevation?

The kinesiology of shoulder elevation with respect to the subacromial arch is characterized by precise concerted action of the deltoid and supraspinatus muscles. These muscles respectively yield compressive and rotational force components to synergistically facilitate successful shoulder elevation. While the deltoid muscle exerts a compressive force that lifts the shaft of the humerus into the subacromial space, the supraspinatus, accompanied by the other cuff muscles, pulls the humeral head inferiorly on the glenoid fossa.[23] Without this coupled action, lack of clearance of the greater tuberosity beneath the acromion

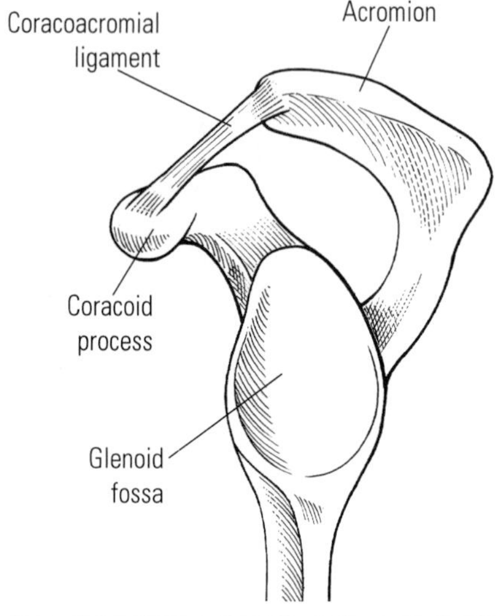

Fig. 10-2 Components of the subacromial arch.

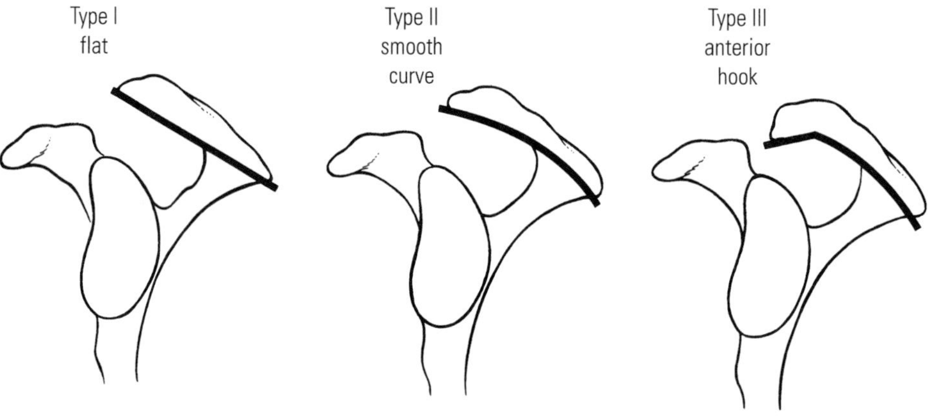

Fig. 10-3 Variations in human acromial posture. (From Rockwood CA, Matsen FA, editors: *The shoulder,* Philadelphia, 1990, Saunders.)

results in upward ramming of the greater tuberosity against the arch and impingement of the interposing cuff tendon or tendons.

6. Can elevation occur if either supraspinatus or deltoid is weak or paralyzed?

Substitution of adjacent muscles compensate for lack of function of either supraspinatus or deltoid muscles so as to facilitate elevation.

- In the absence of strength or as a result of deltoid weakness, the long head of the biceps brachii may partially assume the deltoid's role when the humerus is externally rotated 90° permitting partial abduction; this may occur though the elevation strength is greatly decreased to some 50% of normal power.[24]

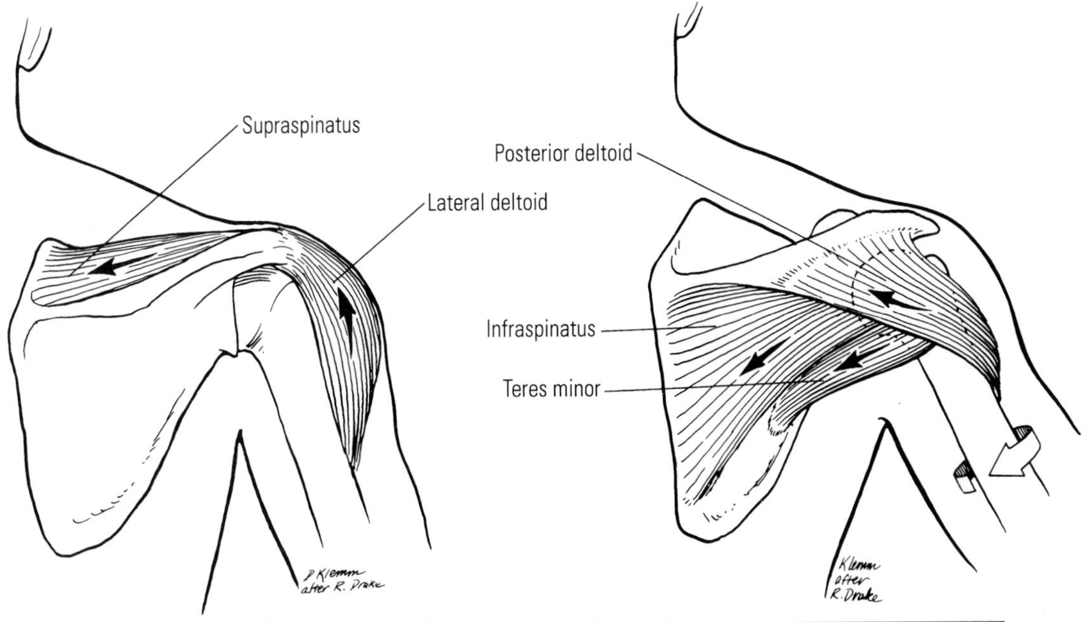

Fig. 10-4 The rotator cuff and deltoid muscle forces at the onset of abduction (0°) and with the arm elevated 90°. The deltoid force changed from a shear to a compressive force. Thus a damaged or weakened supraspinatus muscle causes loss of counterbalance and allows the vertical force of the deltoid muscle to compress the tissue more. (From Bogumill GP: Functional anatomy of the shoulder and elbow. In GIN: Pettrone FA, editor: In *AAOS Symposium on upper extremity injuries in athletes,* St. Louis, 1986, Mosby.)

- In the case of a paralyzed supraspinatus, partial active abduction may be achieved by the three remaining and functioning rotator cuff muscles. Initiation of abduction occurs at about 80% of normal power but is rapidly lost as the 90° mark is approached, and so the arm barely resists the pull of gravity.[7] This rationale serves as the basis of the *positive drop-arm test* (see Fig. 9-3) for detection of tears in the rotator cuff, principally of the supraspinatus tendon.[10] Here the substituting musculature lacks sufficient torque to maintain resistance against gravity or the downward push of the examiner's hand.

7. What is the pathokinesiology accounting for painful arc symptoms?

The deltoid muscle is hinged at its origin and therefore exerts a shear force that forces the humerus upward on the glenoid labrum at 0° abduction.[1] As elevation commences and proceeds to 90°, the deltoid's shear forces are converted to a compressive force that vertically forces the humerus more directly into the glenoid cavity[7] (Fig. 10-4). In the event of a weak or damaged supraspinatus tendon, the loss of the rotational force component results in painful impingement attributable to the imbalance of forces (Fig. 10-5).[7] Toward the end of the range of motion, the deltoid's shear forces translate the humeral head on the glenoid labrum,[7] albeit in a downward direction and corresponding to cessation of pain.

8. What accounts for the painful arc experienced at elevation end range in patients whose impingement has progressed to tendinitis?

The 50° to 130° of shoulder range associated with painful arc may be associated with an ischemic wringing out of the less vascular portion of the supraspinatus tendon.[14] Cyriax[6] hypothesized a rationale to

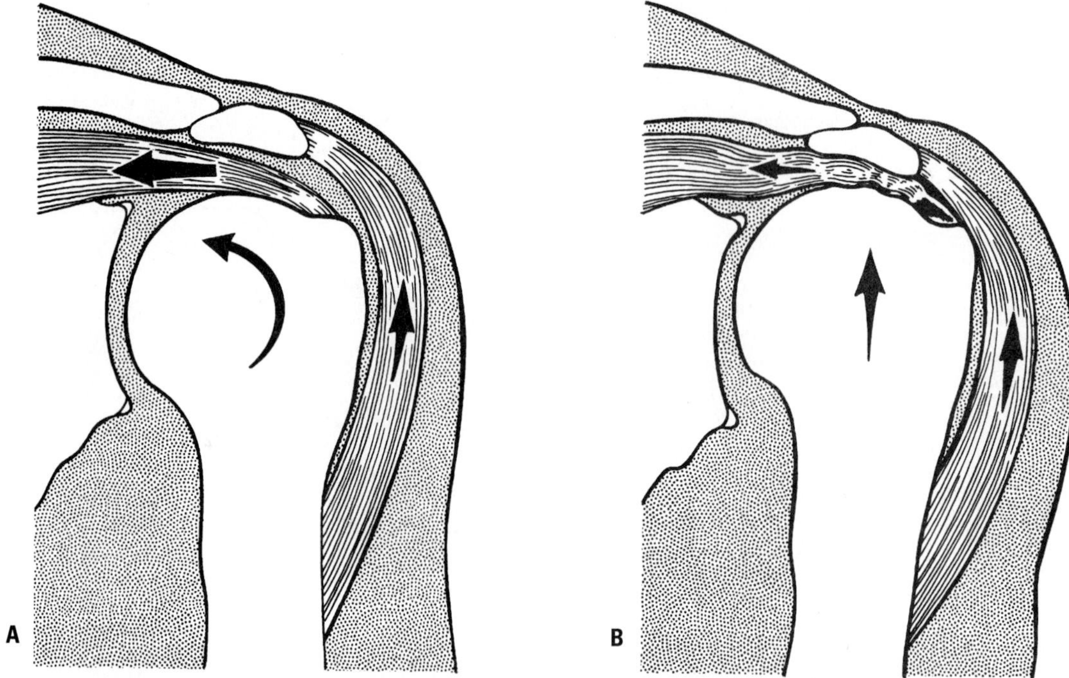

Fig. 10-5 Supraspinatus, exerting a rotational force component, works in synergy with deltoid, which yields a compressive force. Working together, **A,** both muscles facilitate shoulder elevation. **B,** Deep surface tearing of the supraspinatus weakens the cuff's ability to hold the humeral head down and away from the underside of the acromion, resulting in impingement. (From Rockwood CA, Matsen FA, editors: *The shoulder,* Philadelphia, 1990, Saunders.)

explain away *both* the painful arc phenomenon that often occurs as the elevation commences between the 50° to 130° of range and the pain elicited at the very end range of abduction or flexion. Whereas active or passive painful arc is caused by rubbing of the underside of the acromion against a lesion or scar located superficially in the tendon, pain elicited at the end of the range of elevation is caused by passive stretching of a deep distal scar (Fig. 10-6).

- Fig. 10-6, *A,* shows a superficially located lesion at the tenoperiosteal junction; this will elicit a painful arc during active shoulder elevation due to tensile distraction of the superficial tendon lesion.
- Fig. 10-6, *B,* shows a deeply located lesion at the tenoperiosteal junction; this will elicit pain on full passive elevation since the lesion will be pinched between the greater tuberosity and glenoid rim.
- Fig. 10-6, *C,* shows a lesion that has eroded the entire substance of the distal tendon, that is, at the tenoperiosteal junction as well as proximally throughout the entire tendon; this elicits both passive and active painful arc as well as pain from stretching during full passive elevation.
- Fig. 10-6, *D,* shows a lesion located more proximally at the musculotendinous junction, yielding neither a painful arc nor pain on passive elevation.

9. What is the clinical presentation?

Patients with impingement syndrome usually do not present themselves to the therapist or physician acutely but only after their shoulder symptoms have failed to resolve with time, rest, and trying to "work it out." Patients usually complain of functional losses attributable to pain, stiffness, weakness, and

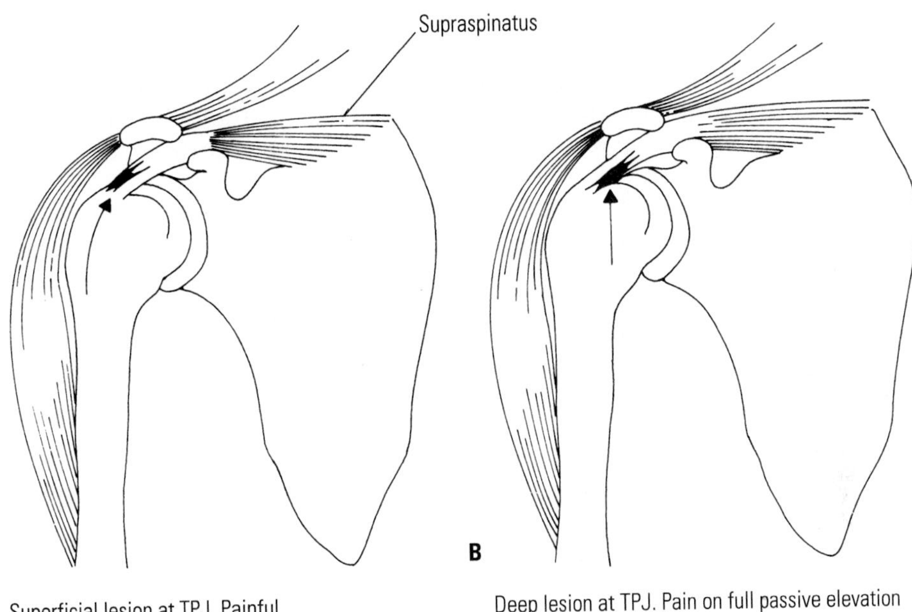

Superficial lesion at TPJ. Painful arc during active elevation

Deep lesion at TPJ. Pain on full passive elevation

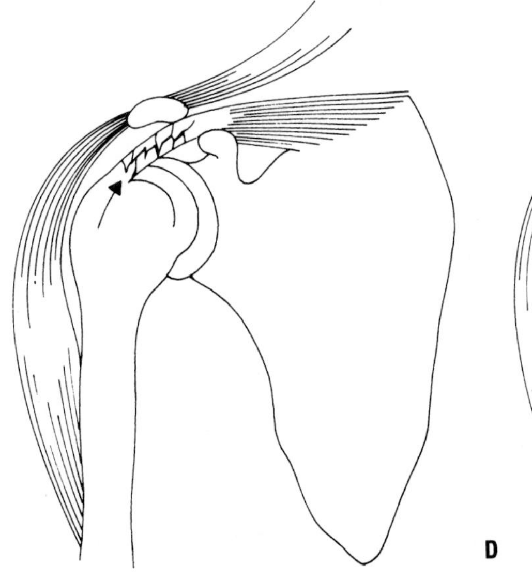

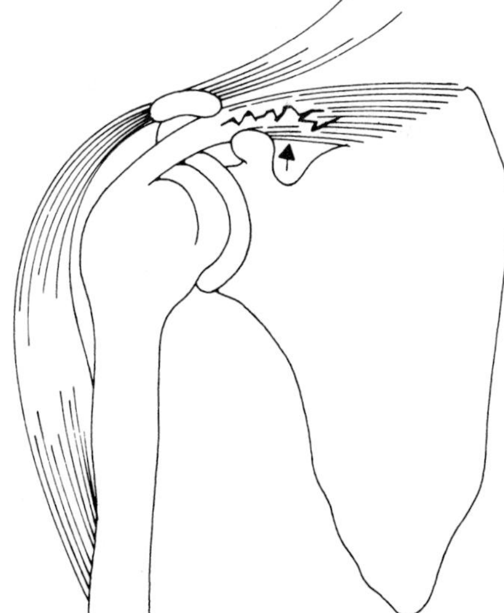

Lesion has eroded entire substance of distal tendon, yielding pain both during passive and active shoulder elevation

Lesion lies at musculotendinous junction—neither a painful passive or active arc of movement

Fig. 10-6 The relationship between the site of lesion, range during which pain is perceived, and whether symptoms occur during passive or active provocation. (From Scully RM, Barnes MR, editors: *Physical therapy,* Philadelphia, 1989, Lippincott.)

"catching" when the arm is used in the flexed and internally rotated position. Symptoms may also include difficulties in sleeping on the affected side and while carrying out routine activities, such as taking a container of milk from the refrigerator. Pain is often felt down the lateral aspect of the upper arm near the deltoid insertion, over the anterior proximal humerus, or in the periacromial area.[16]

Inspection of the shoulder may reveal deltoid or cuff atrophy, particularly if the condition has been chronic. Palpation usually reveals little if any tenderness, which is in considerable contrast to the sharply localized tenderness characteristic of acute calcific tendinitis. The range of motion is often limited, particularly internal rotation and horizontal adduction, affirming some degree of posterior capsule tightness. Passive motion through the 60° to 90° arc of flexion may be accompanied by pain and crepitus, accentuated as the shoulder is moved in and out of internal rotation. Active elevation of the shoulder is usually more uncomfortable than passive elevation. Strength testing of the shoulder may reveal weakness of flexion and external rotation, which may be either the result of disuse or tendon damage. Pain on resisted abduction or external rotation may also indicate that the integrity of the cuff tendons has been compromised.[16]

10. What provocative tests serve as important clinical confirmation?

1. *Neer test,* or *positive impingement sign,* is a sign popularized by Neer and Walsh and reproduces pain and concomitant facial grimace when the arm is forcibly flexed forward by the examiner, jamming the greater tuberosity against the anteroinferior acromial surface (Fig. 10-7).

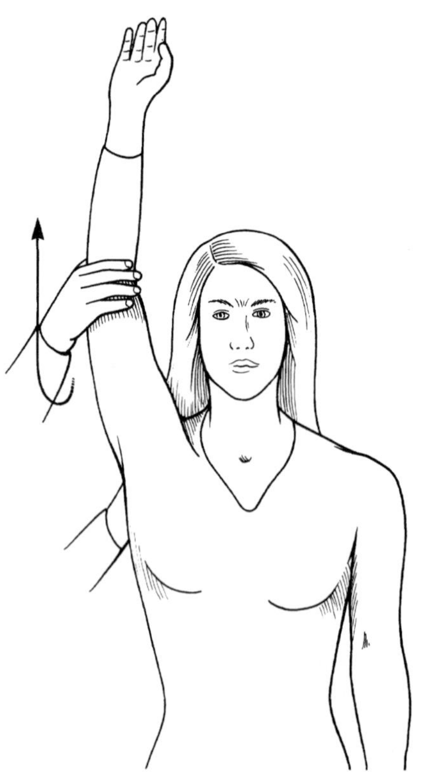

Fig. 10-7 Neer test or positive impingement sign.

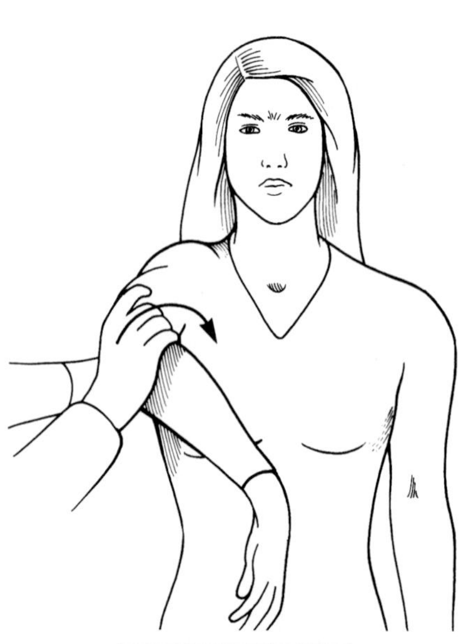

Fig. 10-8 Hawkins test.

2. The *Hawkins test* consists of flexing the humerus to 90° and forcefully internally rotating the shoulder driving the greater tuberosity farther under the coracoacromial ligament. This test is less reliable than Neer's test[8] (Fig. 10-8).

In both maneuvers injection of 10 ml of lidocaine into the subacromial space followed by pain relief helps confirm the diagnosis and rules out other causes of shoulder pain such as acromioclavicular joint sprain and adhesive capsulitis, which are not relieved by injection.[14]

11. Which pattern of capsular tightness of the glenohumeral joint is commonly found with the impingement syndrome?

Commonly associated with the other signs of impingement is stiffness of the posterior glenohumeral joint capsule[16] resulting in limited forward flexion, internal rotation, and horizontal shoulder adduction.[16] With normal shoulder motion, the humeral head remains centered on the glenoid, whereas with a tightened posterior capsule the humeral head is forced upward against the anteroinferior acromion during forward flexion[16] (Fig. 10-9). Thus the impingement process is a self-perpetuating[16] one that is viciously fed by an increasingly failing humeral head depressor mechanism, a tightened posterior capsule that facilitates encroachment, as well as a limited subacromial volume that is decreased by edematous inflammation.

12. What effect does an immobilized scapula have on the impingement syndrome?

The scapula serves as a floating origin for the cuff muscles, maintaining optimum length-tension ratio of those muscles spanning from scapula to humerus throughout the wide range of shoulder movement. A scapula that does not glide freely over the thoracic wall will adversely affect the length-tension ratios,

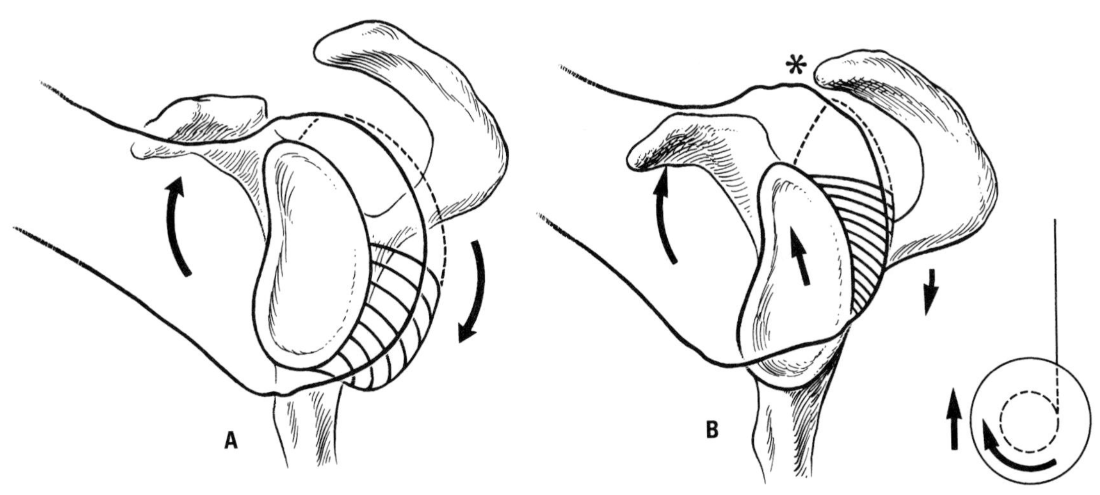

Fig. 10-9 Stiffness of the posterior glenohumeral capsule is commonly associated with signs of impingement. **A,** Normally lax posterior capsule allows the humeral head to remain contered in the glenoid with shoulder flexion. **B,** Stiffness of the posterior joint capsule will aggravate the impingement process by forcing the humeral head upward against the anteroinferior acromion as the shoulder is flexed. This upward transition in association with rotation is analogous to the action of a spinning Yo-Yo climbing a string. (From Rockwood CA, Matsen FA, editors: *The shoulder*, vol 1, Philadelphia, 1990, Saunders.)

resulting in impaired cuff function, hence impaired proximal humeral head depression function. Furthermore, the acromion being both the roof of the arch and a part of the scapula will not be able to elevate high enough to allow optimal clearance of the greater humeral tuberosity.

13. What is the proposed mechanism of the pathologic condition in the young athletic population?

Repetitive microtrauma to the soft tissues housed in the subacromial arch is often attributable to elevation of the glenohumeral joint performed above 80°[7] during sport activities. Classified as an *overuse syndrome,* impingement is most notable with internal humeral rotation[14] during an overhand tennis stroke, the butterfly or crawl swimming strokes, or throwing motion sports. The common traumatic denominator is the proximation of the greater tuberosity to the thick and sharp coracoclavicular ligament.[7]

14. What accounts for the greater percentage of impingement syndrome in butterfly swimmers?

The mechanics of the butterfly stroke, freestyle stroke (Fig. 10-10), and backstroke are similar because they share repeated abduction and internal rotation during the recovery phase. The average competitive swimmer subjects his or her shoulders to approximately 16,000 revolutions per week as compared to the 1000 rev/wk of the professional tennis or baseball player.[11] During the butterfly stroke the humerus is internally rotated during the critical 70° to 120° range of elevation. With pitching, however, the humerus is externally rotated during the windup. This relative external rotation helps clear the greater tuberosity by allowing space for clearance as the humeral head rides beneath the subacromial arch.[7] Additionally, repetitive flexion and internal rotation during swimming may strengthen the pectoralis and the anterior deltoid to

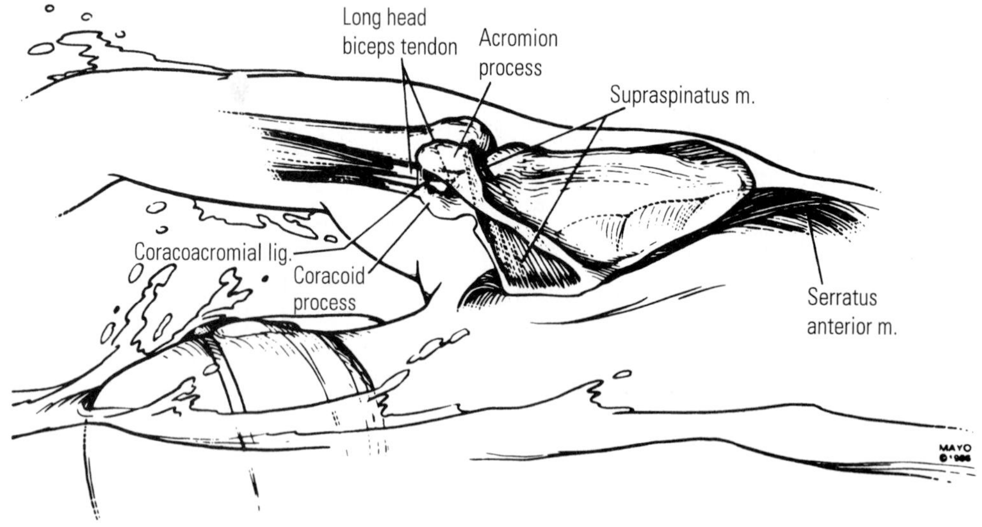

Fig. 10-10 Impingement of supraspinatus and biceps tendons between humeral head and coracoacromial arch can occur with abduction and internal rotation of humerus, as in recovery phase of freestyle stroke. Notice how serratus anterior muscle rotates scapula into abduction as humerus is abducted to allow a greater range of shoulder motion. Scapular rotation also delays impingement of greater tuberosity under coracoacromial arch until humerus is maximally abducted to near 180°. With fatigue or underdevelopment of serratus, humeral impingement may occur at an earlier point in recovery stroke at a lower angle of shoulder abduction. (From Johnson JE, Sim FH, Scott SG: *Mayo Clin Proc* 62:289-304, 1987.)

the point of hypertrophy. With the passage of time, this may pull the humeral head more anteriorly and only serves to further approximate the humerus to the acromion.

15. How do weight lifters become prone to supraspinatus tendinitis?

The disadvantage of overdevelopment of the deltoid and pectoralis muscles, though esthetically pleasing to some, is an altered biomechanics that contributes to pathologic states. Overdevelopment of the anterior chest causes as excessively protracted scapula, which alters normal biomechanics by requiring greater external humeral rotation when one is attempting to position the hand overhead. A tightened pectoralis may cause excessive bicipital tendon tracking against the medial border of the bicipital groove.[7] In addition, excessive deltoid hypertrophy may upset the force couple it shares with the cuff muscles and cause upward pulling of the humeral shaft, infringing on the suprahumeral space.[7] Weight lifters must be reminded not to forget strengthening the cuff musculature, coupled with stretching of tight internal rotators.

16. How do tennis players become vulnerable to supraspinatus tendinitis?

Tennis players (see Chapter 7) can irritate their rotator cuff during the followthrough of an overhead shot, allowing the racket to twist their shoulder into internal rotation and extension lateral to their hip. A more correct movement would be letting the racket finish the overhead stroke across the front of the body. Also, a proper toss during the serve may also greatly decrease the faulty mechanics associated with rotator cuff tendinitis.[7]

17. What is the proposed degenerative mechanism of the pathologic condition in the older population?

One of the many important functions of the rotator cuff is depression of the humeral head so as to prevent upward humeral migration. Depression is paramount to ensuring enough clearance during that all-important 70° to 120° elevation range.[14] It is in this range that the perhaps already avascular or swollen portion of cuff tendon barely clears the roof of the arch, if not actually colliding against it.

With the passage of time, age-related changes in the rotator cuff, whether attributable to ischemic or to other changes, result in eventual cuff failure. This process may be accelerated in athletes such as pitchers and swimmers, who place heavy demands upon their shoulders. With progressive loss of the depressor mechanism, the humeral head migrates ever higher because of the overpowering upward pull of the deltoid. The end stage of this process is one in which protrusion of the humeral head occurs through the cuff muscles as a shoulder equivalent of a *boutonniere lesion.* Here, the cuff tendons have slipped below the equator of the humeral head, resulting in an altered biomechanic pattern in which the action of the rotator cuff is redirected from that of humeral head depression to one of humeral head elevation. Just as in the boutonniere of the finger, the buttonholed cuff is victimized by the conversion of balancing forces into imbalancing forces[16] (see Fig. 9-4).

18. Are the subacromial arch disorders clinically differentiable?

If we understand that the emerging clinical picture is shared by many pathologic states along the continuum of rotator cuff disorders, it is easy to appreciate the great variability of signs and symptoms. However, these finding are not always distinguishable, since tears of the rotator cuff may produce signs and symptoms identical to those found with impingement without rotator cuff tear.[12] Additionally the structures involved are quite small (as compared to the larger soft-tissue structures of the lower extremity) and are packaged tightly together within the subacromial arch, such that provocative movement of one structure, whether active, passive, or resistive, may elicit pain in an adjacent structure by virtue of being in tight proximity.

19. Is there any single model that explains the mechanism of impingement?

Normal shoulder function is dependent on normal function of the humeral head depressors, normal capsular laxity, and adequate subacromial space. There are several models that attempt to explain the basis of impingement. Whatever the mechanism, whether it is Neer's mechanical model, the Pappas et al. theory of proximal humeral migration caused by cuff weakness, architectural variations of the acromion that predispose to susceptibility, or the microvascular model offered by Rathbun and MacNab, these theories may be complementary and interdependent in accounting for impingement in an anatomically confined area.[16]

20. Which occupations are particularly prone to development of impingement syndrome?

Painting, carpentry, warehousing, nursing, longshoring, grocery checking, fruit picking, and tree pruning.[15]

21. What cuff-imaging techniques are available to help diagnose this condition?

Many authorities believe that standard radiographs are of little value and even useless in the assessment of rotator cuff impingement.[27] Nevertheless, radiographs may reveal evidence of some of the conditions associated with impingement syndrome, such as acromioclavicular arthritis, chronic calcific tendinitis, and unfused acromial apophyses before age 21.[5] The last refers to the fact that the acromion arises from three separate centers of ossification—preacromion, mesoacromion, and metacromion[3]—that unite by 22 years of age.[22] When these centers fail to unite, impingement may arise from both downward hinging of the acromion as well as from soft spurs or soft-tissue proliferation at the nonunion site.[18]

Plain radiographs may also show subacromial sclerosis from chronic overloading of the acromial undersurface, known as the "*sourcil*," or "eyebrow," sign. Corresponding sclerosis or cystic changes involving the greater tuberosity may also occur.

Since partial-thickness tears of the rotator cuff may yield an identical clinical picture compared with impingement syndrome, arthrography is a valuable adjunct in the complete evaluation of patients with suspected impingement problems.[4]

Although both shoulder arthrography and arthroscopy may reveal rotator cuff defects involving the deep surface, there is not, as yet, a nonsurgical technique demonstrating midsurface tears of the cuff.[16]

22. What therapeutic management is most appropriate to patients suffering from impingement syndrome? (See pp. 113-118 for an in-depth treatment strategy of stage I rotator cuff lesions.)

The mainstay of *rehabilitative therapy* includes the following:

- Stretching of the posterior glenohumeral joint capsule by mobilization techniques[16]
- Strengthening of humeral depressors
- Maintenance of normal range of motion so as to avoid the onset of adhesive capsulitis[26]
- Strengthening external rotators, extensors, shoulder retractors, and horizontal abductors in swimmers
- Scapulothoracic mobilization
- Emphasizing to patient the importance of consciously externally rotating while elevating the upper extremity
- Resting from activity
- Modifying activities
- Nonsteroidal anti-inflammatory medication
- Modality use to relieve symptoms
- Functional electrical stimulation (FES) to suprascapular fossa to strengthen supraspinatus and other cuff muscle bellies

23. Describe a hypothetical treatment sequence for this patient.

- *Range of motion* activities beginning with passive range of motion and progressing to active range of motion were performed in supine position through the range that elicited pain in the erect posture. Thus abduction, flexion, horizontal adduction, and external rotation were performed above the 120° range.
- *Manual traction* to the glenohumeral joint was applied throughout the range of abduction and external rotation to help reduce any painful catching experienced by the patient. After several weeks, traction was required only in the 90° to 110° range. Upper extremity weight bearing on a Swiss ball also helped through the patient's painful range of motion.
- Grade I and Grade II *joint mobilization* were applied to the glenohumeral joint to stretch the tightened posterior capsule. Gains in the extensibility of this portion of the capsule manifested in improved range of motion and a decrease in the perceived painful arc.
- *Moist heat* was applied to the right shoulder and cervical regions for 10 to 15 minutes at the beginning of each treatment. This was performed to increase tissue extensibility of the region and to prime the glenohumeral joint capsule for mobilization.
- Soft-tissue *massage* to the right upper trapezius, levator scapulae, and deltoid regions are helpful before exercise to facilitate tissue extensibility and promote increased circulation and relaxation.
- *Strengthening* of the force couples of the shoulder and scapula was performed by proprioceptive neuromuscular facilitation principles. Diagonal patterns were initially performed isometrically. The patient then progressed to isotonic exercises using three-pound weights. D1F pattern preceded the D2F pattern particularly when the patient is elevating the shoulder above 90°.

  Selective strengthening of serratus anterior progressed from wall push-ups to counter push-ups, with the arm abducted to 90°. At the end range of elbow extension, an additional push was encouraged to stress the serratus anterior and thereby enhance protraction. Upper trapezius strengthening progressed from 5 to 8 pounds.

  Exercises for shoulder external and internal rotation, flexion, abduction, and extension progressed from isometrics to Thera-Band (see Fig. 9-7) and finally to weights (see Figs. 9-6 and 9-8). Selective strengthening of the rotator cuff was performed with progressively increasing weights (see Fig. 9-5). An Airdyne bicycle was used for shoulder endurance, and strength training progressed from moderate use of the right upper extremity to active propulsion from 5 to 15 minutes.
- *Stretching* of the rotator cuff musculature (see Fig. 9-9) was emphasized as well as the upper and lower fibers of the hypertrophied pectoralis major muscle (Fig. 10-11). Contract-relax techniques proved helpful. The posterior shoulder capsule was stretched by placing the arm in 90° elevation while using the opposite hand to pull the shoulder into horizontal adduction. The inferior capsule may be stretched in the standing position by elevating the arm overhead as far as possible with the elbow flexed and pulling the arm behind the head as far as possible.
- After treatment, *ice* was used for 15 minutes to help retain gains in soft-tissue extensibility. This was terminated after 3 weeks once the patient demonstrated significant gain in painless range of motion and no longer experienced any posttreatment shoulder irritation.[25]
- Application of light *transverse friction* massage just proximal to the insertion of the greater tubercle. Transverse friction disrupts scar tissue and interfibrillary adhesions within the substance of the tendon by forcible broadening of the tendon at its insertion into bone.[6] The induced hyperemia is particularly important here, since hypovascularity may contribute to a rotator cuff tendon disorder.[9] Friction was applied perpendicularly to the span of tendon for 1 to 2 minutes until tenderness subsided, after which pressure was slightly increased for an additional 2 minutes of friction massage. Friction was applied rhythmically at two cycles per second.[9] With successive treatments, pressure and time were gradually

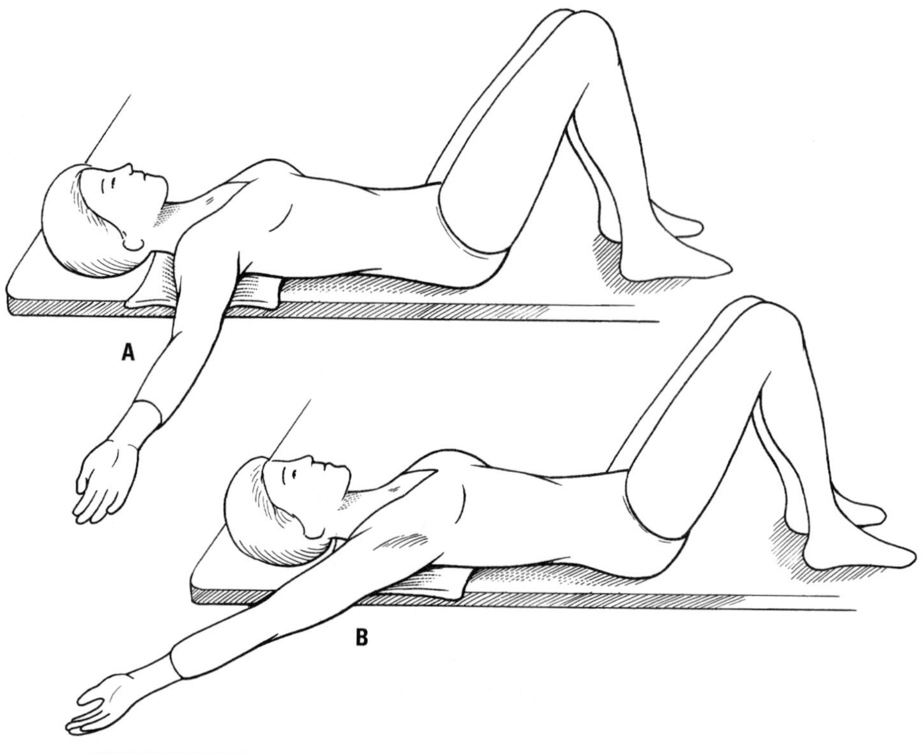

Fig. 10-11 Stretching of, **A,** the upper and, **B,** the lower fibers of the pectoralis major.

increased to 10 minutes. Treatment continued for 10 sessions until the patient reported a decrease in pain.

- The patient was taught *voluntary humeral depression.* The patient was asked to attempt to push her arm caudally, while the therapist provided slight resistance against her elbow for proprioceptive feedback (there was also some scapular depression). The therapist provided verbal reinforcement when the patient successfully performed caudal glide (Fig. 10-12). The patient then progressed to performing caudal glide upon active abduction.[13]
- *Neuromuscular reeducation* was used to decrease impingement and to facilitate normal shoulder biomechanics. The patient was educated regarding proper warm-ups and cooldowns before and after sport activity.
- A comprehensive individualized *home exercise program* was developed for this patient to help maintain the gains made in the clinic and to prevent recurrence of impingement. This program consisted in progressive stretching and strengthening exercises as well as self-mobilization of the posterior glenohumeral capsule (see Fig. 13-6). All home activities were observed by the therapist to ensure proper form.

After 7 weeks of 21 treatment sessions the patient reported a decrease in pain from 5/10 to 1/10 when carrying her briefcase. She has switched to carrying her briefcase to her left shoulder and has lightened her load by carrying only what is absolutely necessary. She is able to perform overhead activities without pain and demonstrates normal muscle length of her pectoralis major muscle. There is no longer a positive impingement sign. Selective tension is positively painful on external rotation 2/10 from 5/10 at the initial

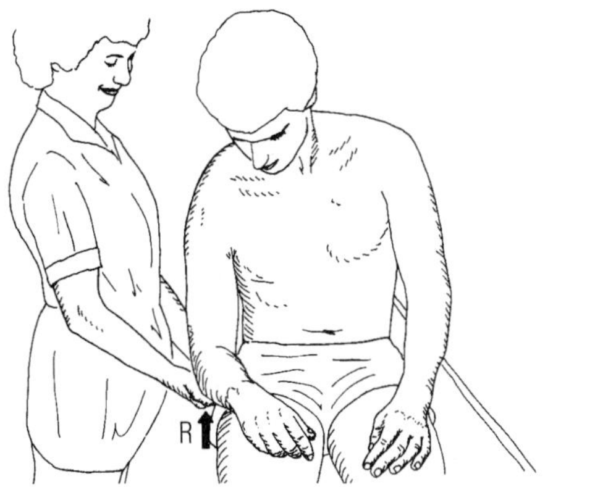

Fig. 10-12 Resistive humeral depression. (From Kisner C, Colby LA: *Therapeutic exercise: foundations and techniques*, ed 2, Philadelphia, 1990, FA Davis.)

evaluation. She swims frequently and has taken several lessons to modify her stroke. She will continue to perform her home exercise program for both shoulders as well as warm-ups and cooldowns as prevention against future impingement. The patient was extremely pleased with the results of therapy.

24. When is surgery appropriate?

Surgery is considered only in those patients who, after having undergone a conservative regimen for a minimum of 6 months,[25] and having explored vocational rehabilitation, continue to experience substantial impingement symptoms.[16] In addition, there must be complete active or passive range of motion in the shoulder joint.[21]

25. What are the three surgical options?

All attempts at surgical treatment of impingement syndrome share the common goal of eliminating the arch of the subacromial tunnel. Surgical procedures in order of increasing severity include the following three:

- Resection of the coracoacromial ligament through a deltoid split.[8]
- Partial acromionectomy (open acromioplasty) involves resection of the anteroinferior acromion with most of the coracoacromial ligament removed. Here, the deltoid undergoes a T-shaped incision that permits inspection of the rotator cuff as well as repair of tears, which are later repaired with sutures or wires. The arm is distracted, so that the subacromial space can be visualized, and a bald spot on the humeral head indicates a rotator cuff tear.[21] After surgery, the arm is placed in a sling and passive range of motion exercise is begun on the fourth day. At 8 postoperative weeks strengthening exercises may be initiated. Other surgeons may prefer active assisted range of motion exercise to be performed immediately the same day as surgery as well as internal and external rotation strengthening also begun immediately. Unless there is concern for the strength of the deltoid reattachment the patient is allowed active shoulder range of motion exercise within the range of comfort. Full recovery may take as long as 4 to 6 months.[21] A radical acromionectomy procedure may worsen a patient's condition and compromise shoulder function.[16]
- With arthroscopic acromioplasty the same amount of bone is removed from the anteroinferior acromion as with an open acromioplasty. Afterwards the arm is placed in a sling for 3 to 8 days followed

by range of motion exercise initially and progressing to cuff-strengthening exercises over time. The rehabilitation period takes up to 3 months.[21]

26. What is the postoperative surgical program?

Rehabilitation usually begins within the first postoperative week,[7] and on the very day of surgery according to some,[16] with passive range of motion below 80° of flexion and abduction. Passive elevation above 80° is delayed for 2 weeks according to the amount of shoulder inflammation present. Active range of motion exercise begins at 2 postoperative weeks so as not to stress the deltoid. Progressive strengthening with minimum resistance followed by isolation of the rotator cuff muscles so as to promote humeral head centralization while the impingement range of 80° to 120° is avoided. Full external rotation range must be gained before overhand activity is attempted so that clearance and not impingement will occur in the suprahumeral space.[7]

27. What is the success rate for returning athletes to competition after surgery?

The low success rate in returning athletes to competition after surgical decompression[27] tends to reinforce the importance of nonoperative management in this population. Strengthening, stretching, and technique modification are the most effective methods for managing impingement in the athlete.[16]

References

1. Bechtro CO: Biomechanics of the shoulder, *Clin Orthop* 146:37, 1980.
2. Bigliani LU, Norris TR, Fischer J, et al: The relationship between the unfused acromial epiphysis and subacromial impingement lesion, *Orthop Trans* 7(1):138, 1983.
3. Chung SMK, Nissenbaum MM: Congenital and developmental defects of the shoulder, *Orthop Clin North Am* 6:382, 1975.
4. Cofield RH, Simonet WT: Symposium on sports medicine: part 2, The shoulder in sports, *Mayo Clin Proc* 59:157-164, 1984.
5. Cuillo J: Swimmer's shoulder, *Clin Sports Med* 5:115-136, 1984.
6. Cyriax J: *Textbook of orthopaedic medicine*, vol 2, ed 11, London, 1987, Bailliere-Tindall.
7. Gould JA III: *Orthopaedic and sports physical therapy*, ed 2, St. Louis, 1990, Mosby.
8. Hawkins RJ, Hobeika PE: Impingement syndrome in the athletic shoulder, *Clin Sports Med* 2(2):394, 1988.
9. Hertling D, Kessler RM: Management of common musculoskeletal disorders, ed 2, Philadelphia, 1990, Lippincott.
10. Hoppenfeld S: *Physical examination of the spine and extremities*, Norwalk, Conn., 1976, Appleton-Century-Crofts.
11. Johnson D: In swimming, shoulder the burden, *Sports Care and Fitness* 1(2):24-30, 1988.
12. Kennedy J, Hawkins R, Krissoff W: Orthopaedic manifestations of swimming, *Am J Sports Med* 6:309-322, 1978.
13. Kisner C, Colby LA: *Therapeutic exercise: foundations and techniques*, ed 2, Philadelphia, 1990, FA Davis.
14. Lillegard WA, Rucker KS: *Handbook of sports medicine: a symptom-oriented approach*, Boston, 1993, Andover Medical Publishers.
15. Luopajarvi T, Kuorinka I, Virolainen M, Holmberg M: Prevalence of tenosynovitis and other injuries of the upper extremities in repetitive work, *Scand J Work Environ Health*, 5(3):48-55, 1979.
16. Matsen FA, Arnitz CT: Subacromial impingement. In Rockwood CA, Matsen FA, editors: *The shoulder*, ed 2, Philadelphia, 1990, Saunders.
17. Morrison DS, Bigliani LU: The clinical significance of variations in acromial morphology. Paper presented at the American Shoulder and Elbow Surgeons, third meeting, San Francisco, 1987.
18. Neer CS II: Anterior acromioplasty for the chronic impingement syndrome in the shoulder: a preliminary report, *J Bone Joint Surg* 54A:41-50, 1972.
19. Neer CS II, Bigliani LU, Hawking RJ: Rupture of the long head of the biceps related to subacromial impingement, *Orthop Trans* 1:111, 1977.
20. Neer CS II: Impingement lesions, *Clin Orthop* 173:70-77, 1983.
21. Netter FH: The CIBA collection of medical illustrations, vol 1, Summit, N.J., 1986, CIBA-Geigy Corp.
22. Petterrson G: Rupture of the tendon aponeurosis of the shoulder joint in antero-inferior dislocation, *Acta Chir Scand* 77(suppl):1-187, 1942.
23. Saunders HD: *Evaluation, treatment and prevention of musculoskeletal disorders*, Minneapolis, 1985, Viking Press.
24. Staples OS, Watkins AO: Full active abduction in traumatic paralysis of the deltoid, *J Bone Joint Surg* (Am) 25:85, 1934.

25. Stroh S: Shoulder impingement, *J Manual and Manipulative Ther* 3(2):59-64, 1995.
26. Thein LA: Impingement syndrome and its conservative management, *J Orthop Sports Phys Ther* 11:189, 1989.
27. Tibone J, Jobe F, Kerlan R, et al: Shoulder impingement syndrome in athletes treated by anterior acromioplasty, *Clin Orthop* 198:134-140, 1985.

Recommended reading

Hawkins RJ, Hobeika PE: Impingement syndrome in the athletic shoulder, *Clin Sports Med* 2(2):391-405, 1983.

Hertling D, Kessler RM: *Management of common musculoskeletal disorders,* ed 2, Philadelphia, 1990, Lippincott.

Kisner C, Colby LA: *Therapeutic exercise: foundations and techniques,* ed 2, Philadelphia, 1990, FA Davis.

Matsen FA, Arnitz CT: Subacromial impingement. In Rockwood CA, Matsen FA, editors: *The shoulder*, Philadelphia, 1990, Saunders.

Stroh S: Shoulder impingement, *J Manual and Manipulative Ther* 3(2):59-64, 1995.

Thein LA: Impingement syndrome and its conservative management, *J Orthop Sports Phys Ther* 11:189, 1989.

11

Chronic Shoulder Discomfort That Progressed to Acute Unrelenting Pain over 4-Month Period

A 46-year-old female homemaker enters your office holding her right upper extremity in a guarded posture with a complaint of acute and worsening throbbing pain of 3 days' duration in her right shoulder that is unrelieved by rest. When questioned, the patient admits to mild pain and tenderness that began 4 months ago, with tenderness over the deltoid muscle and pain elicited when rolling over onto the right shoulder while sleeping. Also there was initially a loss of range of motion as well as a catching and painful sensation whenever the right arm was elevated between 75° to 100°. The patient states that high doses of aspirin have helped ease her pain. She reports a new onset of non-insulin dependent diabetes for 1 year and reports no history of trauma to either shoulder.

Clue:

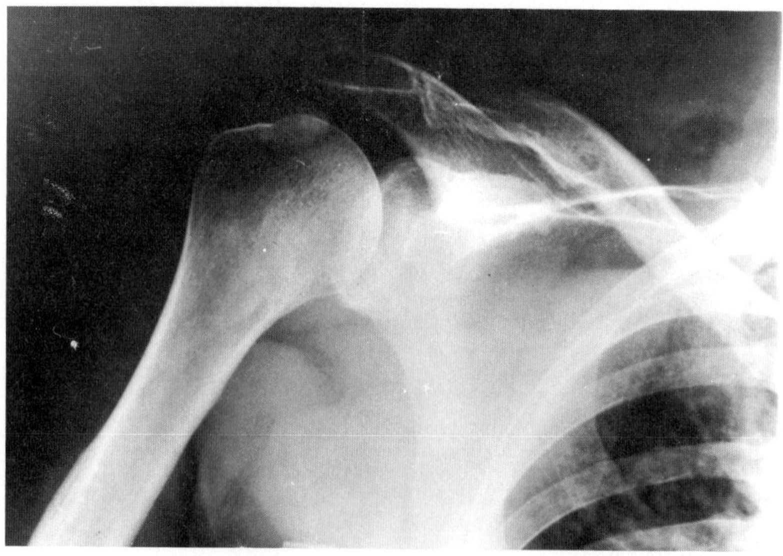

Fig. 11-1 (From Nicholas JA, Hershman EB: *The upper extremity in sports medicine*, ed 2, St. Louis, 1995, Mosby.)

OBSERVATION No redness or sign of atrophy of spinatus muscle bellies.

PALPATION Warmth and extreme tenderness over anterior deltoid area just superior to greater humeral tuberosity.

RANGE OF MOTION Unassessed as patient refuses to move her shoulder.

MUSCLE STRENGTH Untested.

SELECTIVE TENSION Untested.

JOINT PLAY Attempts to assess arthrokinematic motion are met with resistance caused by pain.

UPPER QUADRANT SCREENING Negative results to compression or distraction of the cervical spine.

SENSATION Normal.

1. **What is most likely wrong with this woman?**
2. **What is the cause of this disorder?**
3. **What is the incidence of calcified tendinitis?**
4. **What is the pathogenesis of calcific tendinitis?**
5. **What is the clinical presentation?**
6. **What radiologic views are necessary, and how are apparent calcifications classified?**
7. **How do arthritic changes of this region differ radiologically from calcified tendinitis?**
8. **What is the radiologic appearance of calcific rupture into an adjacent bursa?**
9. **What is the differential diagnosis?**
10. **What rehabilitative therapy is appropriate during the subacute phase?**
11. **What is the appropriate management during the acute phase?**

1. **What is most likely wrong with this woman?**

Fig. 11-1 shows calcification of the insertion of the supraspinatus tendon. *Calcific tendinitis* of the rotator cuff is a common disorder that demonstrates a cyclic nature of calcium deposition and eventual resorption as the tendons heal. While calcium is deposited, the patient suffers only mild to moderate discomfort, whereas during the later resorption phase the shoulder becomes acutely painful.[17] Many pathologic conditions are characterized by a sequential evolution from an acute to a chronic disease state; however, calcific tendinitis does not fit this clinical picture, and these descriptions are perhaps inappropriate in describing this condition. Instead, what we have here is the opposite progression, that is, the patient's subjective report of chronic symptoms preceding acute symptoms. Calcifying tendinitis constitutes a disease entity in its own right[18] and is not related to generalized systemic disease despite the increased frequency of HLA-A1 antigen present in many patients, implying a genetic component to this condition.[15] An association with diabetes mellitus or gout is suspected[5] but has never been proved.[17] Most authors agree that no relationship exists between calcifying tendinitis and external trauma.[17]

2. What is the cause of this disorder?

The cause of calcific tendinitis is unknown, but it is believed that tissue hypoxia is the primary etiologic factor.

Approximately one-half inch proximal to the insertion of the supraspinatus[2] is an area of tendon, dubbed the "*critical zone,*"[10] that corresponds to the area of anastamoses between the osseous and muscular vessels.[11] The vascularity of this area is questioned because certain positions of the upper extremity have a "wringing out" effect resulting from pressure of the humeral head on the tendon when the arm is held in the resting position of adduction and neutral rotation.[13] Additionally there may be an inherent anatomic hypovascularity of the deep substance of the supraspinatus insertion as compared with its superficial aspect.[16] Regardless of which factor is the cause of the disorder, the result is hypoperfusion and tissue hypoxia that leads to a sequence of degeneration, necrosis, and reactive calcification.[17]

3. What is the incidence of calcified tendinitis?

The epidemiology of this disorder varies greatly. Females are more often affected than males, and the right shoulder is usually more often affected than the left.[17] However, cuff tendons of the dominant arm show no greater incidence of involvement than those from the contralateral shoulder.[12] Occupation seems to play some role in the development of this disorder though exactly how is uncertain. Close to 50% of patients in some studies were housewives or persons having clerical jobs. The incidence of calcific tendinitis peaks between 40 and 50 years of age, and bilateral involvement does occur in 15% of patients affected with this disorder.[14] In the athletic population, calcific tendinitis is generally seen in middle-aged athletes.[1]

4. What is the pathogenesis of calcific tendinitis?

Codman and other investigators believe that degeneration of tendon fibers precedes calcification[2] and occurs as a function of the wear-and-tear effect of aging. This hypothesis is supported by the fact that calcific tendinitis seldom affects persons before the fourth decade.[17] On the other hand, there is no evidence that a worker engaged in heavy manual labor will develop calcific tendinitis over time.[17] The tendons of the supraspinatus and the infraspinatus, in fact, undergo an alteration in structure during the middle years,[12] possibly related to chronic trauma, causing the normally orderly parallel collagen bundles composing the tendon to become thin, frayed, irregular, split, ischemic, and necrotic. Eventually the tendons undergo calcification,[17] succumbing to a process that is reminiscent of myositis ossificans. As such, calcific tendinitis is viewed as one possible intermediate pathologic stage along the continuum of cuff tendinopathies that begin with impingement syndrome and terminate with full-thickness rupture of one or more cuff tendons.

On the other hand, the self-healing nature of calcifying tendinitis is not characteristic of a degenerative disease but is rather an evolution of three stages of disease: (1) precalcific, (2) calcific, and (3) postcalcific.[17] Thus, rather than understanding this pathologic condition as two unrelated degenerative disease processes that include both an acute and a chronic calcific tendinitis, we can understand it as a disease cycle (Fig. 11-2) that is inclusive of both manifestations of a singular disease entity.

1. In the initial *precalcific stage*, the predilected area of tendon undergoes histologic change (such as fibrocartilagenous transformation, presumably triggered by tissue hypoxia). This stage is characterized by two phases and incorporates both the acute and subacute and the chronic stages of this disease.

- *Formative phase.* This phase is the reactive deposition of calcium crystals as the body's reaction to chronic trauma, possibly in combination with senescence, that follows tendon degeneration, ischemia, and necrosis. If the patient undergoes surgery at this stage, the deposit appears hard and chalklike. This initial state of deposit formation lacks vascular and cellular reaction.

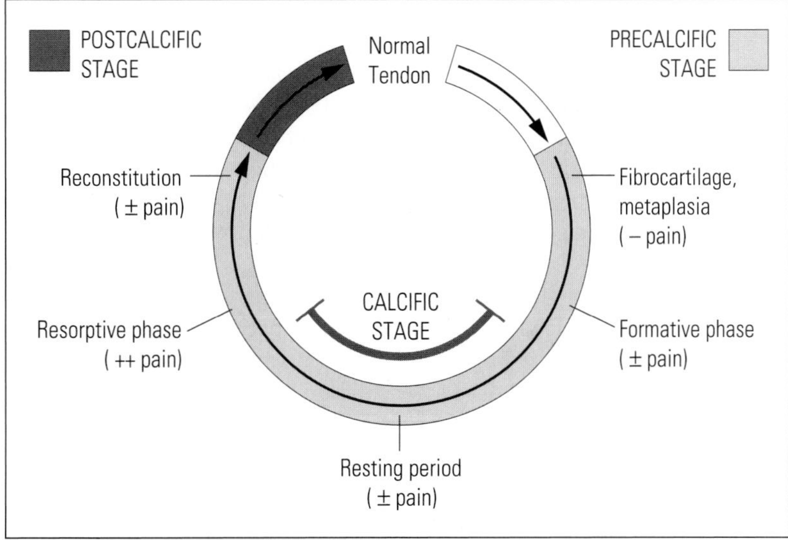

Fig. 11-2 Cycle of pain and inflammation with calcific tendinitis.

- *Resorptive phase.* This phase occurs after a relative period of inactivity of the disease process and is characterized by increased vascularization at the periphery of the deposit that ushers in macrophages, which phagocytose and remove calcium. This combination of vascular proliferation and cell exudation causes pain by raising the intratendinous pressure. This in turn may be further exacerbated by increased tendon volume within the unyielding subacromial arch. Lavage performed at this phase yields a thick, white creamlike or toothpastelike exudate.[17]

2. In the *postcalcific stage* there is remodeling of collagen in alignment with the longitudinal axis of the tendon in the space previously occupied by calcium by fibroblasts and newly developed vascular channels.[17]

5. What is the clinical presentation?

There is a tendency to believe that this disorder begins with acute symptoms and progresses to a chronic state. On the contrary, calcification is often symptomless, or at most just moderately uncomfortable at the beginning, whereas the disappearance of calcification is associated with pain.

Chronic signs and symptoms include pain or tenderness. The most frequent site of pain is referred to the insertion of the deltoid. Patients cannot sleep on the affected shoulder and complain of increased night pain. Decreased range of motion, a painful arc between 70° and 110°,[8] and a sensation of catching when going through an arc of motion are often reported. Supraspinatus muscle belly atrophy is a sign of long-standing calcifying tendinitis.

During the acute resorptive stage pain is so severe that patients refuse to move their shoulders. Pain is described as "throbbing" and is unrelieved by rest. Any attempt at mobilization of the glenohumeral joint will be resisted by the patient who will hold her or his upper extremity close to the body. Symptoms may last up to 2 weeks when acute, 3 to 8 weeks when subacute, and 3 months or more when chronic.

6. What radiologic views are necessary, and how are apparent calcifications classified?

In cases of suspected tendon calcification a radiograph must be taken and should include anteroposterior films in neutral as well as medial and lateral rotation. Supraspinatus deposits are readily visible in neutral rotation, whereas deposits on infraspinatus and teres minor are best seen in internal rotation. Subscapularis tendon calcification is rare and only clearly viewed on radiographs taken with the shoulder in external rotation. Scapular views are helpful in determining whether calcification has caused impingement. A positive finding confirms, at the very least, the presence of an intact cuff and rules out rupture of cuff tendons.[17]

There are two different radiologic appearances of calcific tendinitis, corresponding to the chronic and acute phases of this disease:[17]

- Corresponding to the *formative phase* in which the patient experiences mild or moderate discomfort (that is, chronic or subacute), the deposit appears dense, homogeneous, and with well-defined borders.
- Corresponding to the *resorptive phase* in which the patient experiences acute symptoms, the deposit appears fluffy, fleecy, or cloudlike, with ill-defined borders that are often barely visible (that is, with decreased density) and may extend into the adjacent bursa.[3,4]

7. How do arthritic changes of this region differ radiologically from calcified tendinitis?

Whereas deposits in calcific tendinitis are for the most part localized inside the tendon and may extend into the bursa, calcification seen in arthropathy is in continuity with or extending into the bone. Moreover, the latter are small and stippled in appearance, overlie the greater tuberosity, and are often accompanied by degenerative or articular changes characteristic of osteoarthritis. In addition, the acromiohumeral (that is, subacromial) space may be narrowed.[17]

8. What is the radiologic appearance of calcific rupture into the adjacent bursa?

Ruptures into the bursa appear as a crescentlike shadow overlying the actual calcification, extending over the greater tuberosity, and outlining the extent of the bursa.[9] This appearance may be viewed during the acute stage, corresponding to the resorptive phase of this disease cycle.

9. What is the differential diagnosis?

Differential diagnosis includes the following:

- Dystrophic calcifications are viewed as small stippled deposits seen around the torn edges of the tendon but especially sitting over the greater tuberosity after a complete tear of the supraspinatus or other cuff tendons. This tear appears as narrowing of the interval between the humeral head and the acromion. In contradistinction, calcific tendinitis deposits are situated inside the tendon without contacting the bone.
- Massive calcification as is seen in the Milwaukee shoulder.[6]
- Osteoarthritis.[17]

10. What rehabilitative therapy is appropriate during the subacute phase?

Therapeutic intervention is based on severity of symptoms and radiologic assessement. Patients with subacute symptoms are classified as belonging to the formative phase, unless radiographs show signs of resorption. The goals of therapy in this stage include maintenance of range of motion and strength. The degenerative changes of the rotator cuff that may result in calcific tendinitis are similar to those responsible for rotator cuff tear. As such, it is imperative that management strategy address prophylaxis and treatment so as to prevent recurrence of the rotator cuff disorder (see pp. 113-118).

Rehabilitative therapy during the subacute formative stage may include the following:

- Acetic acid iontophoresis for calcific deposits with the negative electrode over the site of lesion. The positive electrode may be placed on the ipsilateral forearm. The acetate radical replaces the carbonate radical in the insoluble calcium carbonate deposit, forming soluble calcium acetate.[7]

- Ultrasound so as to facilitate mobilization of calcium crystals.
- Phonophoresis with hydrocortisone.
- Corticosteroid injection with lidocaine to inhibit vascular proliferation, local hyperemia, and macrophage activity.
- Maintaining the shoulder in the position of abduction as often as possible. This position may be achieved by placement of the arm on the backrest of a chair or on a seat beside the patient. When supine, a pillow may be placed in the axilla.
- Moist heat.
- Rest.
- Transcutaneous electrical stimulation.
- Pendulum exercises.
- Exercises to increase range of motion, though it is important to avoid exercises that might cause upward humeral migration.
- Superficial heat such as diathermy in a chronic condition before exercises.

11. What is the appropriate management during the acute phase?

Calcific tendinitis may resolve spontaneously, requiring only nonsteroidal anti-inflammatory medications for a week to 10 days during the acute phase of the disease. It is essential for the therapist to prevent the development of frozen shoulder during this phase (see pp. 160-163). Local ice application may be of help before pendulum exercises or glenohumeral joint mobilization. Iontophoresis to decrease pain, using hydrocortisone or lidocaine, may help relieve pain. However, the physician may attempt lavage during the resorptive phase. Here, symptoms are often acute, with radiographs confirming resorbtion. If lavage is unsuccessful, the needling usually helps relieve symptoms by decreasing intratendinous pressure and is followed by an intrabursal corticosteroid injection. The site of pain is then treated with ice massage and pendulum exercises, as well as nonsteroidal anti-inflammatory medications. Once symptoms have decreased, range of motion activities and strengthening may begin.

Surgical removal is the exception and resorted to only when conservative treatment has failed and symptoms interfere with activities of daily living.

References

1. Anderson TE: Rehabilitation of common shoulder injuries in athletes, *J Musculoskeletal Med,* p 24, Dec 1988.
2. Codman EA: *The shoulder,* Boston, 1934, Thomas Todd.
3. DePalma AF, Druper JS: Long term study of shoulder joints afflicted with and treated for calcific tendinitis, *Clin Orthop* 20:61-72, l961.
4. De Seze S, Welfling J: Tendinites calcificantes, *Rhumatologie* 22:5-14, 1970.
5. Gschwend N, Scherer M, Lohr J: Die tendinitis calcarea des Schultergelenks, *Orthopäde* 10:196-205, 1981.
6. Halverson PB, McCarty DJ, Cheung HS, Ryan LM: Milwaukee shoulder syndrome, *Ann Rheum Dis* 43:734-741, 1989.
7. Kahn J: *Principles and practice of electrotherapy,* ed 2, New York, 1991, Churchill Livingstone.
8. Kessel L, Watson M: The painful arc syndrome, *J Bone Joint Surg* 59B:166-172, 1977.
9. Milone FP, Copeland MM: Calcific tendinitis of the shoulder joint, *AJR* 85:901-913, 1961.
10. Moseley HF, Goldie I: The arterial pattern of the rotator cuff of the shoulder, *J Bone Joint Surg* 45B:780-789, 1963.
11. Nixon JE, DiStefano V: Ruptures of the rotator cuff, *Orthop Clin North Am* 6:423-447, 1975.
12. Olsson O: Degenerative changes of the shoulder and their connection with shoulder pain, *Acta Chir Scand* 181 (suppl):1-110, 1953.
13. Rathbun JB, Macnab I: The microvascular pattern of the rotator cuff, *J Bone Joint Surg* (Br) 52(3):540-553, 1970.
14. Rodnan GP, Schumacher HR: *Primer on the rheumatic diseases,* ed 8, Atlanta, Ga., 1983, Arthritis Foundation.
15. Thompson LL: *The Electromyographer's handbook,* Boston, 1981, Little, Brown & Co.
16. Uhthoff HK, Loehr J, Sarkar K: The pathogenesis of rotator cuff tears. *Proc Third International Conference on Surgery of the Shoulder,* Fukuoka, Japan, Oct 27, 1986.

17. Uhthoff HK, Sarkar K: Calcifying tendinitis. In Rockwood CA, Matsen FA, editors: *The shoulder,* vol 1, Philadelphia, 1990, Saunders.
18. Welting J, Kahn MF, Desroy M, et al: Les calcifications de l'épaule, II. La maladie des calcifications tendineuses multiples, *Rev Rhum* 32:325-334, 1965.

Recommended reading

Brewer BJ: Aging of the rotator cuff, *Am J Sports Med* 7:102-110, 1979.

Griffin EJ, Kavselis TC: Physical agents for physical therapists. In *Ultrasonic energy,* ed 2, Springfield, Ill., 1982, Charles C Thomas.

Uhthoff HK, Sarkar K: Calcifying tendinitis. In Rockwood CA, Matsen FA, editors: *The shoulder,* vol 1, Philadelphia, 1990, Saunders.

Acute and Excruciating Shoulder Pain after Intense Bout of Exercise and Relieved by Rest

12

A 55-year-old male presents himself at your office with sudden pain and loss of function of the right shoulder 5 days ago. Symptoms actually began a week ago and were preceded by spending an intense Sunday afternoon helping his wife do her annual spring cleaning during which he performed lots of overhead activity with his dominant right arm. Pain has increased since 5 days ago and now is severe. The shoulder is held away from the body in 30° to 40° abduction. The patient points to the anterolateral arm over the areas of the middle and upper deltoid muscle bellies as the source of his pain. There is a positive history of prior cuff tendinitis some 4 years ago contralaterally, gout in the right hallux 12 years ago, and a history of mild generalized arthritis. The patient recalls no injury and admits to taking six aspirin per day for the past 3 days, which he reports helps alleviate pain. He has no history of any stomach ulcers.

OBSERVATION There is no redness.

PALPATION The shoulder is only mildly warm. There is tenderness over the bicipital groove, over the cuff tendons, but particularly beneath the right acromion process.

RANGE OF MOTION Active and passive elevation is painful at 50° and yields an empty end feel (that is, the patient refuses to let you, the examiner, move the limb any further along the normal range) because the patient begs you to desist from further elevation, despite the fact that you feel that more movement is possible.[5] Rotation in either extreme is painless and is demonstrated at the end of allowable elevation range; hence a noncapsular pattern is observed. Abduction is noted to be more limited than forward flexion.

MUSCLE STRENGTH Appears to be at least in the fair plus range.

SELECTIVE TENSION Painless resisted motion at a specified range that becomes painful only when one is testing through the 50° to 130° range.

SPECIAL TESTS Negative drop arm test, positive impingement sign.

1. **What is most likely the matter with this gentleman?**
2. **What requisite anatomy is essential to understanding this disorder?**
3. **Is subacromial bursitis a primary or a secondary disorder?**
4. **How many bursae exist in the shoulder, and what are their locations?**
5. **What are the specifics of the mechanism in the evolution of this condition?**
6. **What are the signs and symptoms of this condition?**
7. **How are the subdeltoid and subacromial bursae best palpated?**
8. **What do radiographs reveal about this condition?**
9. **How does the migration of calcification from the cuff tendon to the adjacent bursae facilitate beneficial resolution of the disorder?**
10. **How is calcified cuff tendinitis differentiated from bursitis?**
11. **What is the differential diagnosis of shoulder bursitis?**
12. **What rehabilitative therapy is helpful in the treatment and resolution of this pathologic condition?**

1. What is most likely the matter with this gentleman?

Subacromial bursitis of the right shoulder.

2. What requisite anatomy is essential to understanding this disorder?

The *coracoacromial arch* is composed of two scapular processes—the coracoid and the acromion. These scapular components are connected by the roof of the arch—the coracoacromial ligament. Passage of the cuff tendons under this unyielding arch is managed by the presence of the *subacromial bursa*[12] and its extension the *subdeltoid bursa.*[3] These two soft tissues are actually two serosal surfaces (one on the *underside* of the acromion and deltoid, and the other *over* the cuff tendons) lubricated by synovial fluid so that they may intimately slide over each other.[12] The analogy is one of two fluid-inflated balloons pressed against each other and moving relative to each other during shoulder movement. When normally inflated, as during the inflammatory process, the bursa may enlarge to about the size of a golf ball.[11] These membranes are lined with a synovial membrane that can increase or decrease the amount of synovial fluid available on minimal stimulation.[2]

3. Is subacromial bursitis a primary or a secondary disorder?

Although subacromial bursitis may occur as a primary disorder after a blow to the shoulder,[11] it most frequently occurs secondarily to degenerative lesions of the rotator cuff and is part of the continuum of the many rotator cuff disorders.[15] Additionally bursitis may also be viewed as a separate yet related pathologic condition to calcific tendinitis. That is, although bursitis may evolve as a distinct clinical entity in its own right, it may also evolve secondarily to acute tendon calcification.

4. How many bursae exist in the shoulder, and what are their locations?

Most of the body's bursae exist in or around the shoulder complex,[1] and Codman lists up to 12. However, the most commonly present bursa locations include the following (Fig. 12-1):

- — 1. Subacromial and subdeltoid
- — 2. Between the coracoid and the glenohumeral joint capsule
- — 3. Summit of the acromion

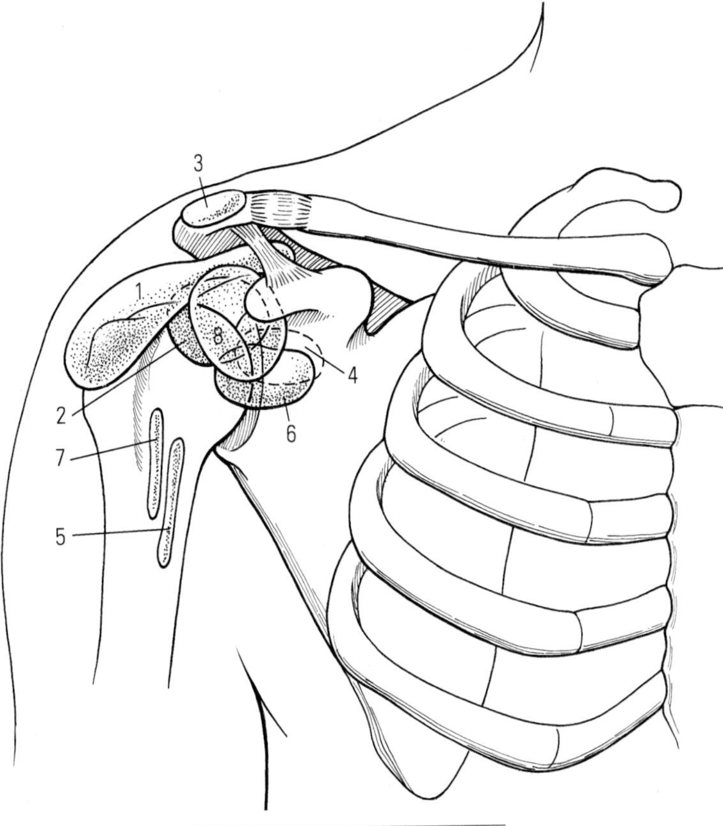

Fig. 12-1 Common shoulder bursae.

- — 4. Between the infraspinatus and the joint capsule
- — 5. Between the teres major and the long head of the biceps
- — 6. Between the subscapularis and the joint capsule
- — 7. Anterior to and posterior to the tendinous insertion of the latissimus dorsi
- — 8. Behind the coracobrachialis muscle[9]

5. What are the specifics of the mechanism in the evolution of this condition?

Shoulder bursitis is a function of the intimate relationship between the supraspinatus tendon and the adjacent bursa within the coracoacromial arch. The disorder may often evolve in the following manner.

Repetitive shoulder movements cause a reactive accumulation of fluid within the bursa in the attempt to attenuate friction. If shoulder movement continues excessively, bursal effusion will maximize, causing tissue tension and pain in the shoulder.[11] Alternately or even simultaneously, bursitis is initiated or worsened in the event that a supraspinatus impingement disorder is already present. Inflammation soon follows and cramps the contents of the subacromial space because of edema accumulation and fibrosis of the tendon. Over time, these changes will spread to include the bursae, which also undergo hypertrophy (proliferative lining) and fibrosis (that is, thickened) so as to interfere with their normal lubrication. The cumulative effect of these changes is to contribute to increasing rather than decreasing friction within the subacromial space.[4]

6. What are the signs and symptoms of this condition?

Bursitis will have a swift onset[15] of extremely severe shoulder pain[14] with dramatic tenderness[16] localized to the insertion of the deltoid at the upper middle thirds of the anterolateral proximal arm.[15] This is in contrast to the more diffuse involvement found with impingement of the supraspinatus or biceps tendon or pain found adjacent to the coracoid process at the medial aspect of the shoulder in subcoracoid bursitis.[16] The patient, usually a man of middle age or older who has done an unusual bout of exercise,[14] experiences a sudden and unprovoked onset of extreme pain within a few days[5] that causes him to seek immediate relief. There is often a history of previous attacks.[9] A *noncapsular end feel* at the end of the range of passive motion with free rotation in either direction is *diagnostic for this disorder.* The clinician may also detect an *empty end feel* with passive movement.[15] If the bursitis is primary and thus not involving the cuff tendons, resistive movement would register painless,[5] implicating a noncontractile structure as the source of pain. This is not the case for resistance testing throughout the range, especially between the 50° to 130° range, where the contracting tendon may compress the inflamed bursa lying between the undersurface of the acromion and the supraspinatus tendon.[15]

The patient maintains the shoulder in an adducted position, which keeps the painful lesion away from the acromial undersurface. Elevation is hindered, abduction more so than forward flexion, and a painful arc between 50° and 130° is present whether movement is active or passive.[14] On palpation there is exquisite local tenderness over the subacromial bursa, which may feel thickened[6] as compared to the contralateral shoulder. Tenderness may also extend as far down as the bicipital groove.[6] Tests for supraspinatus tendinitis and impingement will be positive in this condition.[8]

7. How are the subdeltoid and subacromial bursae best palpated?

The subdeltoid bursa is easily palpated beneath the deltoid muscle (Fig. 12-2). The subacromial bursa is brought within the examiner's reach by moving the shoulder into passive extension, thus rotating both the cuff tendons and the superficial bursa out from under the acromion[6] (Fig. 12-3).

8. What do radiographs reveal about this condition?

Calcific subacromial bursitis and calcific supraspinatus tendinitis may be indistinguishable both radiographically as well as clinically.[1] However, once rupture of calcific material into the bursa has occurred, radiographic study shows a diffuse, lacy, amorphous pattern characteristic of spreading of the calcified mass throughout the bursal cavity.[13]

9. How does the migration of calcification from the cuff tendon to the adjacent bursae facilitate beneficial resolution of the disorder?

During the evolution of a calcific supraspinatus disorder, the calcium expands throughout the substance of the tendon to adhere[10] and irritate[14] the undersurface of the subacromial bursa. This new source of pain serves only to magnify the patient's already throbbing and excruciating pain that is unrelieved by rest.[14] Treatment involves aspiration, under local anesthesia, accompanied by hydrocortisone injection. Although aspiration may not yield calcium, it does, by virtue of multiple punctures, have the effect of allowing the calcium to become dispersed into the bursa where it can be resorbed. On the other hand, if calcific migration is allowed to continue through the bursal membrane, the calcium will eventually

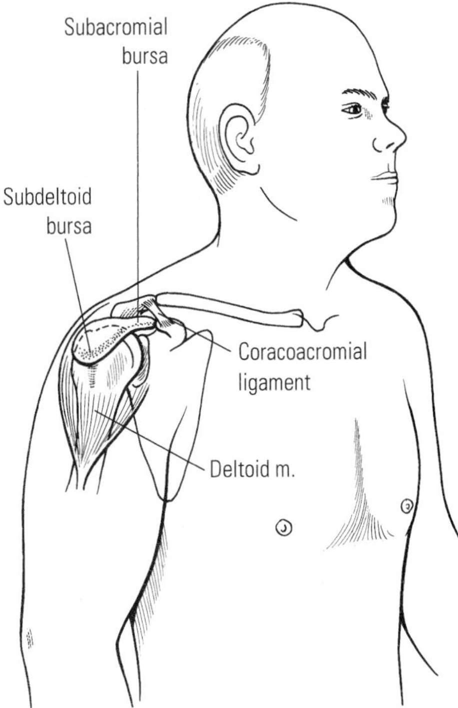

Fig. 12-2 The subdeltoid and subacromial bursae are really one but are separately named according to their adjacent anatomic structures.

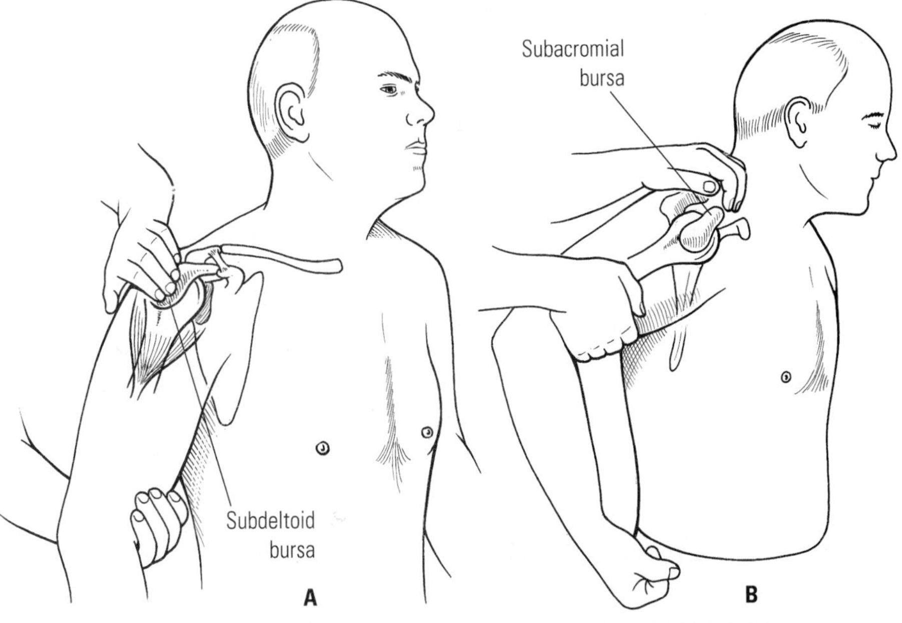

Fig. 12-3 Palpation of the bursa. **A,** Subdeltoid bursa. **B,** Subacromial bursa.

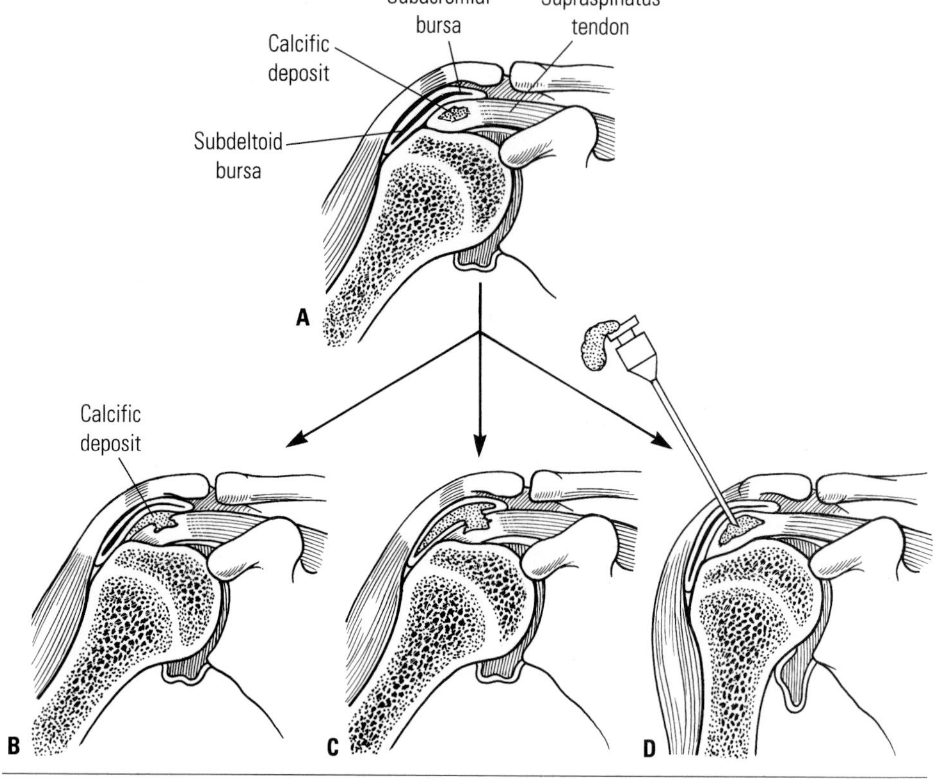

Fig. 12-4 **A,** Calcific deposit in the tendon creates increased cramping within the subacromial space, which further aggravates inflammation and pain. Symptomatic relief when space-occupying calcium no longer concentrates within the subacromial space may occur in one of three ways: **B,** spontaneous upward rupture of the deposit beneath the floor of the bursae; **C,** spontaneous downward rupture of the deposit into the bursa where it may be resorbed; **D,** needle rupture and deposit removal.

rupture the bursa. This *chemical bursitis* is actually beneficial, since the bursa, having a good blood supply, will gradually absorb the calcium, thus allowing symptoms to subside[14] (Fig. 12-4).

10. How is calcified cuff tendinitis differentiated from bursitis?

Although the locale of pain in calcified cuff tendinitis is often indistinguishable from shoulder bursitis because of the proximity of these structures as well as the relatedness of these disorders, the former is distinguishable from the latter by pain unrelieved by rest. Moreover, with shoulder bursitis the patient experiences relatively less pain and will permit evaluation of some shoulder movement.

11. What is the differential diagnosis of shoulder bursitis?

Differential diagnosis includes the following:

- Infection caused by pus producing (pyogenic) organisms, particularly *Staphylococcus aureus*. Infection is suspected in the event of particularly red, warm, and painful swellings.[1]
- Rheumatoid arthritis

- Gout
- Inflammatory arthritis

12. What rehabilitative therapy is helpful in the treatment and resolution of this pathologic condition?

Because shoulder bursitis frequently occurs secondarily to lesions of the rotator cuff, it may be viewed along the continuum of rotator cuff disorders. Because of this, shoulder bursitis may be heir to many of the same limitations inherent to rotator cuff lesions, and management will closely follow treatment of rotator cuff disorder. For a more complete discussion of treatment (see pp. 113-118 and 133-135).

- *Rest.*
- *Ice* to reduce spasm, pain, and inflammation.
- *Phonophoresis* (pulsed ultrasound so as to avoid heat) with hydrocortisone ointment as a coupling agent.
- Codman's *pendulum* and gravity-eliminated rotation *exercises* in the pain-free range to maintain joint capsule mobility; weights should not be used in the acute stage.[15]
- *Nonsteroidal anti-inflammatory medication* in high doses, such as indomethacin, naproxen, or ibuprophen.[1]
- As the acute condition subsides, either *ice or heat* may be used, and a *selective strengthening program* of the rotator cuff muscles is appropriate in short arcs of motion so as to circumvent pain felt at the end of the range of motion. Rotation exercises are best done with the shoulder in approximately 30° to 40° abduction so as to avoid wringing out the supraspinatus tendon.[15]
- Gentle grade I or grade II *joint mobilization* to the glenohumeral joint[7] and shoulder girdle joints so as to stave off the effects of stiffening.
- Sparing *steroid injection* after aspiration in those patients experiencing intensely severe and disabling pain.[14] However, a trial of therapeutic management with nonsteroidal antiinflammatory medication is attempted before injection, since multiple injections have been shown to cause weakening of myotendinous structures and, at best, are treating only inflammation as often evidenced by short-term relief that is followed by gradual return of the disorder. In any event, if pain relief is gained, a serious isolated rotator cuff strengthening program must be launched, as well as appropriate capsular and soft-tissue stretching, with the strategy of treating the aforesaid disorder at its origin, such as the altered biomechanics at the shoulder.[15]
- *Surgical exploration,* excision of calcific deposit, and possibly subtotal acromionectomy are indicated in the occasional completely refractory patient.[13]

References

1. Berkow R: *The Merck manual of diagnosis and therapy,* ed 15, Rahway, N.J., 1987, Merck, Sharp & Dohme Research Laboratories.
2. Bland JD, Merrit JA, Boushey DR: The painful shoulder, *Semin Arthritis Rheum* 7(1):21, 1977.
3. Codman EA: *The shoulder,* Boston, 1934, Thomas Todd Co.
4. Cuillo J: Swimmer's shoulder, *Clin Sports Med* 5:115-136, 1984.
5. Cyriax J: *Textbook of orthopaedic medicine,* vol 1: *Diagnosis of soft tissue lesions,* London, 1982, Bailliere-Tindall.
6. Hoppenfeld S: *Physical examination of the spine and extremities,* Norwalk, Conn., 1976, Appleton-Century-Crofts.
7. Kisner C, Colby LA: *Therapeutic exercise: foundation and techniques,* ed 2, Philadelphia, 1990, FA Davis.
8. Lillegard WA, Rucher KS: *Handbook of sports medicine: a symptom-oriented approach,* Boston, 1993, Andover Medical Publishers.

9. Moffat M: *Lecture and handout series on musculoskeletal therapeutic exercise,* New York, Fall 1989, New York University Department of Physical Therapy.
10. Moore KL: *Clinically oriented anatomy,* ed 2, Baltimore, 1985, Williams & Wilkins.
11. Peterson L, Renström P: *Sports injuries: their prevention and treatment,* London, 1986, Martin Dunitz, Ltd, p 190.
12. Rockwood CA, Matsen FA, editors: *The shoulder,* vol 2, Philadelphia, 1990, Saunders.
13. Rodman GP, Schumacher HR: *Primer on the rheumatic diseases,* ed 8, Atlanta, 1983, Arthritis Foundation.
14. Salter RB: *Textbook of disorders of the musculoskeletal system,* ed 2, Baltimore, 1983, Williams & Wilkins.
15. Saunders ED: *Evaluation, treatment and prevention of musculoskeletal disorders,* Minneapolis, 1985, Viking Press.
16. Schumacher HR, Bomalaski JS: *Case studies in rheumatology for the house officer,* Baltimore, 1990, Williams & Wilkins.

Recommended reading

Rodman GP, Schumacher HR: *Primer on the rheumatic diseases,* ed 8, Atlanta, 1985, Arthritis Foundation.

Salter RB: *Textbook of disorders of the musculoskeletal system,* ed 2, Baltimore, 1983, Williams & Wilkins, p 2141.

Saunders ED: *Evaluation, treatment and prevention of musculoskeletal disorders,* Minneapolis, 1985, Viking Press, p 158.

13 Stiff and Painful Shoulder

A 64-year-old white female presents with a history of a left fractured rib 8 weeks ago while she was sleeping. She reports a history of osteoporosis as well as insulin-dependent diabetes. Her side no longer hurts, yet she complains of a diffuse aching left shoulder pain by day that wakes her at night, especially when she rolls onto the shoulder. When asked, she reports that she is unable to sleep on her left side. Pain is vaguely reported over the area of the deltoid muscle. Dressing and grooming have become nearly impossible because of the pain. There is no complaint of pain to the neck, upper back, elbow, or hand. She complains that she can no longer unbuckle her brassiere from behind, though she can perform most functional activities with her right dominant upper extremity.

OBSERVATION Her left arm appears close against her body in the position of shoulder internal rotation, adduction, and elbow flexion. When she is asked to elevate her left shoulder, she appears to hike her shoulder upward to approximately 40°. There is slight muscle wasting observed over the bellies of the musculocutaneous cuff musculature.

PALPATION There is point tenderness present over the bicipital groove.

ACTIVE AND PASSIVE MOVEMENTS An empty end feel is appreciated. Specific ranges are difficult to measure because of gross limitation of left shoulder movement in virtually all ranges. Approximate ranges are as follows:

- External rotation (ER): 45°
- Abduction: 80°
- Internal rotation (IR): 70°

The following pattern emerges: ER is more limited than abduction which, in turn, is more limited than medial rotation.

JOINT PLAY Anterior and inferior glide are particularly limited, as is lateral distraction. The scapulothoracic (ST) joint feels partially bound because retraction and protraction are grossly limited to one half of their normal range as compared to the contralateral scapula.

RESISTIVE TESTING Left shoulder yields pain when reaching the end range but no pain at midrange.

SENSATION Normal.

REFLEXES Normal.

CLUE An arthrogram of the left shoulder showed a reduced volume of the left glenohumeral joint capsule as well as inapparent axillary fold and biceps brachii sheath.

1. **What disorder is most likely affecting this woman?**
2. **How is frozen shoulder (FS) classified?**
3. **What is the mechanism of contracture formation at the tissue level in secondary FS?**
4. **What anatomy is requisite to understanding the FS disorder?**
5. **What is the result in the clinical course of either type of FS?**
6. **What are the epidemiologic characteristics of FS?**
7. **What is the clinical presentation of FS?**
8. **What are the signs and symptoms of FS?**
9. **What is meant by reverse scapulothoracic rhythm?**
10. **What accounts for pinpoint tenderness over the bicipital groove?**
11. **What is the differential diagnosis?**
12. **How revealing are laboratory investigations?**
13. **What rehabilitative therapy is appropriate to treating this condition?**
14. **What does manipulation or surgery involve, and when is it appropriate?**

1. What disorder is most likely affecting this woman?

Adhesive capsulitis, or *frozen shoulder* (FS), is a distinct clinical syndrome[33] associated with pain and restricted range of active and passive glenohumeral motion.[24] In the majority of cases, frozen shoulder is a self-limiting disorder that resolves with time though leaving some residual loss of motion in up to 70% of all patients.[2] Because of functional loss in 10% to 15% of patients[2] and because there is no consistently effective treatment, a strong case exists for prevention through avoidance of immobilization after trauma or other pathologic state in the shoulder.[16]

2. How is frozen shoulder (FS) classified?

Primary FS Patients having no positive findings in their history, clinical examination, or radiographic review that could explain their pain and a decrease in shoulder motion are classified as having primary FS.[19] These primary idiopathic cases are the most common forms of FS and result from an unknown stimulus that produces profound histologic changes in the capsule that are substantially different from changes produced by simple immobilization.[32] An autoimmune theory has been proposed as the pathomechanics of primary FS, but no conclusive evidence has been found.[5b,37a]

Secondary FS In contrast to the former, secondary FS develops after a variety of antecedent episodes such as accidental injury, surgery of the breast or upper limb, upper limb immobilization, rib fracture, primary cancer or infection, myocardial infarction, cervical disc disease, arthritis, or lengthy duration of intravenous infusion.[18] In most cases, the common denominator is disuse of the upper extremity with the shoulder typically held in internal rotation (IR) and in adduction and with the elbow in flexion. Disuse of the limb in this position places the anteroinferior portion of the glenohumeral (GH) joint such that the capsular attachments approximate and foreshorten with time as adhesions develop.[34]

3. What is the mechanism of contracture formation at the tissue level in secondary FS?

Histologically the GH joint capsule is composed of bundles of type I collagen aligned with the axis of tensile strength of the capsule. In secondary FS restriction is caused by thickening and tightening of the capsule by binding and proliferation of individual collagen fibers (Fig. 13-1).

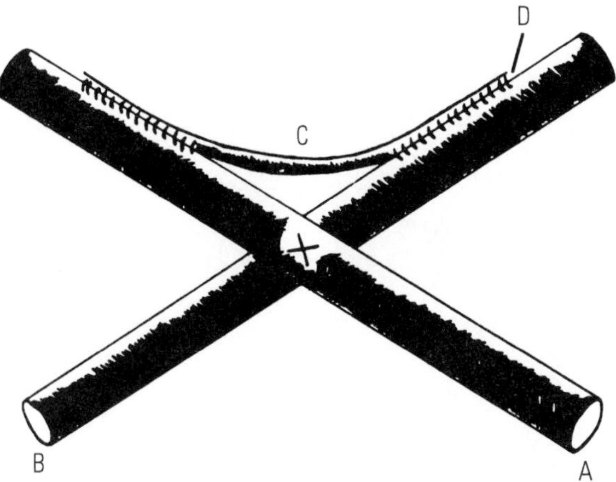

Fig. 13-1 Mechanism of contracture formation at the tissue level. Collagen fibrils, **A** and **B,** come into close contact at point × because of loss of spacing-ground substance. New collagen fibrils, **C,** become fixed by cross-linking, **D,** to inhibit normal gliding. (From Akeson WH, Amiel D, Woo SL-Y: *Biorheology* 17:95-110, 1980.)

4. What anatomy is requisite to understanding the FS disorder?

The GH joint is statically supported by secondary thickenings of the GH joint capsule. The tendons of the rotator cuff adjacent to the joint capsule thicken and support the capsule anteriorly, superiorly, and posteriorly, but not inferiorly (Fig. 13-2, *A*). It is this hiatus that is responsible for the disorder of anteroinferior (that is, subglenoid) shoulder dislocation. In the normal resting position with the arm at the side, it is the oblique orientation of the glenoid fossa that provides a resting shelf for the humeral head. As elevation commences and progresses, the fossa's orientation becomes increasingly vertical as the humeral glides, by analogy, along its runway toward the infraglenoid tubercle. At peak elevation the humeral head is held against an almost vertical fossa as a function of scapular protraction and is prevented from being dislocated inferiorly by the *inferior capsule*—that redundant (double) *axillary fold* of now-tautened ligamentous tissue forming the inferior recess. This inferior capsular ligament will collapse into a lax, pouch-like fold when the arm hangs down in adduction, the slack of which is quickly taken up during elevation because of tautening of this inferior capsule (Fig.13-2, *B*).

5. What is the result in the clinical course of either type of FS?

A low-grade inflammatory response may develop involving the capsule, synovial membrane (synovitis), and musculocutaneous cuff.[24] As a result, adhesions form between all these structures as the normal capsular folds, pouches, and joint cavity become obliterated. The contracted and thickened joint capsule is drawn tightly around the humeral head[25] to eventually become fixed to the bone,[27] and the musculocutaneous cuff muscle bellies become contracted, fixed, and inelastic[22] (Fig. 13-3).

6. What are the epidemiologic characteristics of FS?

Occurring twice as often in females as in males,[24] FS is rarely seen in patients less than 40 and over 70 years of age,[5] except for diabetic patients. Frozen shoulder is more common in the nondominant arm,[14] and about 12% of all patients develop the condition bilaterally.[32] There is a higher than normal association between FS and diabetes mellitus. The incidence of FS in the general population ranges from 2% to 5%

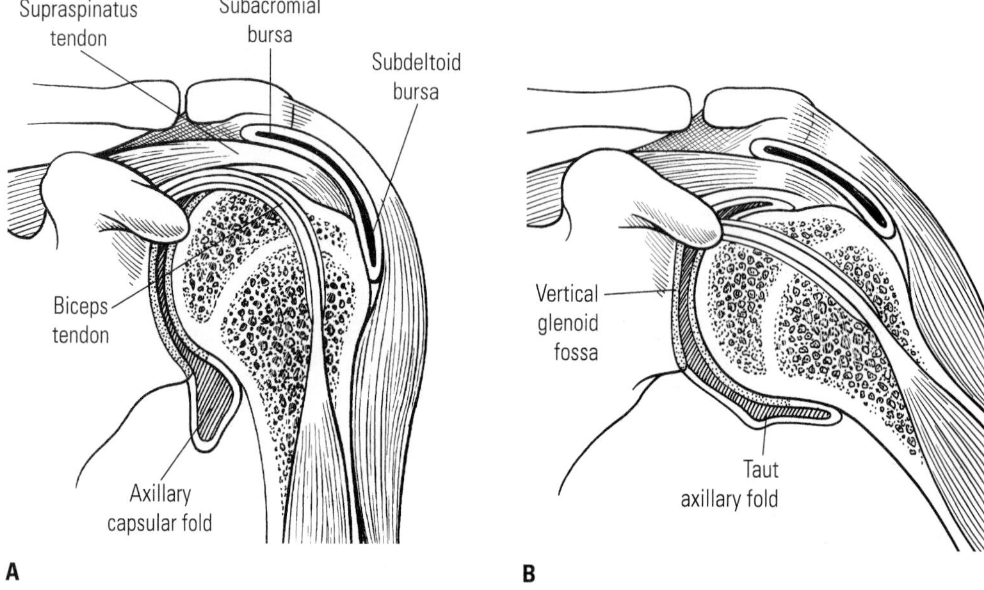

Fig. 13-2 **A,** Coronal section of a left glenohumeral joint showing the inferior capsule unsupported by dynamic constraints. This inferior recess makes a redundant fold with the arm at the side. **B,** As the shoulder is elevated the redundant axillary fold is tautened, providing static support and preventing excessive inferior excursion of the glenohumeral head.

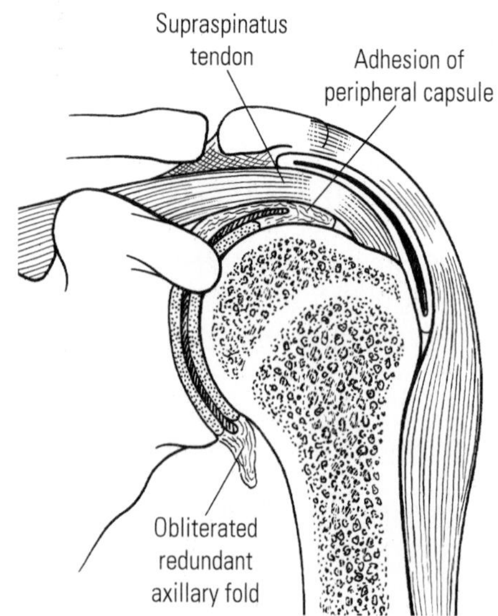

Fig. 13-3 Cross-sectional view of left shoulder shows adhesion development obliterating the redundant axillary fold.

whereas among diabetics, 10% to 20%.[4] Insulin-dependent diabetics have an even higher incidence (36%) of FS as well as a considerably increased frequency of bilateral shoulder involvement (42%).[6]

7. What is the clinical presentation of FS?

Frozen shoulder is a self-limiting disorder lasting 12 to 18 months[10] that classically presents as a cycle of three distinct stages:[33] freezing, frozen, and thawing.[30] These stages are neatly packaged in literature as spanning 6 months each but may actually last shorter or longer because they vary from individual to individual. In patients with secondary FS, these three phases may not always be recognizable.

Stage 1 The *freezing,* or *painful inflammatory, phase* is characterized by acute constant shoulder pain and muscle spasm that restricts movement in all directions, particularly in a *capsular pattern.* The onset is gradual and is experienced as diffuse shoulder pain which the patient has difficulty in localizing anatomically.[33] It is often difficult to obtain a history of any precipitating event. Patients often describe a progressive onset of pain lasting for weeks and months before seeking orthopedic consultation. Pain is usually worse at night and is exacerbated when the patient lies on the affected side. It is during this initial phase that patients are most anxious. As the patient uses the arm less and less, there is usually less discomfort, with the patient taking false satisfaction that he or she is doing the best thing for the shoulder. The duration of this phase is variable, lasting anywhere from 2 to 9 months.[30] The pain during this phase is even elicited during the midrange of movement.

Stage 2 The *frozen,* or *stiff, phase* is characterized by subsiding pain[16] and progressive loss of shoulder movement in a capsular pattern. When elicited, pain is not felt during midrange but rather at end range, such that suddenly reaching out to grab a swinging door or to catch a falling object is vividly described by the patient as being sharply painful. In this stage pain during rest subsides, and discomfort in the form of a dull ache[33] occurs during movement.[16] Functional restrictions increase as immobility sets in, and patients often seek out the clinician[14] at this stage because they are alarmed by their inability to reach out for a telephone, remove a wallet from a back pocket, reach for an object in the back seat of a car, or swing a golf club or tennis racket.[33] The duration of this phase may last anywhere between 4 to 12 months.[30]

Stage 3 The *thawing phase* is characterized by gradual regaining of shoulder movement, as the shrunken and adherent capsule becomes separated from the humeral head. As motion slowly increases, there is a progressive lessening of discomfort, which comes as a great relief to the patient.[33] This occurs when a patient regains functional stages, such as being able to tuck one's shirt or blouse behind the back, wash one's hair, or achieve a more natural golf swing.[2] The time for regaining of shoulder motion is variable and unpredictable. For some this may require a 4- to 6-week period to resolve, whereas for others this may take up to 6 or even 9 months.[33]

8. What are the signs and symptoms of FS?

Limitation of shoulder motion and its imposition on function is usually the symptom that prods the patient to seek initial attention.[14] Motion is guarded with protective muscle spasm as a common feature that accounts for the arm held against the body in shoulder adduction and medial rotation. Because of pain and guarding, the patient often refuses to allow the joint to be moved to where resistance is felt by the examiner (that is, an *empty end feel*). Later on, after pain has subsided and only decreased motion persists, a capsular end feel is imparted by capsular structures limiting the range.[35]

The limitation of passive range of motion found in FS is characteristic of a capsular pattern. Lateral rotation is more limited than abduction, which in turn is more limited than medial rotation. During maximal capsular restriction, glenohumeral (GH) joint measurements average approximately 45° ER, less than 80° of abduction, and less than 70° of medial rotation.[18] Testing for accessory GH joint movements demonstrates tightness (that is, physiologic loss of motion) in the anterior and inferior aspects of the GH joint capsule, correlating to osteokinematic loss of lateral rotation and abduction respectively (capsular pattern); lateral distraction is also limited.[36] There may also be decreased scapulothoracic range because of secondary adhesions developing within that joint.

The pain of FS is present during both activity and rest, with patients frequently complaining of pain at night and being unable to sleep on the affected side.[14] As the condition progresses, pain during rest subsides, and discomfort occurs only during movement. Eventually pain will abate, whereas restriction of motion will persist.[16] There is usually no painful arc of motion.[36]

Pain may vary from a mild to a severe ache and is vaguely distributed over the deltoid muscle area, with *point tenderness at the bicipital groove.*[29] Pain may radiate distally throughout the C5 dermatome or more proximally to the upper back and neck, a symptom probably attributable to compensatory overuse of shoulder girdle muscles such as the trapezius, rather than to referred pain from the shoulder.[29] Disuse atrophy may be evident in the rotator cuff, deltoid, biceps brachii, and triceps brachii muscles.[36] Sensory and reflex testing show normal results.[36]

Resisted movements in the midrange of motion during the early painful stage is usually asymptomatic and leads the examiner to conclude that contractile tissues (such as the bicipital and cuff tendons) are uninvolved.[36] In contradistinction, these (capsular) contractile structures are unlikely to elicit pain on passive movement, whereas inelastic (capsular) soft-tissue structures may produce such pain.

9. What is meant by reverse scapulothoracic rhythm?

In healthy individuals approximately 120° elevation is attributable to the glenohumeral joint, and the remaining motion occurs at the scapulothoracic joint in a 2:1 ratio. There is considerable individual deviation[33] from this 2:1 (GH:ST) ratio among the general populace, with differences varying from person to person. With FS, limitation at the GH joint leads to compensatory movement at the ST joint[29] during attempted elevation resulting in an altered or *reverse scapulothoracic rhythm* or ratio. This is observed as a shoulder-hike[20] or girdle-hunching maneuver[36] (Fig. 13-4).

10. What accounts for pinpoint tenderness over the bicipital groove?

The joint capsule of the GH joint bridges the gap between the lesser and greater tuberosities,[17] known as the *transverse humeral ligament* or bicipital aponeurosis (see Fig. 8-9). The synovial membrane that lines the GH joint capsule invests the tendon of the long head of the biceps as that tendon passes deep to the transverse humeral ligament within the bicipital groove. In fact, this synovial sheath may extend for a distance of 5 cm beyond the transverse ligament inferior to the bicipital groove, especially when the arm is in abduction (such as the position where the least amount of biceps tendon lies within the GH joint; see Fig. 8-9).[23] Thus the synovitis within the GH joint during FS is exposed outside the GH joint at the bicipital groove and is available for provocation during palpation. This may also account for why the biceps tendon sheath is outlined arthrographically in the majority of cases of adhesive capsulitis.

11. What is the differential diagnosis?

Because FS is a symptom complex rather than a specific diagnostic entity, several causative factors are presented:

- *Posterior shoulder dislocation* presents as blocked external rotation and an overall limitation of shoulder motion that is superficially likened to FS. Appropriate history and radiographs, specifically an axillary view, conclusively determines whether the humeral head articulates with the glenoid.[33]
- In cases of *acute tendinitis* or *bursitis* restrictions of both active and passive movements of the GH joint may mimic that of FS. The history of onset should raise suspicion as to the correct diagnosis. Furthermore,

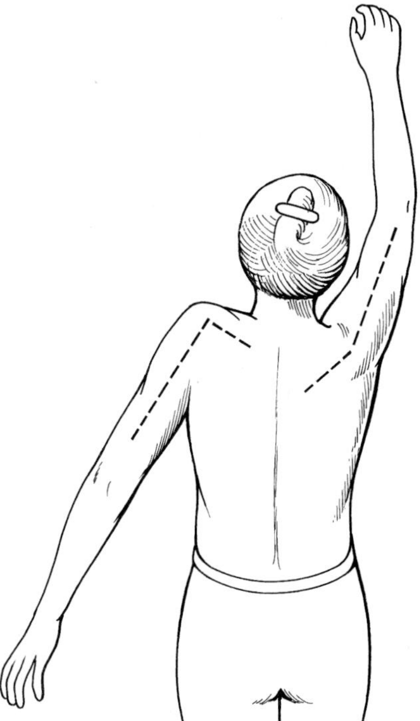

Fig. 13-4 Reverse scapulothoracic rhythm. Broken lines indicate the position of the scapular spine and humeral axis on each side, showing little or no movement in the left shoulder. This "shoulder-hiking" attempt at abduction elevates rather than depresses the humeral head.

although injection of the subacromial bursa will greatly improve passive range of motion (PROM) with the tendinitis-bursitis type of disorder, it will have little or no effect improving the range of motion (ROM) of the FS patient.[33] In addition, resistive muscle testing in midrange will be painless with FS but painfully implicates the biceps brachii or rotator cuff tendons.[8] Furthermore, whereas in FS there is initially painful restriction in every direction, supraspinatus tendinitis is characterized by pain elicited during active movement through a specific arc of movement.[36]

- A large *calcific deposit* may occasionally block active and passive shoulder motion. Shoulder radiographs taken to display the subacromial space, with the humerus in internal and external rotation, should detect such a calcification.[19]
- A painful acromioclavicular (AC) joint may also mimic FS and is suspected when clinical findings reveal localized tenderness over the AC joint. Lidocaine into the AC joint should relieve all symptoms in a primary *AC joint disorder* such as arthritis. In the event of partial pain relief, but without improvement in ROM, the clinician must look beyond the AC joint for the cause of symptoms.[33] AC joint sprain is characterized by a large lump over the lateral end of the clavicle.
- *Osteochondromatosis* or other causes of intra-articular loose bodies may present as a painful stiff shoulder and are identified by the typical locking or catching of the GH joint. Loose bodies may appear on the radiograph.[33]

- Primary or secondary *malignancy* must be ruled out in most patients in their sixth decade or older who present with localized skeletal pain. Radiographic imaging of soft tissues, radionuclide bone scanning, and blood screening are indicated. A biopsy may be considered once a specific lesion is identified.[33]

12. How revealing are laboratory investigations?

Arthrography is the standard diagnostic test for FS.[27] This technique reveals at least a 50% reduction of shoulder joint volume (such as, 5 to 10 ml compared to approximately 20 to 30 ml in healthy shoulders).[32] Other findings include irregular joint outline,[26] tight and thickened capsule,[27] loss of axillary fold, and biceps brachii tendon sheath not evident[24] because of dye absence.[10] Arthrographic findings do not indicate the type of onset (primary or secondary) or the rate and extent of recovery.[3] No abnormality is detected on plain radiographs except mild to moderate bone demineralization (osteopenia)[31] caused by disuse[24] in those patients who have had a prolonged period of disuse.[31] Decreased space between the acromion and the humeral head[32] may also be apparent. Radionuclide bone scanning often slows an increased uptake of contrast material in patients with FS.[37] Hematologic investigations reveal an association between HLA-B27 histocompatibility antigen and patients suffering from FS.[5a]

13. What rehabilitative therapy is appropriate to treating this condition?

The treatment objective in the early stage of FS is to interrupt the cycle of pain and inflammation and facilitate an early "thaw" of the frozen joint. Improvement tends to be characterized by spurts and plateaus.[34] Initially, treatment modalities include:

- *Salicitate analgesics* with or without codeine[33] to allow movement into the painful range.
- *Pendulum* swing and circular swing exercises for 2 to 3 minutes every 1 to 2 hours to be performed into the painful range.[33] Moving tissues engorged with blood and inflammatory exudate stimulates circulation and resorption of cellular debris.[36] Pendulum exercises with attached cuff weights at the wrist permit some range of motion with passive distraction of the glenohumeral joint.
- *Passive range of motion exercise* facilitates improved motion,[21] but may also reduce pain because of a neuromodulation effect on joint mechanoreceptors.[1] The therapist may assist in depressing the humeral head as the patient attempts to elevate, to prevent pinching of subacromial tissue.
- *Iontophoresis* or *phonophoresis* using ions with analgesic and anti-inflammatory properties.
- *Transcutaneous electrical stimulation* to relieve pain.

If after approximately 2 weeks pain continues, an injection of corticosteroid with lidocaine may give significant pain relief.

As the pain subsides, the following therapeutic modalities may be added to the treatment regimen:

- *Active range of motion* in forward elevation with either internal or external rotation into the painful end range so as to prevent adhesion formation.[34] The therapist may passively assist during the end range of movement as he or she may guide the limb further into the range without eliciting spasm or a stretch reflex that accompanies muscle guarding. Initially, active abduction is best carried out while the therapist passively depresses the humeral head so as to avoid pinching subacromial tissue.
- *Strengthening exercises* are very important, since FS often leads to muscle shortening, weakness, and atrophy. Strengthening begins as the range of GH motion returns, and is most effective as short arc exercises using an elastic band within the *pain-free* range.[34] Exercises may initially be isometric because attempts at isotonic activity may be thwarted by reflex inhibition and pain.
- *Joint mobilization* (grades I or II) even into *painful* physiologic range is appropriate because this is not harmful and simply facilitates increased capsular mobility[34] by stretching and breaking adhesions. Good mobilization strategy would include stretching the predominantly tight portions of the capsule that limit motion in a capsular pattern, that is, to stretch the anterior and medioinferior portions of the

capsule so as to facilitate increased range in external rotation and abduction respectively. Mobilization must seek to localize stretch to specific portions of the joint capsule and then gradually to increase intensity without eliciting protective muscle contraction.

Inferior glide is comfortable for patients and very helpful in relieving muscle spasm. Achieving this movement is particularly important, since spasm, present in the acute stage, interferes with normal joint mechanics by causing the humeral head to move superiorly. Inferior glide may be performed with the patient lying prone and with the arm hanging freely off the side of the plinth.[12]

- Gentle self-mobilization exercises may be incorporated in the subacute stage as the patient begins to tolerate capsular stretching. Moving the body in relation to a stabilized humerus is safer for the joint and less painful for the patient to perform[15] (Fig. 13-5, *A*).

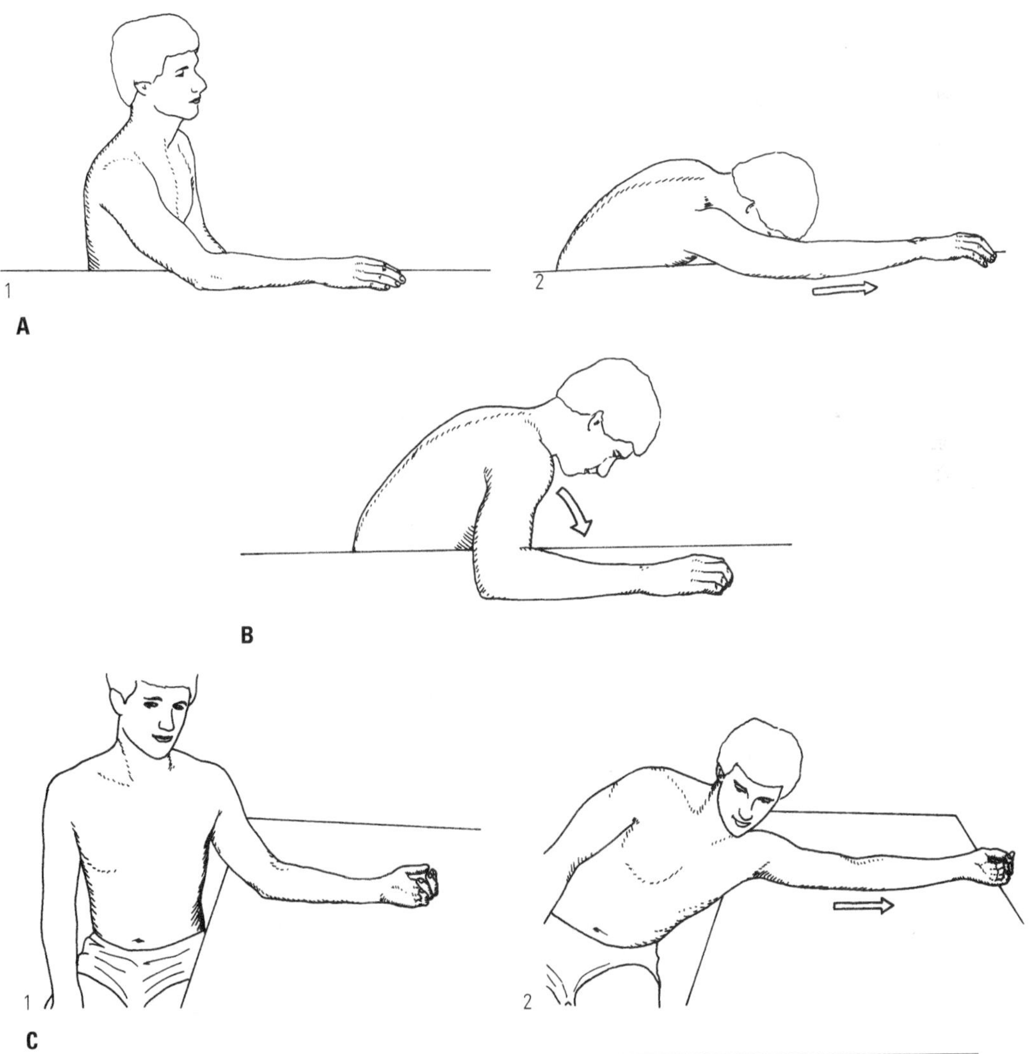

Fig. 13-5 **A,** Beginning, *1*, and end, *2*, positions for self-stretching to increase shoulder flexion with elevation. **B,** End position for self-stretching to increase shoulder external rotation. **C,** Beginning, *1*, and end, *2*, positions for self-stretching to increase shoulder abduction with elevation.

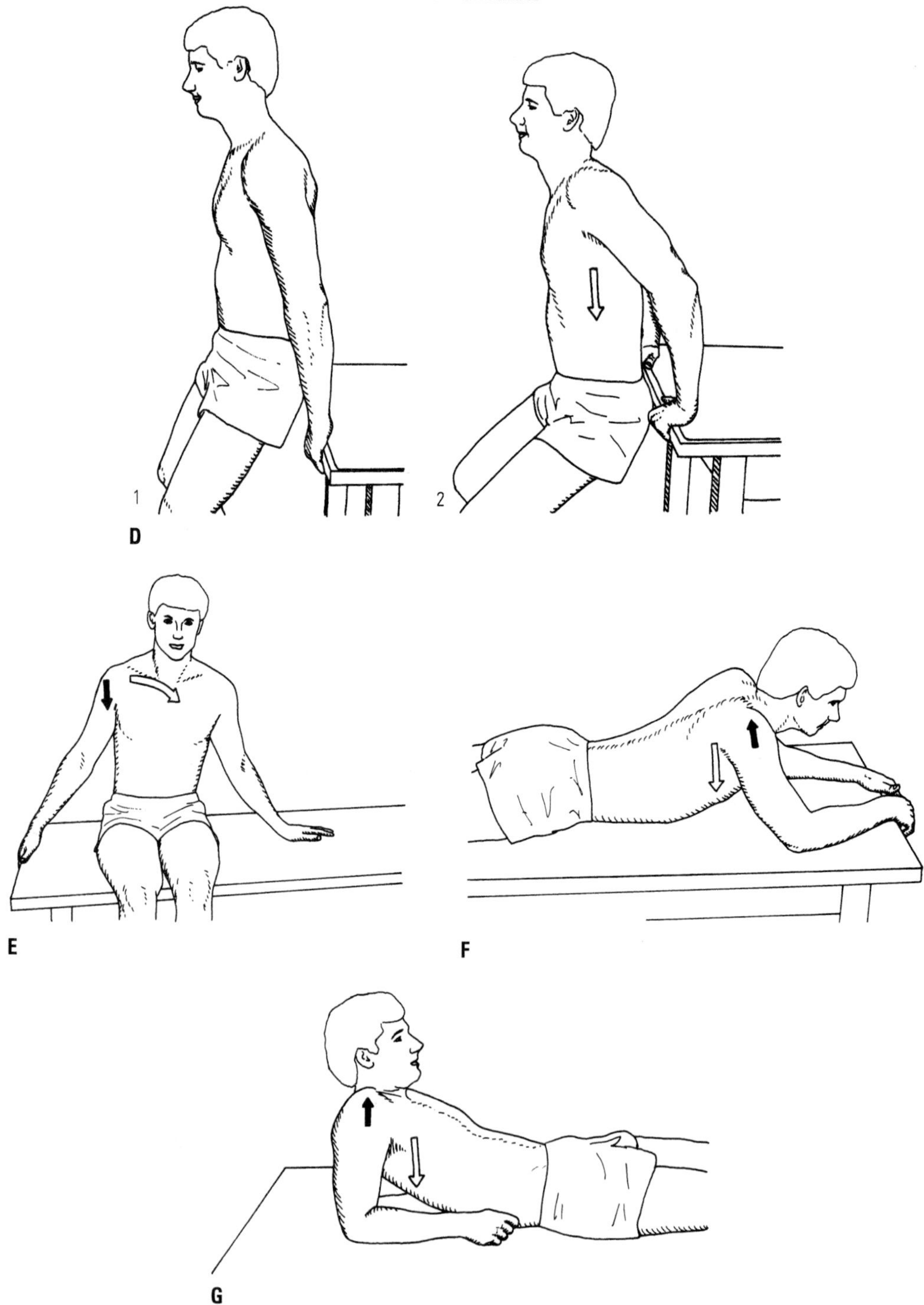

Fig. 13-5, cont'd. D, Beginning, *1,* and end, *2,* positions for self-stretching to increase shoulder extension. **E,** Self-mobilization; caudal glide of the humerus occurs as the person leans away from the fixed arm. **F,** Self-mobilization; posterior glide of the humerus occurs as the person shifts his body weight downward between the fixed arms. **G,** Self-mobilization; anterior glide of the humerus occurs as the person leans between the fixed arms. (From Kisner C, Colby LA: *Therapeutic exercise: foundations and techniques,* ed 2, Philadelphia, 1990, FA Davis.)

- *Moist heat*[33] before mobilization and stretching exercises, provided that inflammation is reduced, is helpful to increasing tissue extensibility. Gains in reclaiming range of motion may be preserved by ice packing with the shoulder supported in the position of maximum abduction and external rotation.[34]
- *Ultrasound* provides a deep heating effect precisely to the muscle-bone interface and is best applied at the anteroinferior capsule with the arm stretched into abduction and ER. Ultrasound also breaks down molecular binding that causes criss-crossed collagen fibers in the joint capsule to adhere to one another.[11] By increasing tissue extensibility, ultrasound is especially useful when used before manual techniques stretching the glenohumeral joint capsule.
- *Stretching* activities include using the good extremity to assist the affected arm up the back progressively achieving greater range of IR. A towel in the opposite hand passed over the opposite shoulder pulling the affected hand up the back may accomplish the same effect. IR stretching may be initiated when one stretches into extension using a stick behind the back. Forward elevation stretch may be performed by assisted elevation of the arm so as to reach up to a solid object just beyond one's reach. Patients stand on tiptoes and then lower themselves and sustain a moderate stretch adjusted to tolerance for 20 to 30 seconds. This stretching is repeated 5 times, and then the arm is assisted down by use of the opposite arm, since freefall from the new upper limit of forward elevation can be very painful.[33] It may be necessary to achieve stretching of the joint capsule before one performs stretches into specific ranges.
- *Wand exercises* to increase range of motion and strength to the shoulder. A Velcro cuff may eventually be added for resistance. (See Fig. 6-5.)
- *Muscular reeducation* to minimize the substitution pattern of left shoulder elevation by means of a right shoulder shrug and right trunk lean. Once normal range is regained, the patient is instructed to palpate the left upper trapezius for muscular activity while performing left shoulder elevation before a mirror. This allows incorporation of visual feedback of trapezius activity and avoidance of right-sided trunk bending.
- *Prevention.* A strong case for prevention may be made because no treatment is consistently effective for management of FS.[16] Many patients receive little or no advice from the emergency room or orthopedic physician regarding the need for early motion. The classic example is of a patient sent home from the doctor wearing a shoulder sling cradling the upper extremity after a finger or wrist fracture.

14. What does manipulation or surgery involve, and when is it appropriate?

Manipulation under anesthesia as treatment of FS is a source of much controversy in orthopedic circles[9] because of complications such as fracture, dislocation, brachial plexus injury, and gross tearing of soft tissue causing further scarring.[35] When it is performed, an assistant stabilizes the scapula while the humerus is abducted until the capsule tears. Some surgeons also perform forced lateral and medial manipulations after abduction, whereas others consider these manipulations too risky because of potential fracture.[10] After injection of corticosteroids, patients begin gentle range of motion exercise in forward elevation, external rotation, and use of a pulley for stretching on the very same day as manipulation.[33] To prevent the ruptured tissues from healing in their former state of retraction, the arm must be abducted at least 90° for 1 to 2 weeks while the patient is recumbent.[27]

Surgery is usually a last resort in those patients who have not responded to conservative treatment or for whom manipulation is contraindicated because of a history of osteoporosis, dislocation, or fracture.[27] The use of systemic steroids has inherent risks for potential systemic complications.[7]

Because there are no serious medical complications of FS, a judgment to accept restricted motion rather than undertake manipulation or surgical release is acceptable. Many patients can learn to function quite well with a moderately restricted range of shoulder motion.[33]

References

1. Barak T, Rosen ER, Sufer R: Mobility: passive orthopaedic manual therapy. In Gould JA, Davies GJ, editors: *Orthopaedic and sports physical therapy*, St. Louis, 1985, Mosby.
2. Binder AI, Bulgen DY, Hazleman BL, Roberts S: Frozen shoulder: a long-term prospective study, *Ann Rheum Dis* 43:361-364, 1984.
3. Binder AI, Bulgen DY, Hazleman BL, et al: Frozen shoulder: an arthrographic and radionuclear scan assessment, *Ann Rheum Dis* 43:365-369, 1984.
4. Bridgman JF: Panarthritis of the shoulder and diabetes mellitus, *Ann Rheum Dis* 31:69-71, 1972.
5. Bruckner FE, Nye CJS: A prospective study of adhesive capsulitis of the shoulder ("frozen shoulder") in a high risk population, *Q J Med* 198:191-204, 1981.

5a. Bulgen DY, Hazleman BL: Letter, *Lancet* 2:760, 1981.

5b. Bulgen DY, Binder A, Hazleman BL, and Park JP: Immunological studies in frozen shoulder. *Journal of Rheumatology* 9(6):893-898, 1982.

6. Conti V: Arthroscopy in rehabilitation, *Orthop Clin North Am* 10(3):709-711, 1979.
7. Cruess RL: Corticosteroid-induced osteonecrosis of the humeral head, *Orthop Clin North Am* 16(4):789-796, 1985.
8. Dandy DJ: *Essential orthopaedics and trauma*, London, 1989, Churchill Livingstone.
9. De Seze S: Les épaules douloureuses et les épaules bloquées, *Concours Med* 96(36):5329-5357, 1974.
10. Grey RG: The natural history of idiopathic frozen shoulder, *J Bone Joint Surg* 60:564, 1978.
11. Griffin J: Physiological effects of ultrasonic energy as it is used clinically, *Phys Ther* 46:18-23, 1966.
12. Hertling D, Kessler RM: Management of common musculoskeletal disorders, ed 2, Philadelphia, 1990, Lippincott.
13. Kaltenborn F: *Course notes*, Kent, Ohio, April 1931.
14. Kessel L, Bayley I, Young A: The upper limb: the frozen shoulder, *Br J Hosp Med* 25:334, 336-337, 339, 1981.
15. Kisner C. Colby LA: Therapeutic exercise: foundations and techniques, ed 2, Philadelphia, 1990, FA Davis.
16. Kuzin F: Two unique shoulder disorders: adhesive capsulitis and reflex sympathetic dystrophy syndrome, *Postgrad Med* 73:207-210, 214-216, 1983.
17. Last RJ: *Anatomy, regional and applied*, ed 5, London, 1972, Churchill Livingstone.
18. Loyd JA, Loyd HM: Adhesive capsulitis of the shoulder: arthrographic diagnosis and treatment, *South Med J* 76:879-883, 1983.
19. Lundberg BJ: The frozen shoulder, *Acta Orthop Scand* 119(suppl):1-59, 1969.
20. Magee DJ: *Orthopaedic physical assessment*, Philadelphia, 1989, Saunders.
21. Maitland GO: Treatment of the glenohumeral joint by passive movement, *Physiotherapy* 69:3-7, 1983.
22. McLaughlin HL: On the frozen shoulder, *Bull Hosp Joint Dis* 12:383-393, 1951.
23. Moseley HF: *Shoulder lesions*. Springfield, Ill., 1945, Charles C Thomas.
24. Netter FM: The CIBA collection of medical illustrations, vol 8: *Musculoskeletal system*, part 2, Summit, N.J., 1990, CIBA-Geigy Corp., p 199.
25. Neviaser JS: Adhesive capsulitis of the shoulder, *J Bone Joint Surg* 27:211-222, 1945.
26. Neviaser JS: Arthrography of the shoulder joint, *J Bone Joint Surg* 44:1321-1330, 1962.
27. Neviaser JS: Adhesive capsulitis and the stiff and painful shoulder, *Orthop Clin North Am* 11:327-333, 1980.
28. Nicholson GG: The effects of passive joint mobilization on pain and hypomobility associated with adhesive capsulitis of the shoulder, *Orthop Sports Phys Ther* 6:238-246, 1985.
29. Post M, editor: *The shoulder: surgical and nonsurgical management*, Philadelphia, 1978, Lea & Febiger.
30. Reeves B: The natural history of the frozen shoulder syndrome, *Scand J Rheumatol* 4:193-196, 1975.
31. Resnick D: Shoulder pain, *Orthop Clin North Am* 14(1):81-97, 1983.
32. Rizk TE, Pinals RS: Frozen shoulder, *Semin Arthritis Rheum* 11:440-452, 1982.
33. Rockwood CA, Matsen FA, editors: *The shoulder*, vol 2, Philadelphia, 1990, Saunders.
34. Saunders HD: *Evaluation, treatment and prevention of musculoskeletal disorders*, Bloomingdale, Minn., 1985, Educational Opportunities.
35. Simon WH: Soft tissue disorders of the shoulder: frozen shoulder, calcific tendinitis, and bicipital tendinitis, *Orthop Clin North Am* 6:521-539, 1975.
36. Wadsworth CT: Frozen shoulder, *Phys Ther* 66(12): 1878-1883, 1986.
37. Wright MG, Richards AJ, Clarke MB: Letter: ^{99m}Tc-pertechnetate scanning in capsulitis, *Lancet* 2:1265-1296, 1975.

37a. Young A: Immunological studies in the frozen shoulder. In: Bailey J. and Kessel L (eds.): *Shoulder surgery.* Berlin-Heidelberg: Springer Verlag, 1982, pp 110-113.

Recommended reading

Grey RG: The natural history of idiopathic frozen shoulder, *J Bone Joint Surg* 60:564, 1978.

Rockwood CA, Matsen FA, editors: *The shoulder*, vol 2, Philadelphia, 1990, Saunders, pp. 837-862.

Wadsworth CT: Frozen shoulder, *Phys Ther*, 66(12):1878-1883, 1986.

Painful Bump over Distal End of Clavicle 14

A 31-year-old father presents with immediate pain and a bump over the left distal end of the clavicle, which happened yesterday when he tried to demonstrate a cartwheel to his 4-year-old son. When asked, he reports that he fell onto his shoulder. The patient volunteers that attempting to touch his right shoulder with his left hand and trying to elevate his shoulder are most painful.

CLUE:

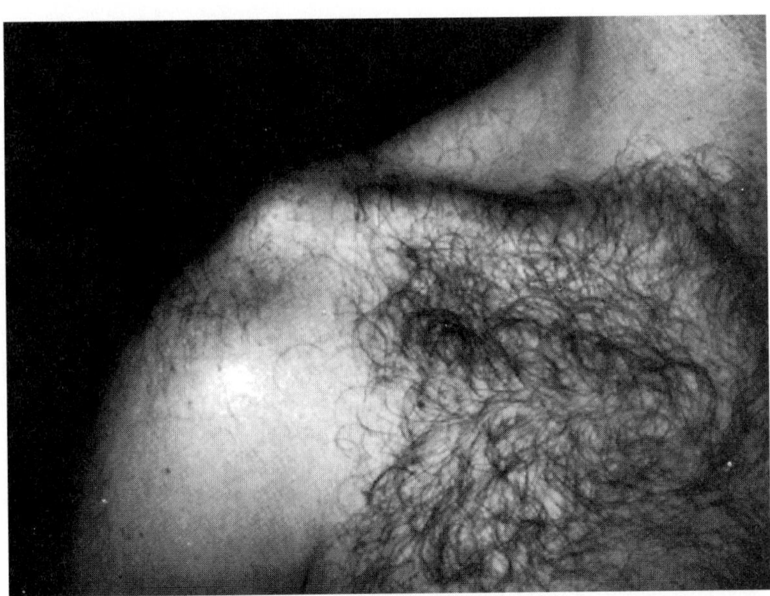

(From Nicholas JA, Hershman EB, editors: *The upper extremity in sports medicine*, ed 2, St. Louis, 1995, Mosby.)

PALPATION There is pain and tenderness, with protruding bump felt over left distal end of clavicle.

PASSIVE RANGE OF MOTION Painful at extremes of motion.

ACTIVE RANGE OF MOTION Full and painful, though left shoulder abduction to 90° and horizontal abduction elicited increased pain. Left shoulder shrugging is also painful.

MUSCLE STRENGTH Left shoulder flexion and abduction to 90° are weakened to good minus.

SELECTIVE TENSION Resistive horizontal adduction is painful.

1. **What is most likely to have happened?**
2. **What is the anatomy of the acromioclavicular (AC) joint?**
3. **What are four bony variations of the AC joint in decreasing order of incidence?**
4. **Is there a disk or meniscus interposed between the articulating ends of the clavicle and the acromion?**
5. **What is the kinesiology of the AC joint?**
6. **What are the pathomechanics of injury?**
7. **What is the clinical presentation?**
8. **What is the classification of injury?**
9. **What therapeutic management is appropriate for first- and second-degree AC joint sprains?**
10. **What is the recommended treatment for third-degree AC joint sprain?**

1. What is most likely to have happened?

A shoulder disarticulation referred to as a shoulder separation involving the acromioclavicular joint. When untreated, the injury may result in permanent residual deformity, weakened shoulder abduction,[7] and eventual traumatic arthritis.

2. What is the anatomy of the acromioclavicular (AC) joint?

The AC joint is a planar (that is, gliding) synovial joint. The flat lateral flare of the scapular spine known as the "acromion process" articulates with the lateral end of the convex clavicle. Stability of this joint is primarily provided by the *AC joint capsule and ligament complex*. Providing *anteroposterior stability* of the AC joint, this complex is the first structure to absorb an impact in the event of injury. A *secondary static stabilizer* is the *coracoclavicular ligament*, consisting of a *medial conoid band* and a *lateral trapezoid portion* (Fig. 14-1), which together provide *vertical plane stability*. These latter two ligaments, by virtue of the orientation of span, enable the clavicle to hold the scapula and upper limb[6] in what is colloquially described as a "broad shoulder." The third source of stability to the AC joint is the dynamic contribution of the trapezius and deltoid attachments to the superior aspect of the AC ligaments.

3. What are four bony variations of the AC joint in decreasing order of incidence?

Bony variations of the AC joint are presented according to their increased frequency within the population.

- Distal end is oblique and overrides a congruous obliquity of the acromion.
- Articular surfaces are vertical and congruous.
- Articular surfaces are incongruous.
- Distal surface is oblique and underrides a congruous acromial articular surface.[5]

4. Is there a disk or meniscus interposed between the articulating ends of the clavicle and the acromion?

The wedge-shaped intra-articular disk (Fig. 14-2) has been found to be missing in approximately 80% of the population. Before 20 years of age, segments of human population possess menisci or an intra-articular disk

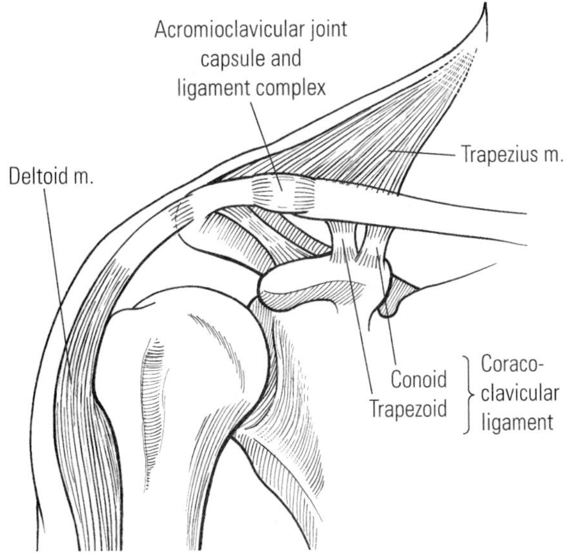

Fig. 14-1 Acromioclavicular joint stability provided by primary, secondary, and tertiary joint stabilizers.

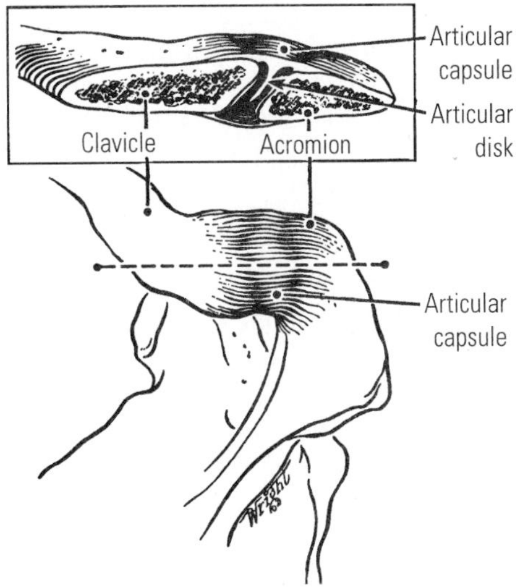

Fig. 14-2 Superior view of the right acromioclavicular joint. *Inset,* Coronal section of the joint showing a wedge-shaped intra-articular disk. (From Moore KL: *Clinically oriented anatomy,* ed 2, Baltimore, 1985, Williams & Wilkins.)

interposed between the acromion and the clavicle. After 30 years of age, many people show degenerative changes of these structures.[5]

5. What is the kinesiology of the AC joint?

The kinesiologic function of the AC joint must be understood in the context of clavicle function. The clavicle undergoes long axis rotation between both the AC and the sternoclavicular (SC) joints. Because of its

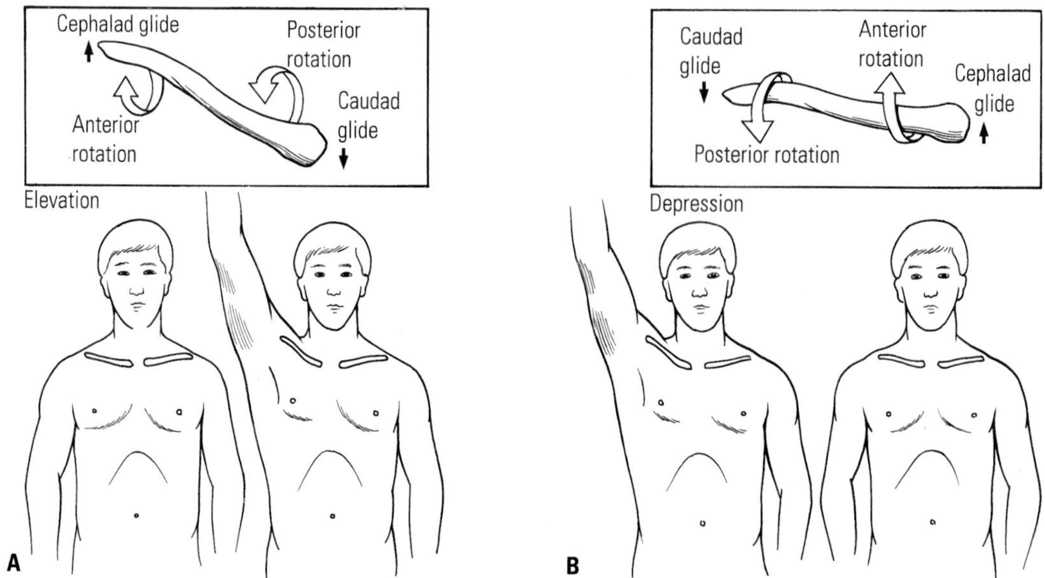

Fig. 14-3 Medial and lateral clavicular movements corresponding to shoulder elevation and depression. **A,** Shoulder elevation is accompanied by the latter end of the clavicle undergoing elevation and anterior rotation; the opposite motions occur at the medial end. **B,** Reverse motion sequence occurs. Thus, the two ends of the clavicle move vertically, albeit inversely to each other, like a mechanical crank. This, as well as inverse rotations on either end, occur as a direct function of the crank-like shape of the clavicle.

gentle S shape the clavicle acts as a mechanical *crank.* What this means is that motion at one end will cause a reverse motion at the other end. During shoulder elevation, there is cephalad glide of the clavicle with anterior rotation at the acromial end, and caudal glide (depression) with posterior rotation at the sternal end of the clavicle. The opposite motions occur during shoulder depression. This may be confirmed by simultaneous palpation and observation of both the medial and lateral ends of the clavicle while the shoulder is moved through its range of flexion and depression (Fig. 14-3).

6. What are the pathomechanics of injury?

This injury is common in contact sports resulting from a hard fall onto the point of the shoulder (Fig. 14-4) as when a hockey player is "driven into the boards." This is the same mechanism as that involving injury to the upper brachial plexus that rends the shoulder and neck apart because of a great force of impact. The caudalward force drives down the acromion, though the clavicle does not descend along with it because it is strongly anchored in place by the trapezius and sternomastoid muscles; instead the stabilizing ligaments are tensed and may sprain if the force of injury exceeds their inherent strength.

7. What is the clinical presentation?

The patient presents with a large lump over the lateral end of the clavicle that is tender and severely painful at the exact site of the joint.[13] The observed protuberance occurs because the shoulder falls away from the clavicle unsupported by the weight of the upper limb so that the acromion passes inferior to the

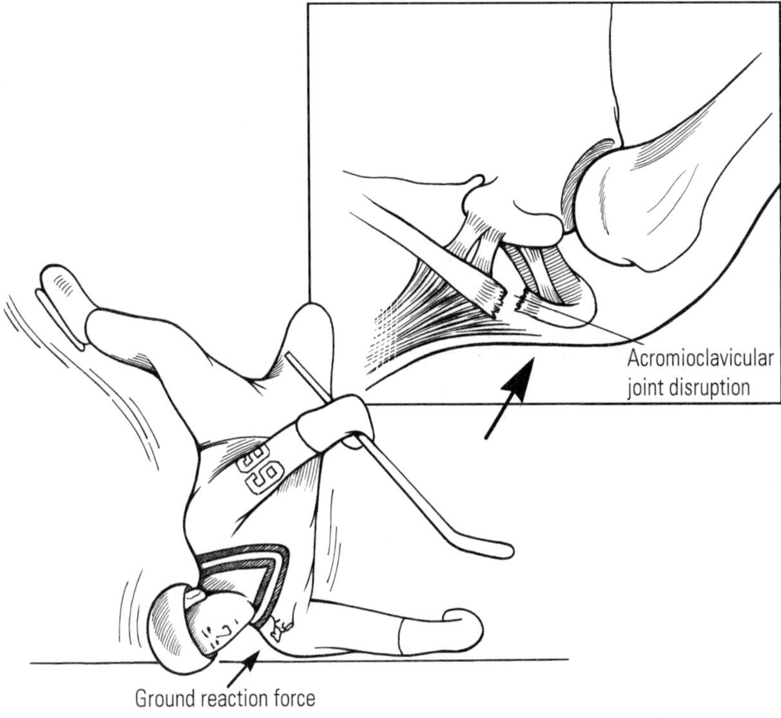

Fig. 14-4 Acromioclavicular joint sprain. Mechanism of injury.

lateral end of the clavicle. In addition, the clavicle is pulled upward by the unopposed action of the trapezius and sternomastoid muscles.[7] The result is a *stair-step deformity*[3] (see p. 165) best viewed when the arm is allowed to hang at the side. Although resistive motions, except for horizontal adduction, do not hurt, passive movements, especially at the extremes of motion are quite painful. The most painful movement is passive adduction across the front of the upper thorax; active horizontal adduction is also painful.[3] Active motion above 90° of shoulder motion will cause pain. The clavicle hangs freely, and the precise and interrelated components of shoulder function are altered so that abduction will be compromised. Pain is in fact attributable to injury to the deltoid muscle, especially on abduction, where the free end of the lateral clavicle rams up painfully into the interior of the deltoid.

8. What is the classification of injury (Fig. 14-5)?

Type I, first degree, mild injury A mild force stretches the AC joint capsule and ligament complex but does not disrupt the fibers of the joint. There is no palpable instability here.

Type II, second degree, moderate injury A moderate force disrupts the AC joint capsule and ligament complex fibers and may partially stretch or tear the coracoclavicular ligament complex. Moderate antero-posterior (A-P) instability and possible mild vertical plane instability is referred to as *subluxation* of the AC joint. Here the characteristic "step" becomes obvious and is made even more visible if the patient is given a weight to hold in each hand.

Type III, third degree, severe injury A severe force drives the scapula and its two processes downward, disrupting both the acromioclavicular and the coracoclavicular ligaments. The muscular attachments may

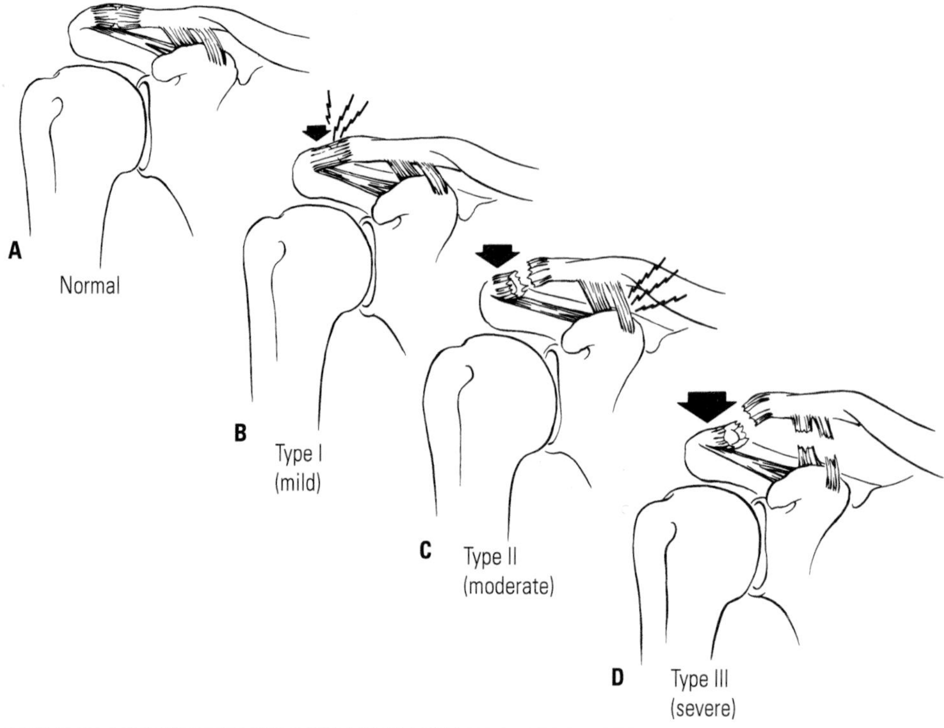

Fig. 14-5 These schematic drawings illustrate the ligamentous injuries that occur to the acromioclavicular joint. **A,** Normal anatomic relationships. **B,** In type I injury, a mild force is applied to the point of the shoulder, which stretches only the acromioclavicular articulation but does not disrupt the fibers of that joint. **C,** In type II injury, a moderate force applied to the point of the shoulder displaces the acromion process distally, disrupts the acromioclavicular ligaments, and may partially stretch the coracoclavicular ligaments. **D,** In type III injury, the severe force applied to the point of the shoulder drives the acromion and accompanying coracoid process downward, disrupting both the acromioclavicular ligaments. (From Pettrone FA, editor: *AAOS symposium on upper extremity injuries in athletes,* St. Louis, 1986, Mosby; modified from Allman FL: *J Bone Joint Surg* 49A:774, 1967. In Rockwood CA, Green OP, editors: *Fractures in adults,* ed 2, Philadelphia, 1984, Lippincott.)

have also been compromised. Pronounced A-P instability with vertical-plane instability is termed *dislocation*, since the AC joint surfaces have lost all contact. A gap may be viewed on a stress A-P radiograph and is emphasized if the patient stands while a weight is suspended from the wrist.[3]

9. What therapeutic management is appropriate for first- and second-degree AC joint sprains?

Grade I No immobilization is needed in a first-degree sprain and treatment may be with ice massage and progressive active range of motion as pain allows. Strengthening exercises should begin as the pain decreases[3] and should emphasize trapezius and deltoid strengthening to help stabilize the AC joint. Unrestricted activity is usually permitted some 7 to 10 days after the injury.[5]

Grade II

- Immobilization using an immobilizer that holds the humerus superiorly and the clavicle inferiorly[3] so as to approximate the torn ends. This position permits approximation of scar tissue so as to provide maximum stability once healing is complete.

- Cross-fiber massage to the capsule or ligaments to organize scar-tissue alignment.[4]
- Mobilization to the glenohumeral (GH), scapulothoracic (ST), and sternoclavicular (SC) joints to forestall the effects of stiffening.
- Intermittent ice.
- Gentle range of motion begun early on[3] within pain-free limits.
- As the pain decreases, wean patient off immobilization and increase activity.
- Nonpainful strengthening exercises, especially to deltoid and trapezius muscles.
- Unrestricted activity is usually achieved 2 to 3 weeks after the injury.

After a moderate sprain, some degree of residual subluxation of the AC joint may occur,[3] and may become evident when the patient later feels difficulty when working with the arms in front of the body (as when writing on a blackboard, operating a keyboard, or carrying a tray).[2]

10. What is the recommended treatment for third-degree AC joint sprain?

Treatment of type III injury is controversial and has two approaches:

Conservative approach Kenny-Howard sling halter[1] for 4 to 6 weeks,[3] ice, and isometrics to tolerance. Range of motion exercises after immobilizer is removed and progressive strengthening when mobilization is permitted are indicated. The deltoid and trapezius work should not be emphasized because this may apply disruptive force to the AC joint capsule and ligament complex.

Surgical approach

1. Open reduction, capsular repair, and *internal fixation* by insertion of a threaded wire through the acromion, across the AC joint, and well into the clavicle. The wire is removed after 6 weeks.[7] After surgery, isometrics are performed as pain permits, while active range of motion exercise begins 2 to 4 weeks after the operation, followed by progressing to active strengthening 4 to 6 weeks after the operation.[3]
2. Open reduction by *screw fixation* of the clavicle to the coracoid process and transfer of the tip of the coracoid and attached pectoralis minor muscle to the clavicle.[3] The arm is then immobilized in a sling with early gentle active range of motion exercises and isometrics followed by AROM exercises to 90°, usually after 7 to 10 days. Progressive strengthening begins 4 to 6 weeks after the operation.[7]

References

1. Cyriax J: *Textbook of orthopaedic medicine*, vol 1: *Diagnosis of soft tissue lesions*, London, 1982, Bailliere-Tindall.
2. Dandy DJ: *Essential orthopaedics and trauma*, Edinburgh, 1989, Churchill Livingstone.
3. Gould JA III: *Orthopaedic and sports physical therapy*, ed 2, St. Louis, 1990, Mosby.
4. Kisner C, Colby LA: *Therapeutic exercise: foundations and techniques*, ed 2, Philadelphia, 1990, FA Davis.
5. Moffat M: Lecture and handout series on musculoskeletal therapeutic exercise, Fall 1989, New York University Department of Physical Therapy, New York University Medical Book Store.
6. Moore KL: *Clinically oriented anatomy*, ed 2, Baltimore, 1985, Williams & Wilkins.
7. Salter RB: *Textbook of disorders of the musculoskeletal system*, ed 2, Baltimore, 1983, Williams & Wilkins.

Recommended reading

Bearden JM, Hughston JC, Wheatley GS: Acromioclavicular dislocation: method of treatment, *J Sports Med* (4):5-17, 1973.

Bowers KD: Treatment of acromioclavicular sprains in athletes, *The Physician and Sports Medicine* 2(1):79-89, 1983.

Malone T, McPoil T, Nitz AJ: *Orthopaedic and sports physical therapy*, ed 3, St. Louis, 1996, Mosby.

Moffat M: Lecture and handout series on musculoskeletal therapeutic exercise, Fall 1989, New York University Department of Physical Therapy. New York University Medical Book Store.

Rockwood, CA, Young DC: Disorders of the acromioclavicular joint. In Rockwood CA, Matsen FA: *The shoulder,* vol 1, ed 2, Philadelphia, 1990, Saunders.

Fall on Point of Shoulder, Causing Sagging of Upper Extremity, Loss of Shoulder Function, and Much Pain on Movement

15

A 34-year-old adult male was riding his dirtbike over a mountain trail when the front wheel of his bike dipped suddenly into a gully, causing the rider to pitch forward over the handlebars to land on the point of his right shoulder. The patient acutely presented the following appearance (Fig. 15-1).

The patient now presents himself to you 3 weeks later in a swathe-and-sling binder with a prescription from the local orthopod for "therapy." The patient informs you that he works in a heavy industry plant that requires him to hoist heavy objects and to pull down on large heavy machine levers.

1. **What is most likely to have occurred to this man's shoulder?**
2. **How is the clavicle embryologically unique as compared to other long bones?**
3. **What is the biomechanical significance of the strutlike design of the collarbone?**
4. **What is the most common pattern of clavicle fracture?**
5. **What is the mechanism involved in fracture of the middle third of the clavicle?**
6. **What is the classification of clavicle fractures?**
7. **What is the typically observed deformity after fracture of the clavicle?**
8. **What concomitant internal injuries may accompany fractures of the medial third of the clavicle?**
9. **What kind of pulmonary insult may occur to the lung or lungs during fracture of the medial clavicular section?**
10. **What type of nerve injury is suspected after fracture of the medial third of the clavicle?**
11. **What major vascular injury may concurrently occur with fractures of the medial third of the clavicle?**
12. **What other skeletal injuries may accompany clavicle fracture?**
13. **What mechanism accounts for clavicle fracture in newborns?**
14. **What is the clinical presentation of birth fracture of the clavicle?**
15. **What mechanism most often accounts for clavicle fractures in children?**
16. **What radiography is appropriate when one suspects clavicular fracture?**
17. **What is the medical management of clavicle fracture?**
18. **How long does the clavicle require to heal after fracture?**
19. **How soon after clavicle fracture may active and resistive activity commence?**

1. What is most likely to have occurred to this man's shoulder (Fig. 15-1)?

Clavicle fracture.

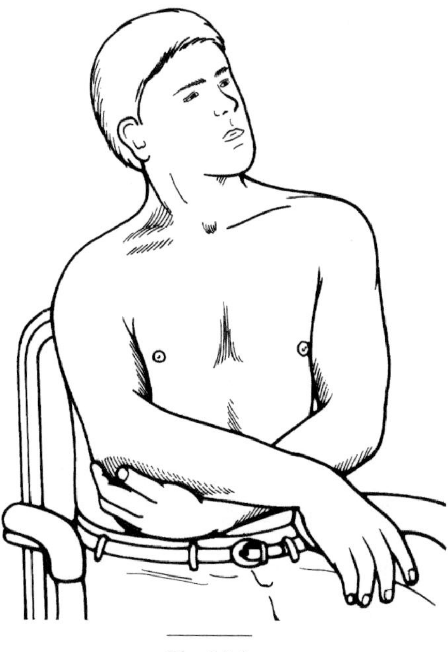

Fig. 15-1

2. How is the clavicle embryologically unique as compared to other long bones?

The clavicle is embryologically unique in being the first bone in the body to ossify and the only long bone to ossify by intramembranous ossification without going through a cartilaginous stage.[10] Cosmetically, the crank-shaped clavicle bespeaks grace yet conveys strength in its slender swanlike appearance. Its name is derived from the Latin word *clavis* 'key,' the diminutive of which is *clavicula*.[17] Although appearing nearly straight when viewed from the front, it actually appears as an S-shaped or *crank-shaped* bone when viewed from above (Fig. 15-2).

3. What is the biomechanical significance of the strutlike design of the collarbone?

The clavicle is the sole bony strut linking the trunk to the shoulder girdle and arm. The significance of this is twofold:

- In the domestic cat, the clavicle, unlike in man, is free at both ends and perforce does not link the sternum and humerus (Fig. 15-3). Uniquely adapted to land on its forelegs, the cat will therefore not fracture its clavicle since its clavicle absorbs the impact energy of landing by moving to a limit set by restraining soft tissue.

Man's clavicle, however, is adapted for carrying weights because of its firm attachment to the sternum medially and the acromion and coracoid processes laterally by ligaments (Fig. 15-4), the tensile strength of which exceeds that of bone.[7] The impact absorbed by a fall onto an outstretched arm is thus transmitted up the length of the clavicle to either dissipate or cause fracture at that bone's weakest point, the middle third.

- The clavicle is mechanically analogous to the cantilever (Fig. 15-5). A cantilever is a beam supported only at one end while projecting freely at the other end. The mechanical advantage gained by this lever system is the ability to carry loads significantly greater than its own weight. Airplane wings, for

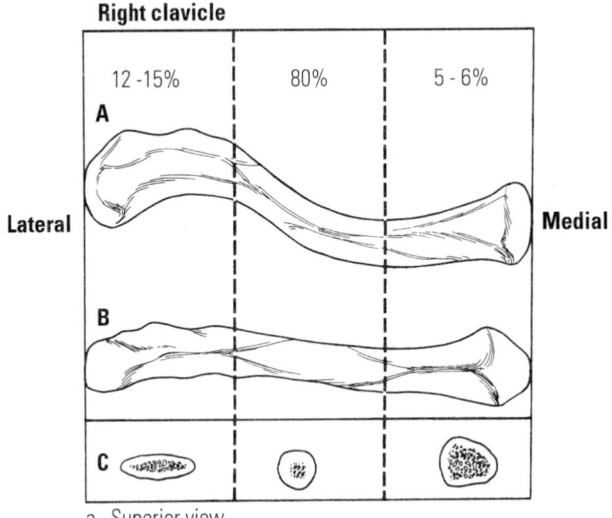

Fig. 15-2 The clavicle appears as an S-shaped double curve when viewed from above, *a.* It appears nearly straight when viewed from in front, *b.* The outer end of the clavicle is flat in cross-section but becomes more tubular in the medial aspect, *c.* (From Craig EV: Fractures of the clavicle. In Rockwood CA, Matsen FA, editors: *The shoulder*, vol 1, Philadelphia, 1990, Saunders.)

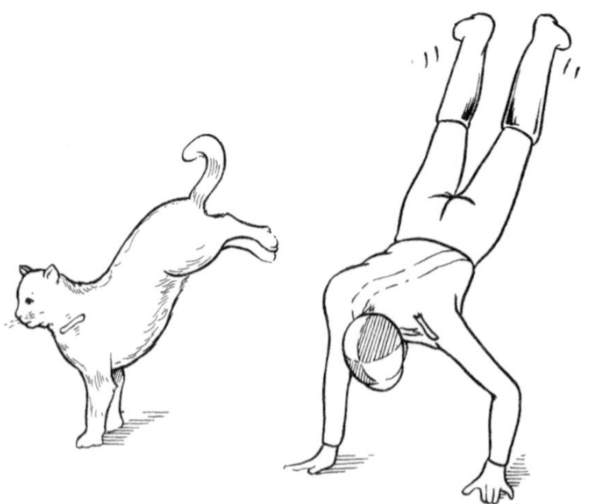

Fig. 15-3 Falls on the outstretched arms. The cat, unlike man, does not fracture its clavicle because it does not link the sternum and humerus as in man. (From Dandy DJ: *Essential orthopaedics and trauma*, Edinburgh, 1989, Churchill Livingstone.)

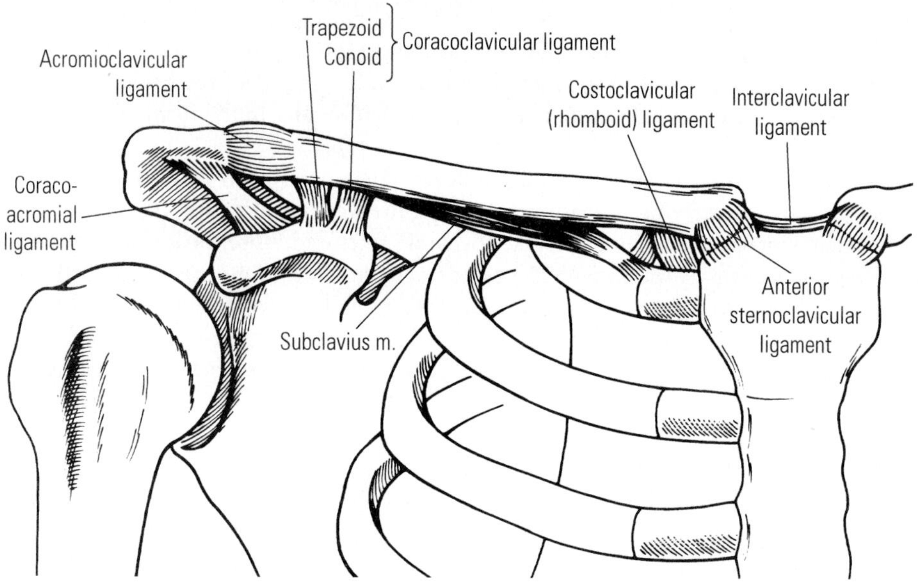

Fig. 15-4 The clavicle is securely bound by ligaments at both the sternoclavicular and the acromioclavicular joints. It is the only bony strut from the torso to the upper extremity.

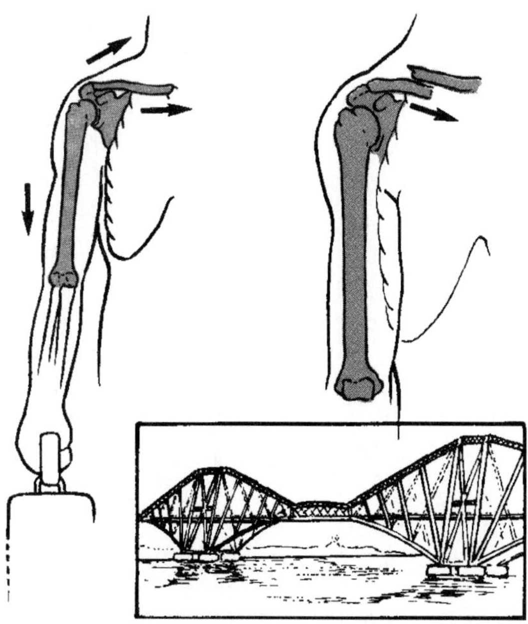

Fig. 15-5 Cantilever action of the clavicle. When the clavicle is broken, the shoulder is not supported and moves downwards and medially. Inset: *Cantilever bridge.* (From Dandy DJ: *Essential orthopaedics and trauma,* Edinburgh, 1989, Churchill Livingstone.)

example, that have no props or struts to brace them are examples of cantilevers that tolerate considerable forces of air lift. A cantilever bridge has two towers on opposite sides of the river, and each tower supports beams that meet in the middle of that bridge. If half of the bridge were dismantled, say, by an explosive, the other half could still carry as much weight, in the form of trucks, trains, and automobiles, as before.

By linking the arm to the axial skeleton by a cantilever system, the weight of the body serves as a counterweight that permits the carrying of loads greater than the weight of the arm itself.[7] This capability is diminished or made impossible when the clavicle becomes fractured, since the length of the lever arm is subsequently decreased. Muscle spasm pulls the outer fragment beneath the inner one, further diminishing its length. In light of this it then becomes obvious why individuals with cleidocranial dysostosis (congenital absence of the clavicle, Fig. 15-6) may exhibit weakness when supporting overhead loads; it is precisely the overhead position that calls upon the leverlike function of the clavicle to prop weighted objects away from the body.

4. What is the most common pattern of clavicle fracture?

Group I clavicle fracture refers to a break of the middle third of that bone and is the most common pattern of fracture (80%)[18,20] in both adults and children.[8] Aside from stability imparted to the proximal and medial ends of the clavicle by ligamentous and muscular attachments, the cross-sectional diameter of the clavicle differs along the length of its shaft such that the middle third of that bone is most vulnerable to injury. Whereas the flat outer third of the clavicle is ideally suited to the myriad attachments of muscles and ligaments, the tubular medial third has a cross section that best protects those branches of the brachial plexus lying behind the

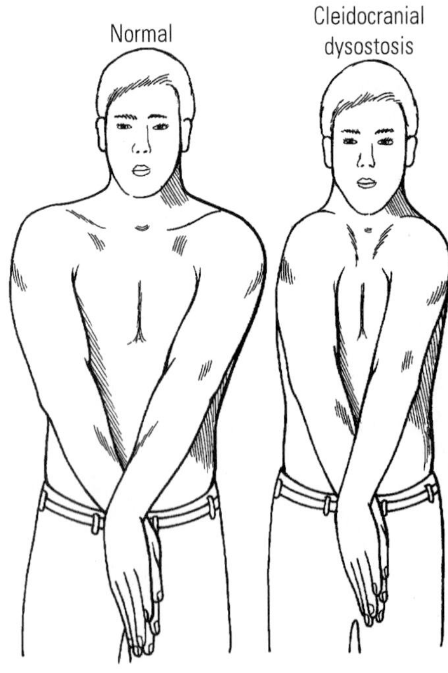

Fig. 15-6 Cleidocranial dysostosis.

clavicle. The vulnerable central section, however, is not just free of any stabilizing attachments but is also in fact the thinnest cross section of that bone and perforce the weakest, especially to axial loading.[15]

5. What is the mechanism involved in fracture of the middle third of the clavicle?

The classic mechanism of fracture to the middle third of the clavicle is from a fall onto an outstretched arm and is best understood by the counterpoint idea of the three-point force system. The *indirect force* travels up along the shaft of the humerus until it encounters two counterpoints: one at the glenohumeral joint and one at the sternoclavicular joint (Fig. 15-7). Force dispursal will then, one would hope, occur along the length of the shaft of the clavicle but will result in a *spiral fracture* of the middle third in the event that disruptive forces exceed intrinsic bone strength.[8] Injury may also occur from a *direct force* as occurs from a blow directly over the middle third of the clavicle, resulting in a fracture (Fig. 15-8). Injury may

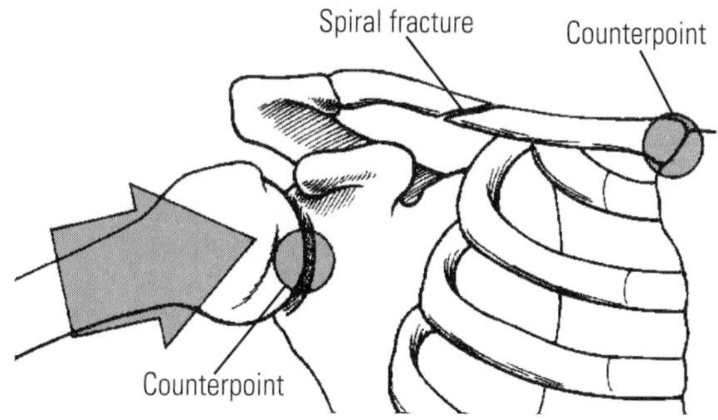

Fig. 15-7 An indirect force encounters counterpoints at the glenohumeral and sternoclavicular joints causing a spiral fracture at the middle third of the clavicle. (Modified from DePalma AF: *Surgery of the shoulder*, ed 3, Philadelphia, 1983, Lippincott.)

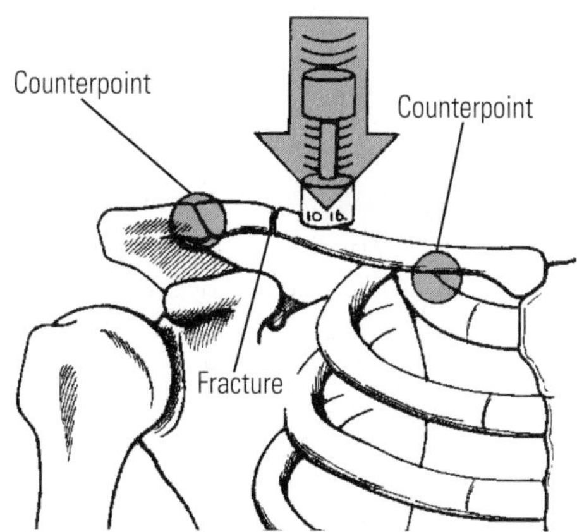

Fig. 15-8 A direct force applied over the middle third of the clavicle causing a fracture to occur at the juncture of the middle and outer thirds. (Modified from DePalma AF: *Surgery of the shoulder*, ed 3, Philadelphia, 1983, Lippincott.)

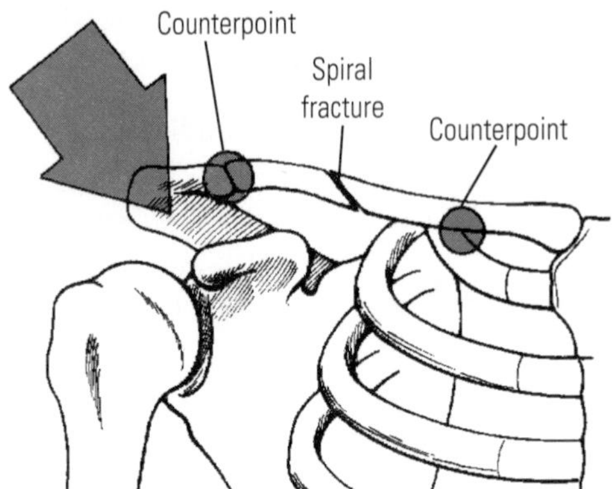

Fig. 15-9 A direct force applied onto the point of the shoulder forcing the clavicle downward against the first rib and resulting in a spiral of the middle third. (Modified from DePalma AF: *Surgery of the shoulder,* ed 3, Philadelphia, 1983, Lippincott.)

also occur from a direct fall onto the point of the shoulder, which also results in a spiral fracture of the middle third (Fig. 15-9).

6. What is the classification of clavicle fractures?

Although fractures of the clavicle have in the past been classified according to fracture configurations (that is, greenstick, oblique, transverse, and comminuted),[24] the common classification is now according to the location of fracture. This approach is more reflective of a comprehensive view, if one takes into consideration the mechanism of injury, clinical presentation, and alternative treatment methods.[4]

Both group II and group III fractures refer to breakage at the distal and medial thirds of the clavicle respectively. These groupings are further subdivided according to the integrity of ligamentous structures supporting the clavicle at the sternoclavicular joint medially and the acromioclavicular joint laterally. With children, these injuries are often epiphyseal fractures. With adults, these injuries often have sequelae of degenerative joint changes and associated posttraumatic arthritis.

7. What is the typically observed deformity after fracture of the clavicle?

The deformity of a fractured clavicle has the following observable presentation: the (distal fragment of the) affected shoulder appears lower and droops forward and inward, whereas the proximal fragment is displaced upward and backward, causing a tent-like tautening of the overlying skin. This displacement of segments occurs as a function of the specific muscle attachments on different portions of the clavicle. Attaching to the distal third of the clavicle, the upper trapezius cannot bear the weight of the upper extremity unconnected to the axillary skeleton after fracture, and so gravity causes sagging of the entire upper extremity and the outer fragment as a unit. Additionally, the lateral fragment is adducted by the pectoralis major; this adduction causes the lateral fragment to override the medial fragment and gives the appearance of a shortened clavicle. The inner fragment is elevated by the sternocleidomastoid muscle (Fig. 15-10).

The head and chin are tilted away from the fracture site to relax the pull of the sternocleidomastoid. Or the patient may angle his or her head toward the injury, attempting to relax the pull of the trapezius on the outer fragment. The patient may often splint the sagging arm against the body while holding the affected elbow with the other hand.[4]

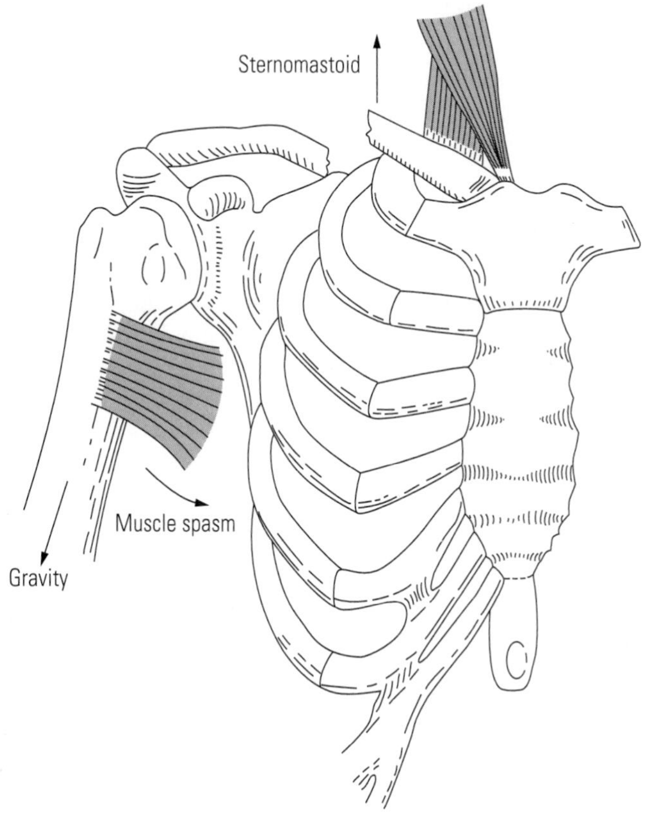

Fig. 15-10 Deformity accompanying a clavicle fracture. (From Ellis H: *Clinical anatomy*, ed 7, Oxford, 1983, Blackwell Scientific Publications.)

8. What concomitant internal injuries may accompany fractures of the medial third of the clavicle?

Injuries to the lungs, brachial plexus, or subclavian and axillary vessels may occur from accompanying fractures of the first rib or of the medial third of the clavicle. Although the usual adult clavicular shaft fracture is oblique in nature, excessive forces may instead cause a dangerous comminuted fracture. If the middle spike projects from superior to inferior, the clinician must be alerted to the potential for associated pulmonary or neurovascular injuries. Generally, manipulation of fracture fragments, regardless of fracture pattern, is inadvisable without x-ray studies of the position of those fragments.[27]

9. What kind of pulmonary insult may occur to the lung or lungs during fracture of the medial clavicular section?

Because the apical pleura and lobes of the upper lung lie adjacent to the clavicle, a shard from a severely displaced fracture may puncture the pleura and result in pneumothorax or hemothorax.[20] As such, the anteroposterior radiographic view should include the upper lung fields taken in the upright position with particularly close attention paid to the lung outline. It is essential to auscultate for asymmetry as well as the decrease of breath sounds to rule out pneumothorax.

10. What type of nerve injury is suspected after fracture of the medial third of the clavicle?

The neurovascular bundle emerges from the thoracic outlet under the clavicle atop the first rib.[19] The portion of the medial cord of the brachial plexus that gives rise to the ulnar nerve crosses the first rib directly under the medial third of the clavicle, and is at risk for injury.[4] The other two cords of the plexus are too far laterally and posteriorly to be injured after fracture.

11. What major vascular injury may concurrently occur with fractures of the medial third of the clavicle?

The subclavius muscle and the thick cervical fascia act as a barrier to direct injury of the vessels. If initial displacement of fracture fragments has not injured the vasculature, they are unlikely to become further injured, since their migration (secondary to muscle spasm) often pulls them out of harm's way.[4]

The anterior curve of the medial two thirds of the clavicle provides a rigid arch beneath which the great vessels pass as they move from the thoracic outlet down toward the axilla.[25] Fracture of the medial third of the clavicle may result in one of the following four severe vascular phenomena:

- A laceration resulting in life-threatening hemorrhage is suggested by an upper limb that is cold, pulseless, and pale and by the presence of a bruit[26] or a difference in pressure[29] between both arms.
- Arterial thrombus and occlusion may lead to distal ischemia.
- Damage to the arterial wall may lead to aneurysm formation and late embolic phenomena.
- Venous thrombosis may lead to late pulmonary embolism.[4]

If a major vessel injury is suspected, an arteriogram should be performed.[29] In the rare event of a tear of a large vessel, surgical exploration is required.[4]

12. What other skeletal injuries may accompany clavicle fracture?

Associated skeletal injuries may include sternoclavicular or acromioclavicular separations or fracture dislocations through these joints.[3,13]

13. What mechanism accounts for clavicle fracture in newborns?

Several factors account for clavicular fracture at birth, the most significant being presentation of the infant. In cephalic presentation of the vaginally delivered newborn, compression of the leading clavicle against the maternal symphysis pubis occurs.[16] With breech delivery, direct traction may occur as the obstetrician, trying to depress the shoulders and free the arm in the delivery of the head, inadvertently fractures the clavicle.[23] No incidence of fracture is reported in babies delivered by cesarean section.[1] Other contributing factors causing clavicular fractures in newborns include size (≥52 cm),[11] birth weight (3800 to 4000 g), inexperience of the physician, and midforceps deliveries.

The infant's mother might notice that her baby cries after being picked up and appears to be hurt.[2] The baby does not seem to use his or her arm naturally and cries if the arm is moved during activities such as dressing. The mother may notice swelling or crepitus or take the baby to the pediatrician because of the "sudden appearance of a lump;"[6] this lump is caused by fracture callus and typically appears 7 to 11 days after fracture.[5] On palpation, one may feel a tender, uneven border of the clavicle, which is asymmetrical when compared to the contralateral side.

14. What is the clinical presentation of birth fracture of the clavicle?

Clinical presentations of the clavicle are twofold:

- The fracture may be clinically inapparent, and a crack may or may not be heard during delivery.[2] Close examination may reveal an asymmetry of the clavicle contour or a shortening of the neck line.[4]
- The fracture may be clinically apparent (pseudoparalysis) as a form in which the child exhibits some degree of unilateral upper extremity paresis on attempted volitional movement or during elicitation of

the Moro reflex.[9,22] Here, clavicular fracture must be differentiated from the following conditions: Erb's palsy, separation of the proximal humeral epiphysis, and acute osteomyelitis of the clavicle or proximal humerus. A clavicle fracture may coexist with brachial plexus injury.[23]

15. What mechanism most often accounts for clavicle fractures in children?

The mechanism of injury for clavicle fractures in children is identical to that of adults and may occur from a fall onto the point of the shoulder or upon an outstretched hand from a changing table, high chair, or bunk bed. Unlike the adult, trauma often results in a greenstick or incomplete fracture rather than a displaced fracture. As with other fractures of long bones, clavicular fractures may be a sign of trauma in the physically abused child.[4]

16. What radiography is appropriate when one suspects clavicular fracture?

X-ray evaluation of the shaft of the clavicle is best viewed in two projections:

- An anteroposterior view that typically reveals the upward displacement of the proximal fragment as well as caudal displacement of the distal fragment secondary to muscle spasm.
- A 45° cephalic tilt view permits more accurate assessment of the anteroposterior relationships of the two fragments.[4]

Fractures of the distal third of the clavicle are easily missed with the above-mentioned views and are easily passed off as acromioclavicular sprains. The reason is that the standard exposure overexposes the distal end of the clavicle. When suspect, fractures of the distal third are confirmed by employment of one third of the exposure used for the shoulder joint.

Often the novice clinician will not know that these views should be ordered and misdiagnose the injury as an AC sprain based on abnormal standard views as well as the absence of a classic presentation, which may be absent in distal fractures of the clavicle. However, the presence of pain and tenderness on movement some 10 to 14 days after the injury is cause for suspicion of fracture. Standard radiographs at this time will reveal either a line of bony absorption along the clavicular shaft or callus formation at the site of fracture.

17. What is the medical management of clavicle fracture?

With adolescents and adults, provided that no displacement of fracture fragments has occurred, treatment is by supporting the weight of the arm in a broad sling or a posterior figure-of-eight bandage[4] (Fig. 15-11) for 3 weeks.[6] Lack of consistent immobilization may contribute to increasing the likelihood of nonunion; thus immobilization must continue, at the very least, until clinical union has occurred and, there is doubt, even beyond that time. The principle behind this bandage is to raise the distal fragment and depress the inner fragment while simultaneously enabling the ipsilateral elbow and hand to be used in activities of daily living, thus helping stave off adhesion development and loss of range in that extremity.[4]

When there is displacement and overriding of fracture ends, an attempt must be made to reduce the fracture and restore the normal length of the clavicle; local anesthesia may be required. Then, with the fracture reduced, a posterior figure-of-eight bandage with plaster reinforcement or even full-shoulder immobilization in a spica cast is appropriate.[4]

Treatment for newborns consists in simply immobilizing the arm to the infant's trunk for 2 weeks, after which the fracture is sufficiently healed to permit painless volitional movement.[4]

18. How long does the clavicle require to heal after fracture?

The healing period for fracture of the middle third of the clavicle is as follows: infants heal within 2 weeks, children within 3 weeks, young adults heal within 4 to 6 weeks, and adults usually require 6 weeks or longer.[20] Although the fracture site may clinically unite as early as 3 weeks in the adult, radiologic union

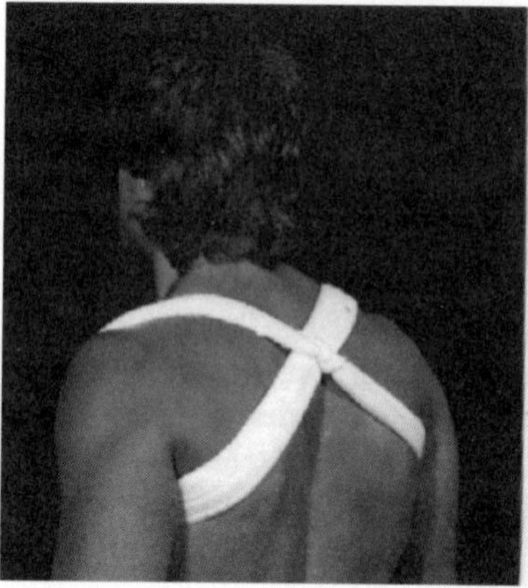
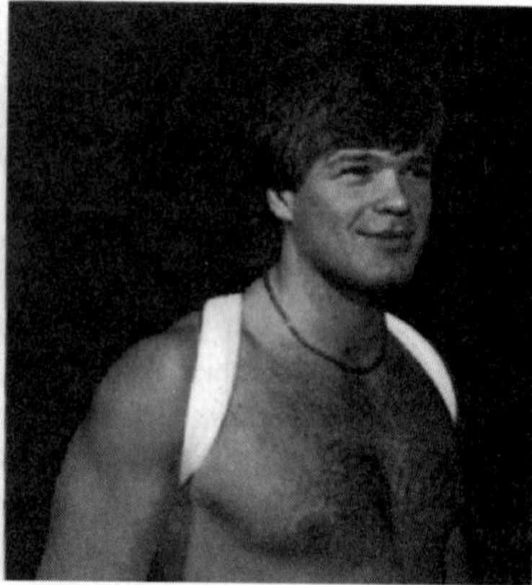

Fig. 15-11 Figure-of-eight bandage. (From Peterson L, Renström P: *Sports injuries: their prevention and treatment,* London, 1986, Martin Dunitz, Ltd.)

may not appear until 12 weeks or longer. Nonunion of unoperated clavicle shaft fracture, defined as failure to show radiographic progression of healing for 4 to 6 months, is rare.[4]

19. How soon after clavicle fracture may active and resistive activity commence?

The clinically relevant question for the therapist treating a patient with a 3- to 4-week-old clavicular fracture is: Will active or resistive exercises serve to stress the fracture site? This question is especially relevant to the 90° to 180° range of shoulder elevation when the clavicle is maximally stressed vis-à-vis its cantilever function.

The guidelines are as follows: During the period of clinical union active range of motion is permitted up to 90° for shoulder elevation as well as passive range of motion above 90°, provided that there is absence of any motion of fragments or tenderness at the fracture site. Glenohumeral joint and scapular mobilization and also shoulder shrugging for the purpose of decreasing the dangers of immobilization are appropriate. After radiologic union, an active range of motion greater than 90° is permitted with the gentle introduction of resistance exercises.

References

1. Balata A, Olzai MG, Porcu A, et al: Fractures of the clavicle in the newborn, *Riv Ital Pediatr.*
2. Batemen JE: *The shoulder and neck*, Philadelphia, 1978, Saunders.
3. Butterworth RD, Kirk AA: Fracture dislocation of sterno-clavicular joint: case report, *Virginia Med Month* 79:98-100, 1952.
4. Craig EV: Fractures of the clavicle. In Rockwood CA, Matsen FA, editors: *The shoulder*, vol 1, Philadelphia, 1990, Saunders.
5. Cummings WA: Neonatal skeletal fractures: birth trauma or child abuse? *J Can Assoc Radiol* 30:30-33, 1979.
6. Dameron TB Jr, Rockwood CA: Fractures of the shaft of the clavicle. In Rockwood CA, Wilkins KE, King RE, editors: *Fractures in children*, Philadelphia, 1984, Lippincott.
7. Dandy DJ: *Essential orthopaedics and trauma*, Edinburgh, 1989, Churchill Livingstone.
8. DePalma AF: *Surgery of the shoulder*, ed 3, Philadelphia, 1983, Lippincott.
9. Freedman M, Gamble J, Lewis C: Intrauterine fracture simulating a unilateral clavicular pseudoarthrosis, *J Assoc Radiol* 33(1):37-38, 1982.
10. Gardner E: The embryology of the clavicle, *Clin Orthop* 59:9-16, 1968.
11. Gitsch VG, Schatten C: Frequenz und potentielle Faktoren in der Genese der geburtstraumatisch bedingten Klavicula Fraktur, *Zentralbl Gynäkol.*

12. Javid H: Vascular injuries of the neck, *Clin Orthop* 28:70-78, 1963.
13. Kanoksikarin S, Wearne WN: Fracture and retrosternal dislocation of the clavicle, *Aust NZ J Surg* 48:95-96, 1978.
14. Klier I, Maayor PB: Laceration of the innominate internal jugular venous junction: rare complication of fracture of the clavicle, *Orthop Rev* 10:81-82, 1981.
15. Ljunggren AE: Clavicular function, *Acta Orthop Scand* 50:261-268, 1979.
16. Madsen ET: Fractures of the extremities in the newborn, *Acta Obstet Gynecol Scand* 34:41-74, 1955.
17. Mosely HF: The clavicle: its anatomy and function, *Clin Orthop* 58:17-27, 1968.
18. Neer CS II: Fractures of the clavicle. In Rockwood CA, Green DP, editors: *Fractures in adults*, Philadelphia, 1984, Lippincott.
19. Reid J, Kennedy J: Direct fracture of the clavicle with symptoms simulating a cervical rib, *Br Med J* 2:608-609, 1925.
20. Rowe CR: An atlas of anatomy and treatment of midclavicular fractures, *Clin Orthop* 58:29-42, 1968.
21. Salter RB: *Textbook of disorders and injuries of the musculoskeletal system*, ed 2, Baltimore, 1983, Williams & Wilkins.
22. Sanford HN: The Moro reflex as a diagnostic aid in fracture of the clavicle in the newborn infant, *Am J Dis Child* 41:1304-1306, 1931.
23. Tancher S, Kolishev K. Tanches P, et al: Etiology of a clavicle fracture due to the birth process, *Akush Ginekol* 24(2):39-43, 1985.
24. Taylor AR: Nonunion of fractures of the clavicle: a review of 31 cases, Proc British Orthopaedic Association, *J Bone Joint Surg* 51B:568-569, 1969.
25. Telford ED, Mottershead S: Pressure at the cervicobrachial junction: an operative and an anatomical study, *J Bone Joint Surg* 30B:249, 1948.
26. Tse DHW, Slabaugh PB, Carlson PA: Injury to the axillary artery by a closed fracture of the clavicle, *J Bone Joint Surg* 62A:1372-1373, 1980.
27. Van Vlack HG: Comminuted fracture of the clavicle with pressure on brachial plexus: report of a case, *J Bone Joint Surg* 22A:446-447, 1940.
28. Widner LA, Riddervold HO: The value of lordotic view in diagnosis of fractured clavicle, Rev *Interam Radiol* 5:69-70, 1980.
29. Yates DW: Complications of fractures of the clavicle, *Injury* 7(3):189-193, 1976.

Recommended reading

Craig EV: Fractures of the clavicle. In Rockwood CA, Matsen FA, editors: *The shoulder*, vol 1, Philadelphia, 1990, Saunders.

Peterson L, Renström P: *Sports injuries: their prevention and treatment*, London, 1986, Martin Dunitz, Ltd.

Painful Bump over Proximal Section of Clavicle

16

A 21-year-old well-built broad-shouldered man presents with acute pain over his right medial clavicle after a football tackle during which eight other men piled on top of him at a preseason training game. Your friend, an athletic trainer by profession, immediately examines this person, and the following clinical picture emerges. The player cradles his right arm with his left upper extremity and tilts his head toward his right side. He complains of considerable pain.

CLUE:

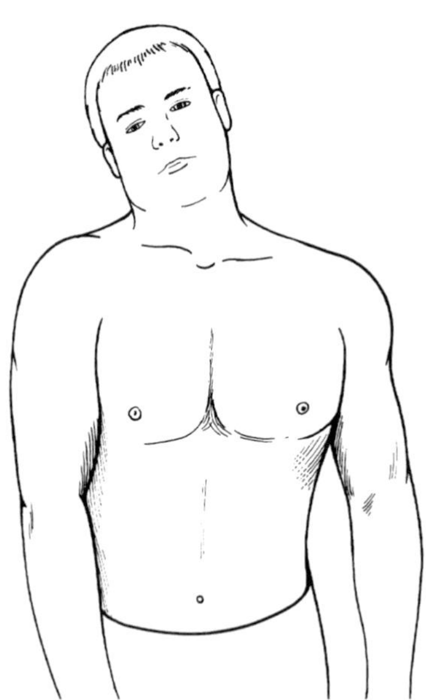

OBSERVATION Prominence over the medial end of the clavicle is noticed. The right shoulder appears to be shortened and thrust forward when compared to the uninvolved side. The clavicle appears less prominent than on the left side.

PALPATION There is a palpable anteriorly projecting bump over the middle of the clavicle that is tender and feels warm to the dorsum of the examiner's hand.

RANGE OF MOTION Appears to be limited, but exactly how much is masked by muscle guarding in all directions.

MUSCLE STRENGTH Difficult to test secondary to pain.

PULSES Normal as is color to distal end of right extremity.

NOTE Discomfort increases when the patient is placed in supine and refuses to lie back entirely; thus his right scapula is slightly lifted off the grass.

1. **What is most likely to have occurred in this athlete?**
2. **What requisite anatomy is relevant to fully understanding this injury?**
3. **Describe sternoclavicular (SC) joint incongruity.**
4. **Describe the ligamentous stability of the SC joint.**
5. **What is the first line of ligamentous defense against SC joint disruption?**
6. **What are the functions of the intra-articular disk ligament and the interclavicular ligament?**
7. **Describe the costoclavicular and SC ligaments and their function.**
8. **What is the kinesiology of the SC joint?**
9. **What is the range of motion of the SC joint?**
10. **What direct force mechanisms cause posterior SC joint injury?**
11. **What indirect force mechanisms cause anterior SC joint injury?**
12. **What is the classification of SC joint injury?**
13. **Why is diagnosis predicated on clinical evidence rather than on radiologic evidence?**
14. **What is the medical treatment of subluxation or dislocation when not life threatening?**
15. **What therapeutic intervention and advice is appropriate?**

1. What is most likely to have occurred in this young athlete?

Anterior dislocation *separation* of the sternoclavicular (SC) joint is an uncommon injury that may occur after a blow or fall to the front of the shoulder that drives the medial inner end of the clavicle forward and the lateral outer end backward.[10] Excessive forces are transmitted along the long axis of the clavicle (serving as a first line of defense), where they may dissipate or fracture the clavicle near the junction of that bone's middle or lateral third.[6] If the clavicle fails to transmit or absorb these forces, injury may then occur more medially at the SC joint.

2. What requisite anatomy is relevant to fully understanding this injury?

When thinking about the SC joint, it is important to realize that the entire mass of the shoulder girdle, including the scapula, attaches to the axial skeleton at the SC joint. This linkage sequence begins from sternum to clavicle and from clavicle to scapula by way of the coracoid and acromion and from scapula to humerus by way of the ligamentous connections off the coracoid process. This *coracohumeral ligament*, an anterior medial structure that anastomoses with the hoodlike tendons of the cuff muscles, affords checking against excessive external rotation together with the *glenohumeral ligament*. Additionally, the joint cavity of the SC joint is oblique and contains a meniscus, or disk of sorts.[8] The most common causes of SC dislocation are vehicular accidents and sport injuries in that order.[7]

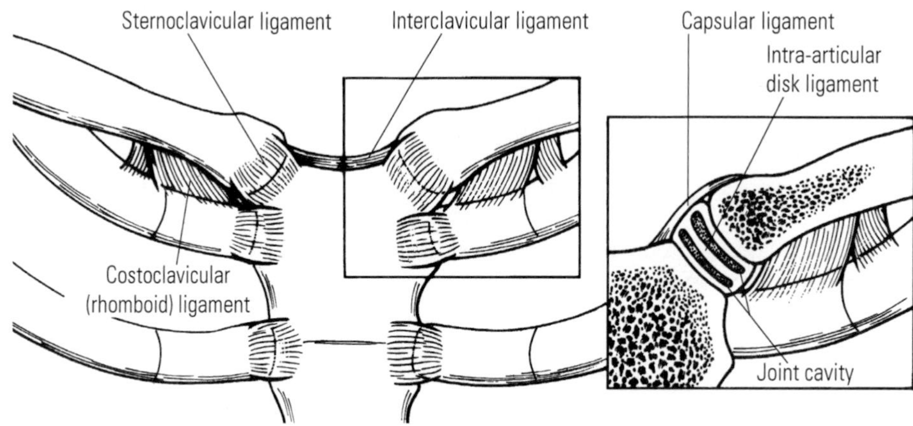

Fig. 16-1 Ligamentous stabilizers of the sternoclavicular joint.

3. Describe sternoclavicular (SC) joint incongruity.

The SC joint is a diarthrodial joint composed of a large medial concave surface from front to back and as a convex surface vertically on its clavicular end that articulates with the curved notch of the manubrium of the sternum.[3] The joint is of a saddle variety the joint surfaces of which are so incongruent as to give the SC joint the distinction of having the least amount of bony stability of all major body joints.[9]

4. Describe the ligamentous stability of the SC joint.

Because of considerable joint incongruity, integrity at the SC joint is principally afforded by surrounding ligaments. These ligaments include the capsular ligament, the intra-articular disk ligament, costoclavicular (rhomboid) ligament, sternoclavicular ligament, and interclavicular ligament, all of which contribute toward maintenance of normal shoulder poise (Fig. 16-1).

5. What is the first line of ligamentous defense against SC joint disruption?

The *capsular ligament*, covering the anterosuperior and posterior aspects of the SC joint, represents thickenings of the joint capsule that are more prominent anteriorly.[9] These thickenings serve as a first line of defense, since they are the most important structures preventing medial upward displacement caused by downward disruptive force upon the distal end of the clavicle.[1]

6. What are the functions of the intra-articular disk ligament and the interclavicular ligament?

The *intra-articular disk ligament* passes through the SC joint while going from the first rib to the sternum and, as such, divides the joint into two separate joint spaces. This ligament acts as a checkrein against medial displacement of the inner clavicle. The interclavicular ligament connects the superomedial aspects of each clavicle with the capsular ligaments and upper sternum.[9] This band, homologous to the wishbone in birds,[3] assists in maintenance of shoulder poise (such as holding up the shoulder).[9]

7. Describe the costoclavicular and SC ligaments and their function.

The *costoclavicular ligament*, together with the *sternoclavicular ligament*, strongly anchor the medial end of the clavicle to the sternum. The former ligament is short and strong, consisting of an anterior and a posterior fasciculus with a bursa interposed between the two fasciculi.[1] The fibers composing these two fascicular components cross and have a twisted (cruciate) appearance.[4] The anterior fascicular fibers rising from the anterior medial surface of the first rib are directed upward and laterally[9] so that their kinesiologic function is to resist excessive upward clavicular rotation.[1] In contrast, the posterior fascicular fibers are shorter in span and arise just lateral to the anterior fibers on the first rib and are directed upward and medially[9] so as to check excessive downward clavicular rotation.[1] Thus the costoclavicular ligaments, analogous to the knee cruciate ligaments, provide stability to the SC joint during clavicular rotation (such as shoulder elevation and depression). Additionally, this two-part ligament is in many ways similar to the two-part configuration of the coracoclavicular ligament stabilizing the acromioclavicular joint on the lateral end of the clavicle.[9]

8. What is the kinesiology of the SC joint?

The costoclavicular ligament acts as a pivot for the clavicle, which seesaws about this fixed point[2] as the outer end of the clavicle elevates and depresses with shoulder flexion/abduction and extension/adduction. This motion and the importance of the various supporting ligaments are illustrated by the following thought experiment[9] (Fig. 16-2).

9. What is the range of motion of the SC joint?

The SC joint, like the saddle joint in the thumb, is freely movable with motions in almost all planes, including rotation. During normal shoulder rotation the clavicle and therefore the medial articulation of that long bone, such as the sternoclavicular joint, are capable of 30° to 35° of elevation or depression, 35° of combined forward and backward movement, and 45° to 50° of long-axis rotation[9] (Fig. 16-3).

10. What direct force mechanisms cause posterior SC joint injury?

Force applied to the anteromedial aspect of the clavicle causes the clavicle to become pushed posteriorly behind the sternum and into the mediastinum.[9] Posterior (retrosternal) dislocation (Figs. 16-4 and 16-5) is rare and dangerous,[10] and if it is suspected, both airways and peripheral pulses must be assessed, since the posterior protruding clavicle may compress both the trachea and the great vessels behind it.[5] Ways in which this injury may occur include a head-on vehicular collision in which the steering wheel pushes directly on the sternum and the heart, a kick delivered to the front of the middle of the clavicle, action of a person being run over by a vehicle, action of a person being pinned between a vehicle and a wall, and compression when an athlete lying on the ground is jumped upon. The jumper's knee lands directly over the medial third of the clavicle. Because of our anatomy, barring a javelin or some other projectile entering through the back and leaving anteriorly, it would be most unusual for a direct force to produce an anterior SC dislocation.[9]

11. What indirect force mechanisms cause anterior SC joint injury?

The most common mechanism of injury causing SC dislocation by indirect force occurs by anterior SC dislocation[9] (Figs. 16-6 and 16-7). An indirect force occurs when the shoulder is laterally compressed while simultaneously rolled backward, resulting in ipsilateral anterior dislocation. If the shoulder, however, is rolled forward, ipsilateral posterior dislocation will occur. A football pile-on in which the player falls to the ground and lands on the lateral area of his shoulder commonly results in indirect forces contributing to a pathologic condition. Before the player can get out of the way, several other players pile on top of both of his shoulders, applying significant compressive force on the clavicle down toward the sternum in one of two patterns. If during the compression the landed lateral part of the shoulder is rolled backward, the clavicle will lever backward

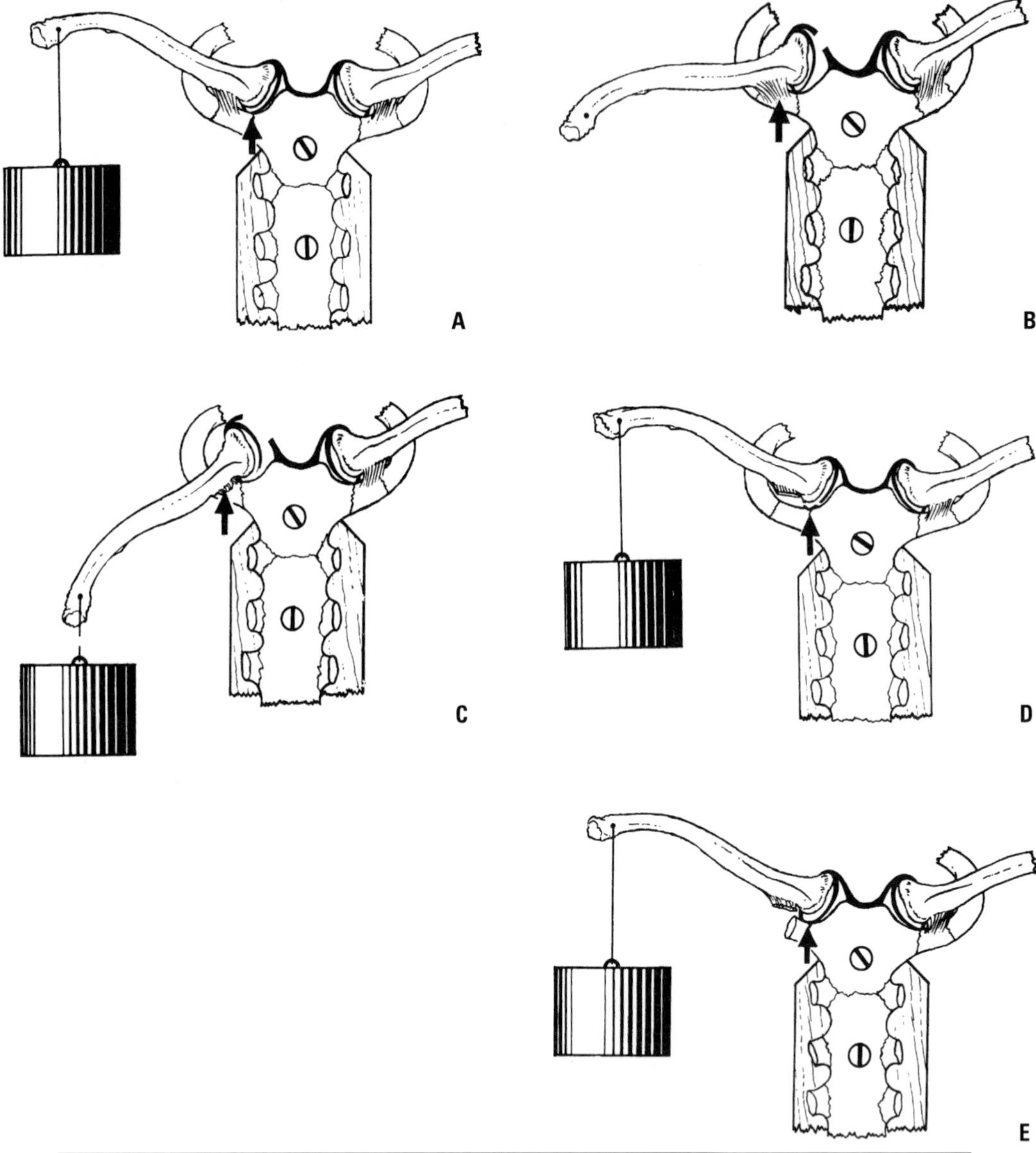

Fig. 16-2 Thought experiment demonstrating the importance of the various ligaments around the sternoclavicular joint in maintaining normal shoulder poise. **A,** The lateral portion of the clavicle is maintained in an elevated position through the sternoclavicular ligaments. The *arrow* indicates the fulcrum. **B,** When the capsule is completely divided, the lateral portion of the clavicle descends under its own weight without any loading. The clavicle will seem to be supported by the intra-articular disk ligament. **C,** After division of the capsular ligament, it was determined that a weight of less than 5 pounds was enough to tear the intra-articular disk ligament from its attachment on the costal cartilage junction of the first rib. The fulcrum was transferred laterally so that the medial third of the clavicle hinged over the first rib in the vicinity of the costoclavicular ligament. **D,** After division of the costoclavicular ligament and the intra-articular disc ligament, the lateral end of the clavicle could not be depressed as long as the capsular ligament was intact. **E,** After resection of the first medial costal cartilage along with the costoclavicular ligament, there is no effect on the poise of the lateral end of the clavicle as long as the capsular ligament remains intact. (From Bearne JG: *J Anat* 101:159-170, 1967.)

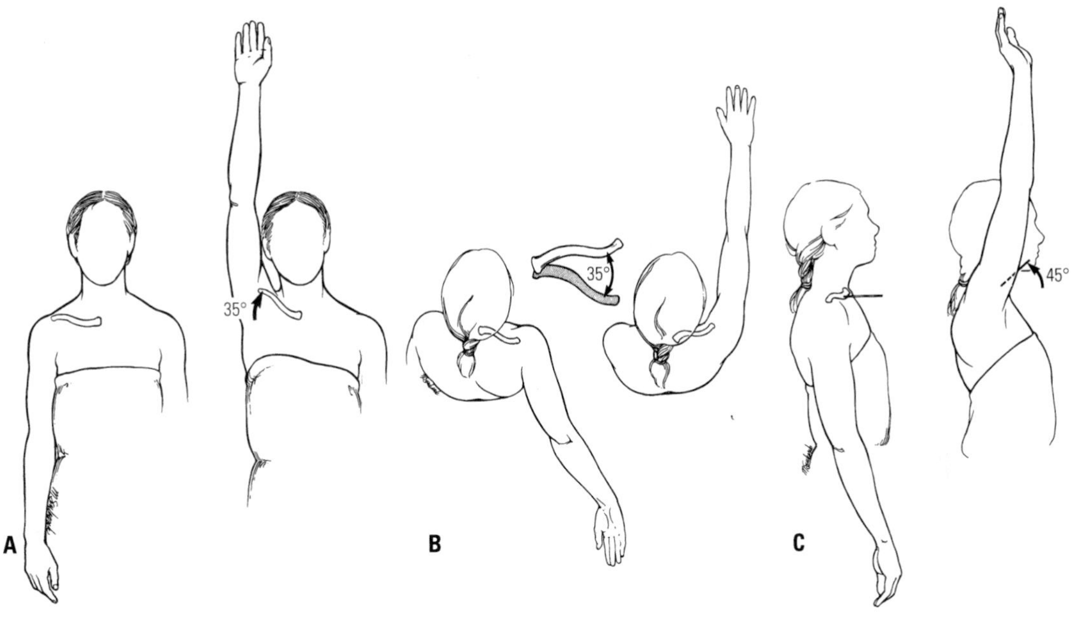

Fig. 16-3 Motions of the clavicle and the sternoclavicular joint. **A,** With full overhead elevation the clavicle elevates as far as 35°. **B,** With adduction and extension the clavicle is displaced anteriorly and posteriorly by 35°. **C,** The clavicle rotates on its long axis over a range of 45° as the arm is elevated to the full overhead position. (From Rockwood CA, Matsen FA, editors: *The shoulder,* vol 1, Philadelphia, 1990, Saunders.)

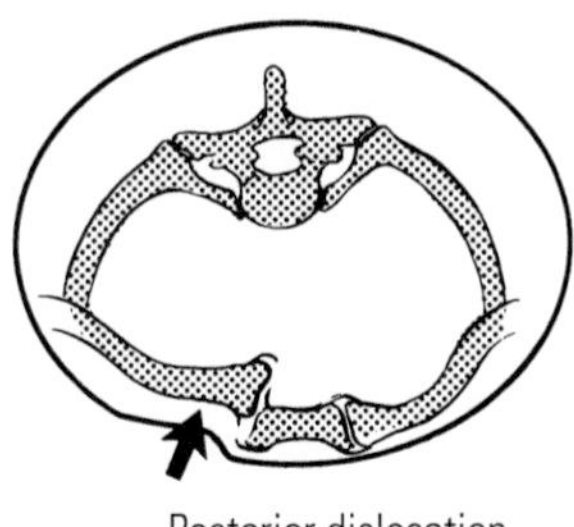

Fig. 16-4 Posterior dislocation of the sternoclavicular joint. A cross-sectional view through the thorax. (From Rockwood CA, Green DP, editors: *Fractures,* ed 2, Philadelphia, 1984, Lippincott.)

producing an anterior dislocation medially, where the clavicle meets the SC joint; whereas, if the shoulder is rolled forward, the force directed down onto the clavicle yields a posterior dislocation of the SC joint. Other types of indirect forces causing SC joint dislocation include a cave-in on a ditch digger with lateral shoulder compression by falling dirt; lateral compressive forces on the shoulder when an individual becomes pinned between a vehicle and a wall; and a person's falling onto an outstretched abducted arm, which serves to drive the shoulder medially in the same manner as lateral compression of the shoulder does.[9]

12. What is the classification of SC joint injury?

Mild sprain All the ligaments are intact, and the joint is stable. There is mild to moderate pain, particularly on upper extremity movement. Although the joint may be slightly swollen and tender, there is no instability noted.[9]

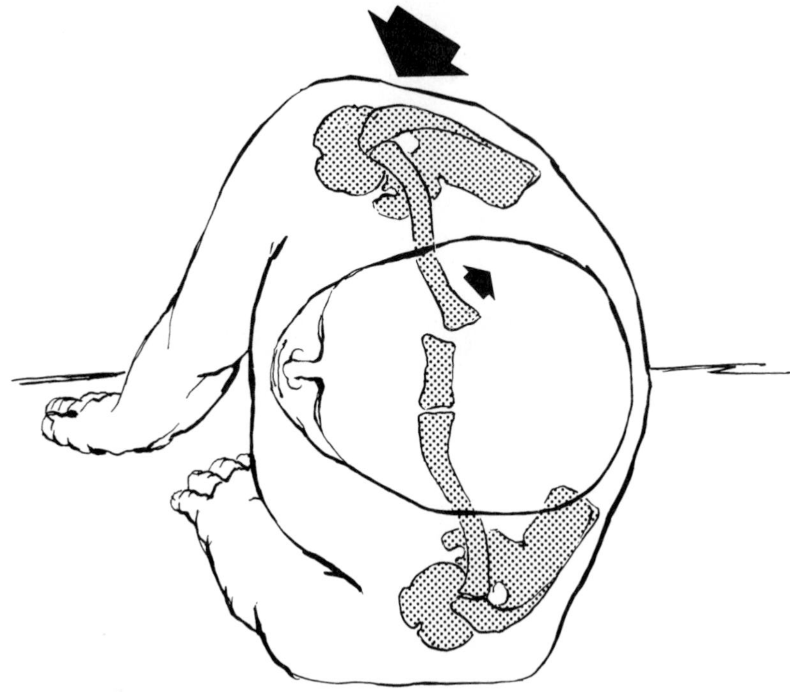

Fig. 16-5 Mechanisms that produce anterior or posterior dislocations of the sternoclavicular joint. If the patient is lying on the ground and a compression force is applied to the posterior lateral aspect of the shoulder, the medial third of the clavicle will be displaced posteriorly. (From Rockwood CA, Green DP, editors: *Fractures,* ed 3, Philadelphia, 1984, Lippincott.)

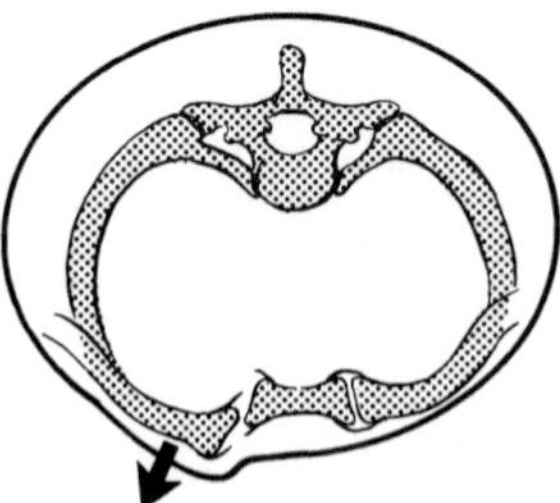

Fig. 16-6 Anterior dislocation of the sternoclavicular joint. A cross-sectional view through the thorax. (From Rockwood CA, Green DP, editors: *Fractures,* ed 3, Philadelphia, 1984, Lippincott.)

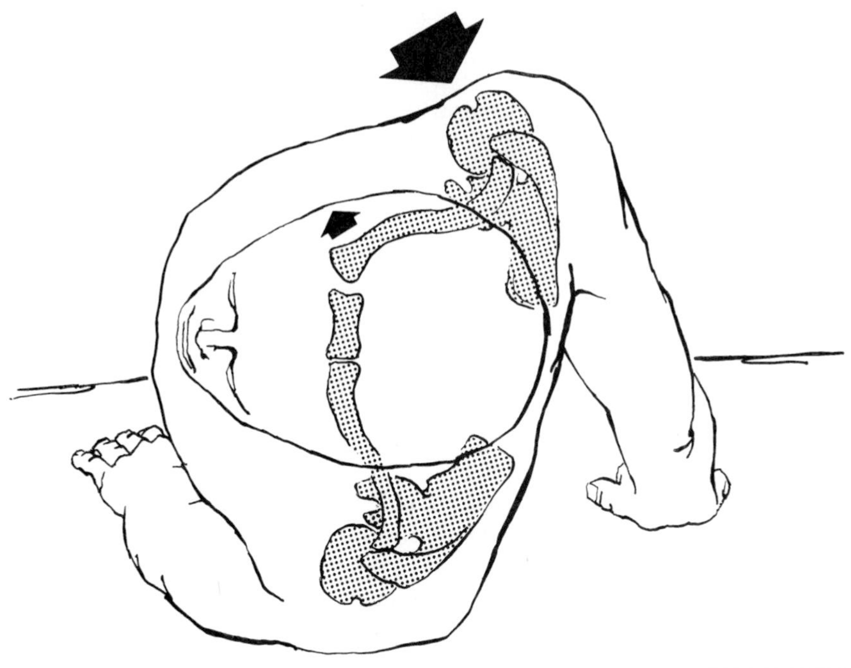

Fig. 16-7 When the lateral compression force is directed from the anterior position, the medial third of the clavicle is dislocated posteriorly. (From Rockwood CA, Green GP, editors: *Fractures*, ed 2, Philadelphia, 1984, Lippincott.)

Moderate sprain There is anterior or posterior subluxation of the SC joint because of partial disrupture or severe stretch of the capsule, intra-articular disk, and costoclavicular ligament. Swelling is noted and pain is intense, especially with any arm movement.[9]

Severe sprain There is complete disruption of the SC ligaments with dislocation being either anterior or posterior. Severe pain is present and is increased by any arm movement, though especially when the shoulders are laterally pressed together. Discomfort is increased when the patient is placed in the supine position; it will be noted that in this position the involved shoulder will not lie back flat on the table. The patient will usually support the injured arm across the trunk with the uninvolved arm. The affected shoulder appears to be shortened and thrust forward when compared with the normal shoulder. In addition, the head may be tilted toward the side of the dislocated joint.[9] Whereas an anterior SC joint injury shows a visibly prominent medial clavicle that can be palpated anterior to the sternum, the anterosuperior fullness of the chest normally imparted by the superior outline of the clavicle is less prominent and visible with posterior SC joint dislocation. Additionally, with posterior dislocation the corner of the sternum becomes more easily palpated as compared with the normal contralateral SC joint. There is greater pain experienced with posterior dislocation, and the patient may complain of shortness of breath, experience a choking sensation, feel tightness of the throat, experience decreased circulation of the ipsilateral arm, be in a state of shock, or possibly have a pneumothorax.[9]

13. Why is diagnosis predicated on clinical evidence rather than on radiologic evidence?

Aside from a history of injury, this condition is more readily diagnosed clinically by local tenderness and prominence of the medial third of the clavicle than by radiographic determination. The reason is that even with specially recommended oblique views distortion may occur from clavicles being superimposed one over the other.[9]

14. What is the medical treatment of subluxation or dislocation when not life threatening?

Dislocation, if present, may be reduced by local pressure over the dislocated end of the clavicle,[10] and the reduction can be maintained by immobilization of a figure-of-eight bandage.[5] In the event of moderate sprain with subluxation, reduction is achieved by the physician drawing the patient's shoulders backward as if reducing and holding a clavicular fracture, followed by a clavicle strap or figure-of-eight strap to hold the reduction in place.[9]

15. What therapeutic intervention and advice is appropriate?

In the event of a *mild sprain*, application of ice for the first 12 to 24 hours, followed by heat, has proved to be helpful. The upper extremity is immobilized for 3 to 4 days in a sling with gradual return to everyday activities thereafter. With *moderate sprains*, ice is appropriate for the first 12 hours, followed by heat for 24 to 48 hours, as well as immobilization. For both mild and moderate sprains nonsteroidal anti-inflammatory medications and rest are appropriate.[5] Selective strengthening of coracoclavicular-ligament dynamic synergists (that is, the pectoralis minor and subclavius muscles) is a treatment strategy that, by virtue of increased tone and hypertrophy, diminish disruptive forces and further strain to the already frayed fibers of the SC ligamentous supports. When only mild to moderate sprain has occurred, the injured athlete can resume sporting activity relatively early, even if pain and other symptoms remain for several months.[8]

References

1. Bearn JG: Direct observations of the function of the capsule of the sternoclavicular joint in clavicular support, *J Anat* 101(1): 159-170, 1967.
2. Dandy DJ: *Essential orthopaedics and trauma*, Edinburgh, New York, 1989, Churchill Livingstone.
3. Grant JCB: *Method of anatomy*, ed 7, Baltimore, 1965, Williams & Wilkins.
4. Gray H: *Anatomy of the human body*, ed 28 (CM Guss, editor), Philadelphia, 1966, Lea & Febiger.
5. Lillegard WA, Rucker KS: *Handbook of sports medicine: a symptom-oriented approach*, Boston, 1993, Andover Medical Publishers.
6. Moore KL: *Clinical oriented anatomy*, ed 2, Baltimore, 1985, Williams & Wilkins.
7. Nettles JL, Linscheid R: Sternoclavicular dislocations, *J Trauma* 8(2): 158-164, 1968.
8. Peterson L, Renström P: *Sports injuries: their prevention and treatment*, London, 1986, Martin Dunitz, Ltd.
9. Rockwood CA, Matsen FA, editors: *The shoulder*, vol 1, Philadelphia, 1990, Saunders.
10. Salter RB: *Textbook of disorders of the musculoskeletal system*, ed 2, Baltimore, 1983, Williams & Wilkins.

Recommended reading

Rockwood CA: Disorders of the sternoclavicular joint. Rockwood CA, Matsen FA: *The shoulder*, vol 1, Philadelphia, 1990, Saunders.

Diver Accident with Acute Pain and Deformity in Shoulder

17

A 50-year-old man jumped head first off a high diving board, with arms overhead, landing in deep water directly on upturned palms. The swimmer immediately felt something "out of place" in his left shoulder and could not use that shoulder because of pain. He yelled for help and treaded to safety where he was assisted out of the pool and then cradled his right upper extremity with his left arm, sling style.

Clue:

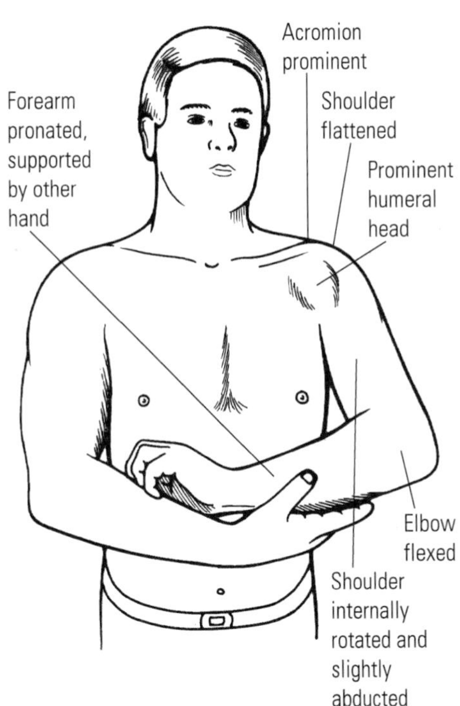

1. **What is most likely to have occurred in this man's shoulder?**
2. **How do we understand the role of the glenohumeral joint in terms of kinesiologic stability and mobility?**
3. **What osseous anatomy is relevant to an understanding of shoulder dislocation?**

4. **How does size, shape, and tilt of the glenoid fossa affect glenohumeral joint stability?**
5. **What contribution does atmospheric pressure have on glenohumeral joint stability?**
6. **What are the dynamic glenohumeral joint stabilizers?**
7. **What are ligamentous and capsular restraints that contribute to glenohumeral stability?**
8. **What predisposing motion causes this injury?**
9. **What neural, vascular, tendinous, or skeletal structures might be damaged along with this injury?**
10. **What other joints or bones could be damaged by a fall onto an outstretched hand and pronated forearm?**
11. **What are the four kinds of anterior dislocation?**
12. **What is the clinical presentation of anterior dislocation?**
13. **What special tests are appropriate?**
14. **What are the three kinds of posterior dislocation?**
15. **What is the mechanism of posterior dislocation, and how is this managed?**
16. **Why is posterior dislocation more likely than anterior dislocation after electric shock?**
17. **What is the clinical presentation of posterior dislocation?**
18. **What radiographs are appropriate in detecting dislocation?**
19. **What medical treatment is appropriate in the treatment of anterior dislocation?**
20. **What are some common forms of reduction?**
21. **What is the postreduction management?**
22. **What is the difficulty in managing chronic anterior traumatic dislocations?**
23. **What accounts for the high incidence of recurrent dislocation?**
24. **What is the mechanism of recurrent dislocation?**
25. **What is "apprehension shoulder"?**
26. **What is recurrent instability with an atraumatic onset?**
27. **How is recurrent instability categorized, and how is it managed?**
28. **What nonoperative management is appropriate after shoulder dislocation?**
29. **What is surgical management in those patients for whom operative treatment is advisable?**
30. **What postoperative therapeutic management is appropriate?**

1. **What is most likely to have occurred in this man's shoulder?**

Anterior (subcoracoid) glenohumeral joint dislocation (Fig. 17-1) is the most common (>90%)[16] of all four[17] possible glenohumeral (GH) dislocations. The shoulder joint is the most commonly dislocated major body joint.[17]

2. **How do we understand the role of the glenohumeral joint in terms of kinesiologic stability and mobility?**

It is important to understand that with every joint system there is a unique trade-off between stability versus mobility. For example, the hip joint sacrifices mobility, that is, circumduction in lieu of stability, whereas the GH joint sacrifices stability for mobility, hence the greater likelihood of GH joint dislocation. The glenohumeral joint evolved from being an essentially weight-bearing joint of a foreleg into a limb that functions mostly in an open kinetic chain and exhibits a wide range of movement capabilities. Thus the GH joint is better suited for mobility and is an example of yet another adaptive change that, despite the price of lost proximal stability, opened the door to unparalleled distal prehensile dexterity. The carpometacarpal joint of the human thumb is the virtuoso of prehension that permitted an opposition capa-

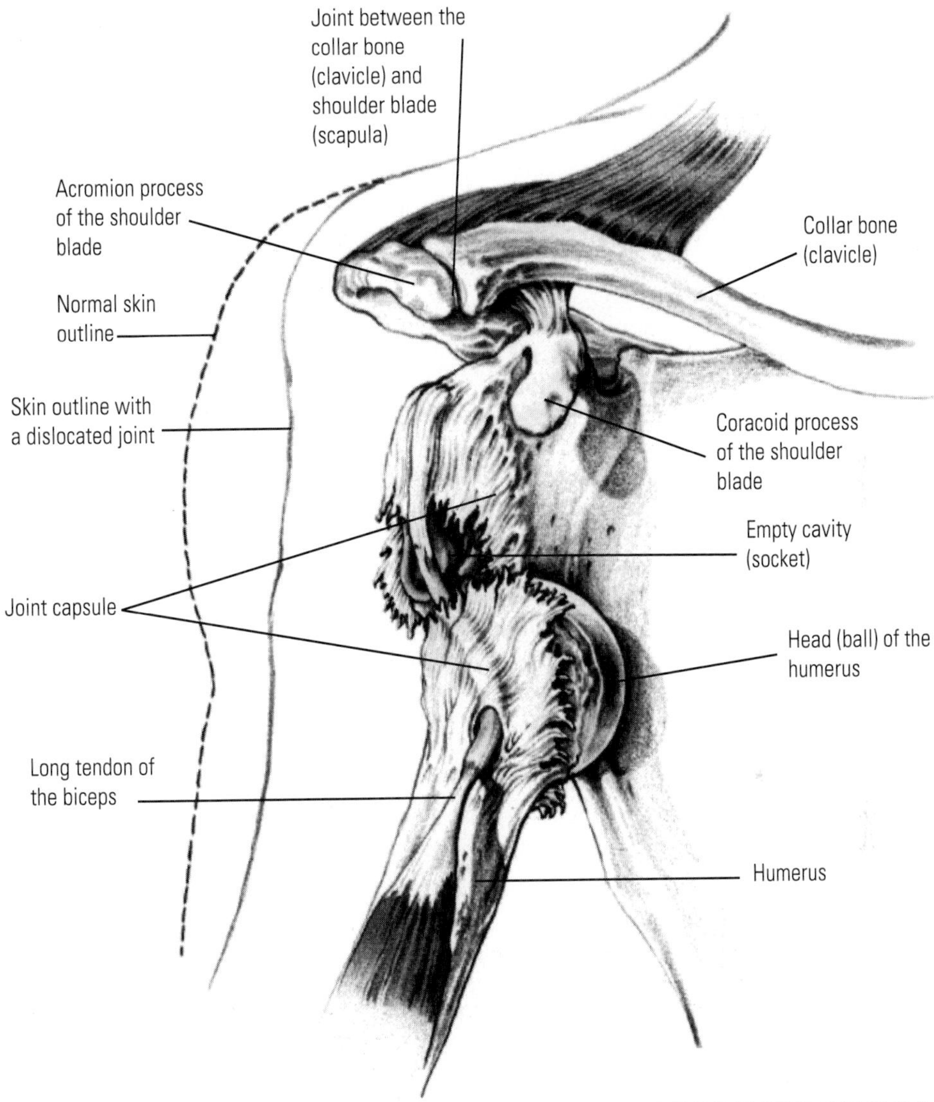

Fig. 17-1 Subcoracoid (anteroinferior) dislocation of the glenohumeral joint with tear of the glenoid labrum and joint capsule. (From Peterson L, Renström P: *Sports injuries: their prevention and treatment,* London, 1986, Martin Dunitz, Ltd.)

bility virtually unparalleled in primates. Ironically, once freed of the quadruped posture, the upright posture enabled man to develop from the most defenseless of all creatures into the most powerful of creatures as a direct function of man's ability to fashion and use weapons and tools.*

*Interestingly, manipulations of the thumb are represented by a larger portion of the cerebral motor homunculus than in the total control of the chest and abdomen.

3. What osseous anatomy is relevant to an understanding of shoulder dislocation?

The small and shallow glenoid fossa of the scapula articulates with the relatively large spherical head of the humerus but provides little coverage for the head, especially when the shoulder is (1) adducted, flexed, and internally rotated; (2) abducted and elevated; or (3) adducted at the side with the scapula rotated downward.[4,29,35] Despite this relative lack of coverage, the normal shoulder kinesiology precisely constrains the head to within 1 mm of the center of the glenoid cavity throughout its wide arc of movement.[12,24] Whether the arm resists the gravitational pull of the limb for long periods of time by just hanging at the side, lifting large resistive loads, or even a professional baseball pitcher's ability to throw a ball at speeds approaching 100 miles per hour, the shoulder incredibly holds together. It is curious then that shoulder instability is not more common than it really is. The reason for this is that glenohumeral joint stability results from a hierarchy of *passive* and *active stabilizing mechanisms.* Minimal loads such as the gravitational pull of the upper limb are resisted by passive mechanisms such as concavity of the glenoid and labrum, finite joint volume, and surface tension provided by joint fluid (synovia). Larger loads such as serving a tennis ball or picking up a child are facilitated by the action of various shoulder muscles.[17]

4. How does size, shape, and tilt of the glenoid fossa affect glenohumeral joint stability?

There is considerable variation in the radii of curvature of the glenoid fossa. The glenoid (acting as a shelf) faces anteriorly at an angle of about 45° to the coronal plane, which places it behind the humeral head for most uses of the shoulder.[17] Obviously, GH joint stability is directly affected by the size, shape, and tilt of the glenoid fossa. The depth and hence stability of this bony fossa are enhanced by contributions of the articular cartilage and glenoid labrum (a thickened capsular attachment to the glenoid rim). Together, they provide an element of plasticity that serves to enhance the quality of GH coupling, similar to the "feathered" edge of a contact lens.[17]

5. What contribution does atmospheric pressure have on glenohumeral joint stability?

The normal shoulder joint is sealed by a joint capsule that prevents outside fluid from entering. There is minimal free fluid[17] (less than 1 ml) with the GH joint that is imbued with a slightly negative pressure of –4.0 mm Hg.[33] An analogy may be drawn when one attempts to pull up the plunger of a plugged syringe that is held upside down; a relative vacuum is created, and it resists upward displacement of the plunger. Similarly the shoulder joint is stabilized by a limited joint volume, and as long as that volume remains in a closed space with minimal free fluid, the joint surfaces cannot be easily distracted or subluxed. Small translations of the humerus on the glenoid (that is, joint play) are permitted as they are balanced by fluid flow in the opposite direction.[17]

When the gap between the articular surfaces becomes very small, intermolecular forces of surface tension, cohesion, and adhesion provide continued coupling of the humerus to the glenoid.[17] *Surface tension* refers to the tendency of the surface of a liquid to contract its surface area so that as little energy is expended as possible to maintain that shape. This is clarified when we consider liquid drops, whether they be molten metal, plain water, or drops of oil; all these examples, like an inflated balloon, assume that configuration having the least surface per given volume: the sphere. The familiar example of two wet microscope slides pressed together illustrates these forces; the two slides readily slide on each other but cannot easily be pulled apart by forces applied at right angles to their flat surfaces. "Tension" refers to the elastic quality of a liquid surface that resembles a membrane under tension. It is surface tension that permits razor blades or sewing needles to "float" when placed on a water surface and permits water bugs to move across the surface of the water.

Adhesion refers to the attraction between unlike substances (liquid to solid, such as joint fluid to bone), whereas *cohesion* refers to the attraction of like substances (joint fluid to joint fluid). These intermolecular forces account for capillary action responsible for bringing water to the roots of plants, for the flow of blood through capillary vessels, for the oil to rise in a lamp wick, or for causing water in a dipped corner of a sugar cube to quickly spread throughout the entire lump.

The addition of excess fluid into the GH joint works to nullify both the joint volume effect and the intermolecular effect. For example, the addition of blood into the joint due to an intracapsular fracture may result in inferior subluxation.[17] Thus we may venture that in the unopened state of the joint, the weight of the limb is almost entirely borne by atmospheric pressure.[14]

Interarticular forces may also be overwhelmed by the application of traction, as for example in the cracking sound of the metacarpophalangeal joint as that joint cavitates. Subatmospheric pressure within the joint releases gas (80% CO_2) from joint solution, and that release is accompanied by a sudden jump of the finger caused by joint separation. The finger does not fall away because the finger is relatively light and does not overwhelm the restraining soft tissue, which keeps it attached to the hand. Once a joint has been cracked it will not do so until about 20 minutes later when all the gas has been reabsorbed.[26,36]

6. What are the dynamic glenohumeral joint stabilizers?

Dynamic GH joint stability is provided by a cowl of muscles[3] composed of the rotator cuff. By virtue of these tendons blending with the GH capsule and ligaments, selective contraction of these muscles adjust the tension of those static structures, producing "dynamic" ligaments.[2] Second, by contracting simultaneously, these muscles press the humeral head into the glenoid socket, securing it into the center of that fossa.[24] Third, by way of selective contraction so as to resist displacing forces, as when the lateral deltoid initiates shoulder abduction, supraspinatus (primarily) and the long biceps tendon actively resist upward displacement of the humeral head relative to the fossa.[21,34] When the pectoralis major and the anterior deltoid elevate and flex the shoulder, they tend to push the humeral head posteriorly out the back of the fossa. This displacement is selectively resisted by the combined contractile efforts of subscapularis, infraspinatus, and teres minor muscles.[17]

Additionally, the glenoid fossa has an upward, lateral, and forward orientation that serves as a seat or shelf for the humeral head. This bony source of stability is provided by the normal muscle tone of the shoulder protractors, the serratus anterior and upper trapezius. In the event of decreased tone, as may occur after a stroke, dynamic stability is lost, and the humeral head simply slides down and off the now almost vertical fossa.

7. What are ligamentous and capsular restraints that contribute to glenohumeral stability?

There are five scapulohumeral ligaments (Fig. 17-2) serving as important static shoulder stabilizers when they are under tension. These ligaments provide a passive *checkrein* function that serve as the last guardian of shoulder stability after all other passive and dynamic mechanisms have been overwhelmed.[17] The anteromedial and anteroinferior glenohumeral ligaments serve to restrain the humeral head during abduction[22] and external rotation[35] of the shoulder respectively, whereas the posterorinferior and posterosuperior capsule serve to restrain the humeral head from posterior dislocation.[32] Inferior to the GH joint, at the axilla, these ligaments manifest as redundant and crenated ligaments that help hold the humeral head against the glenoid. Considerable variation exists in the size of these ligaments, which may explain why certain shoulders appear more unstable.

8. What predisposing motion causes this injury?

The intrinsic instability of the shoulder is increased when shoulder abduction is superimposed on external rotation and extension.[31] These movements yield forces that challenge the anterior capsular ligaments, the glenoid rim, and rotator cuff mechanism and, if sufficient in magnitude, propel the humeral head

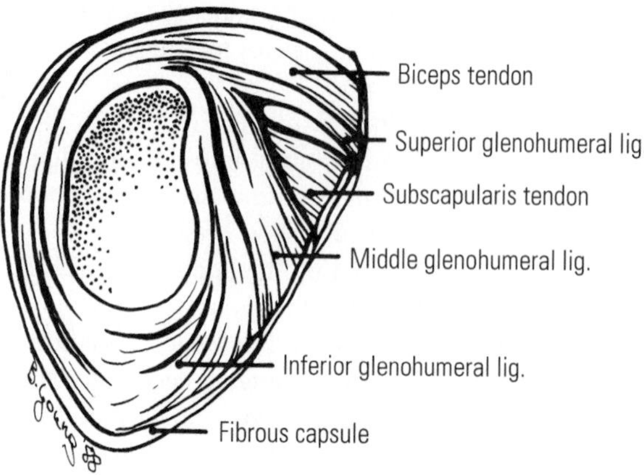

Fig. 17-2 Scapulohumeral ligaments. The coracohumeral and posteroinferior glenohumeral ligaments are not shown. (From Rockwood CA, Matsen FA, editors: *The shoulder*, vol 1, 1990, Philadelphia, Saunders.)

along a path of least resistance toward the inferior glenoid where it may subluxate. As a result, the fibrous ligamentous capsule may be partially torn (sprained), the glenoid labrum may become partially or completely detached from the glenoid (Bankart lesion),[31] or the rotator cuff[15] is damaged. The last may occur because the tendons of the rotator cuff blend in with the capsule as they insert onto the humeral tuberosities.[17] The most common mechanism of injury occurs after a forward fall in which our protective extension response protects our head at the expense of injury elsewhere. Had our swimmer positioned his hand forward instead of upward in extension, he would have provided himself a more streamlined shape and would have avoided landing on the volar surfaces of his hand. In the elderly, this same mechanism of injury fractures the humeral neck rather than dislocates the joint because the bones, having become brittle, are weaker than the ligaments.[3] Anterior dislocation is common in downhill skiing injuries,[1a] in grand mal seizures, and after racket sports when the arm is quickly brought back to meet an oncoming ball, and it may also occur from a ball or blow directly onto the posterolateral aspect of the shoulder.

9. What neural, vascular, tendinous, or skeletal structures might be damaged along with this injury?

Complications of traumatic anterior dislocation include the following:

- Compression *fractures* of the humeral head (Hill-Sachs lesion), fractures of the anterior glenoid lip, and fractures of the acromion or of the coracoid processes associated with superior shoulder dislocation after an extreme forward and upward force on the adducted arm.[17] The greater humeral tuberosity may avulse in tandem with anterior dislocation, especially when the patient lands on outstretched arms, or from a blow or fall onto the shoulder, particularly in older patients. Although the fragment readily unites in good position, the supraspinatus tendon may pull it away. The healed fragment may then wedge in the subacromial arch and obstruct elevation.[3]
- *Cuff tears* may accompany anterior and inferior GH dislocation, especially if the mechanism of injury was a fall onto the lateral aspect of the shoulder.[10] The frequency of this complication increases with age, and its incidence exceeds 30% in patients greater than 30 years of age and is over 80% in patients older than 60. Rotator cuff tears may present as pain or weakness on testing of external rotation or abduction.[17]

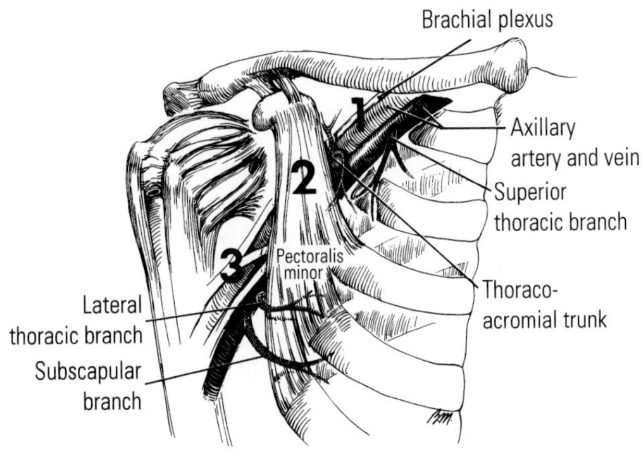

Fig. 17-3 The axillary artery is divided into three parts by the pectoralis minor muscle; the second part is behind it, and the third part is lateral to it. (From Rockwood CA, Green DP, editors: *Fractures*, ed 2, Philadelphia, 1984, Lippincott.)

- *Vascular injuries* most frequently occur in elderly patients with stiffer, more fragile vessels.[17] Injury may occur in the axillary artery, the axillary vein, or the branches of the axillary artery (Fig. 17-3) and most often occur after inferior dislocation. This complication most commonly occurs during closed reduction of an old anterior dislocation mistaken for an acute injury.[17] The vessel is brittle and cannot tolerate the required traction involved in reduction. The radial pulse should be checked and its presence recorded after every reduction, whether chronic or acute. The patient must be closely monitored because this dangerous situation may require emergency surgery.[17]
- *Neural injuries.* The brachial plexus and axillary artery lie immediately anterior, inferior, and medial to the GH joint.[9] The axillary nerve originates at the posterior cord of the brachial plexus, and the anterior branch of this nerve (that is, the circumflex humeral) wraps directly around the humeral wall in the area of the surgical neck.[3] Thus this nerve has no padding and is predisposed to injury from a hard blow to the area, from a fracture of the upper humerus, or after anterior shoulder dislocation. Anterior dislocation may cause traction strain to this nerve in that portion of nerve lying in close relation to the underside of the GH joint articular capsule[20] (Fig. 17-4). Injury most commonly causes a traction neurapraxia resulting in partial or complete paralysis of the deltoid muscles.[17] Although there is usually complete recovery, the nerve should undergo electromyographic studies after injury and then 3 weeks later.[3] Since the deltoid muscle cannot be adequately assessed, it is not enough to simply rely on testing the sensory area over the middle of the deltoid because this method is unreliable.[20] Sensation may also be compromised in the distribution of the musculocutaneous nerve (lateral antebrachial cutaneous nerve) supplying the lateral surface of the forearm. Subsequently, if no change has occurred between the two examinations, the nerve is explored and repaired.[3] Lower brachial plexus injuries may also occur and should be suspected if there has been a concomitant violent abduction strain.

10. What other joints or bones could be damaged by a fall onto an outstretched hand and pronated forearm?

Other types of injury occurring after a fall onto an outstretched hand with the forearm pronated include posterior GH joint dislocation, clavicular fracture, humeral head fractures in senescent adults, supracondylar fractures in children or anterior elbow dislocation in adults, dislocated radial head, fractures of

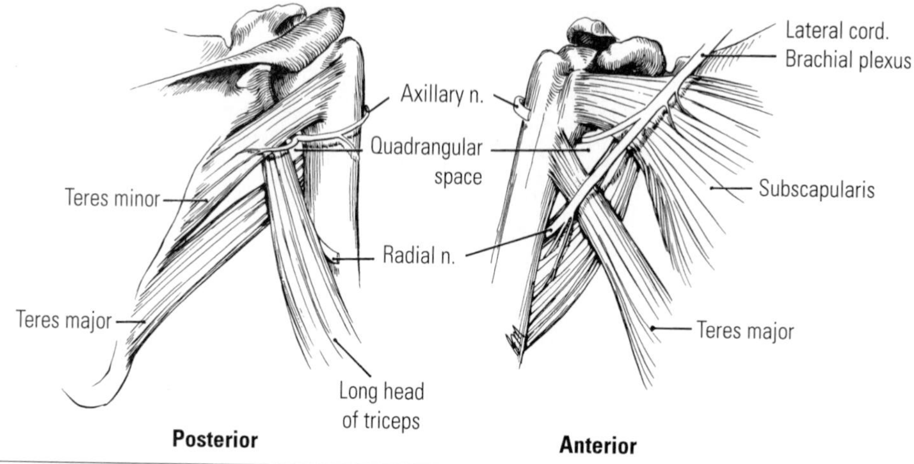

Fig. 17-4 Relations of the axillary nerve to the subscapularis muscle, the quadrangular space, and the humeral neck. With anterior dislocations the subscapularis is displaced forward, and such displacement creates a traction injury to the axillary nerve. The nerve cannot move out of the way because it is held above by the brachial plexus and below where it wraps around behind the neck of the humerus. (From Rockwood CA, Green DP, editors: *Fractures*, ed 2, Philadelphia, 1984, Lippincott.)

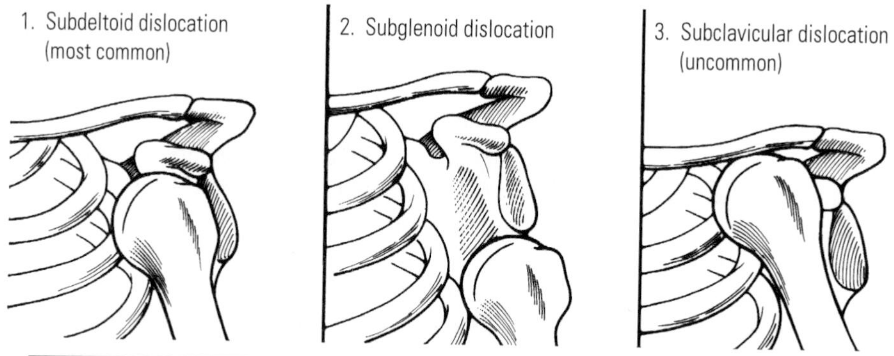

Fig. 17-5 Anterior glenohumeral joint dislocation. *1,* Subcoracoid dislocation is the most common. *2,* Subglenoid dislocation. *3,* Subclavicular dislocation is uncommon.

the radial head, fractures of the capitellum, Colles's fracture, scaphoid fracture, and lunate dislocation.[30] This list highlights the orthopedic principle in which the same injury mechanism produces age-specific injuries.[19]

11. What are the four kinds of anterior dislocation?

Classification of anterior dislocation (Fig. 17-5):

- ***Subcoracoid.*** The humeral head is displaced anteriorly with respect to the glenoid and is inferior to the coracoid process. This is the most common type of anterior dislocation.
- ***Subglenoid.*** The humeral head lies anterior and below the glenoid fossa.
- ***Subclavicular.*** The humeral head lies medial to the coracoid process, just inferior to the lower border of the clavicle.
- ***Intrathoracic.*** The humeral head lies between the ribs and thoracic cavity.

- Subclavicular dislocation is uncommon, whereas intrathoracic dislocation is rare. These two forms of dislocation are usually associated with severe trauma.[17]

12. What is the clinical presentation of anterior dislocation?

The acute anteriorly dislocated shoulder is very painful (that is, sharp stabbing pain), and muscles are in spasm in the attempt to stabilize the joint. The dislocated humeral head may be palpable anteriorly or inferiorly in the armpit.[5] In the posterior part of the shoulder, a cavity may be palpated below the acromion where the humeral head usually resides. The arm is held in slight abduction and external rotation. Anterior dislocation usually yields a shoulder that is incapable of complete internal rotation and abduction.[17]

The characteristic profile (on p. 193) presents as a flat lateral shoulder contour that produces a straight drop in line of the shoulder from the tip of the acromion[5] to the lateral humeral epicondyle, known as the *positive Hamilton's ruler test.*[3] A square shoulder[31] with apparent indentation beneath the

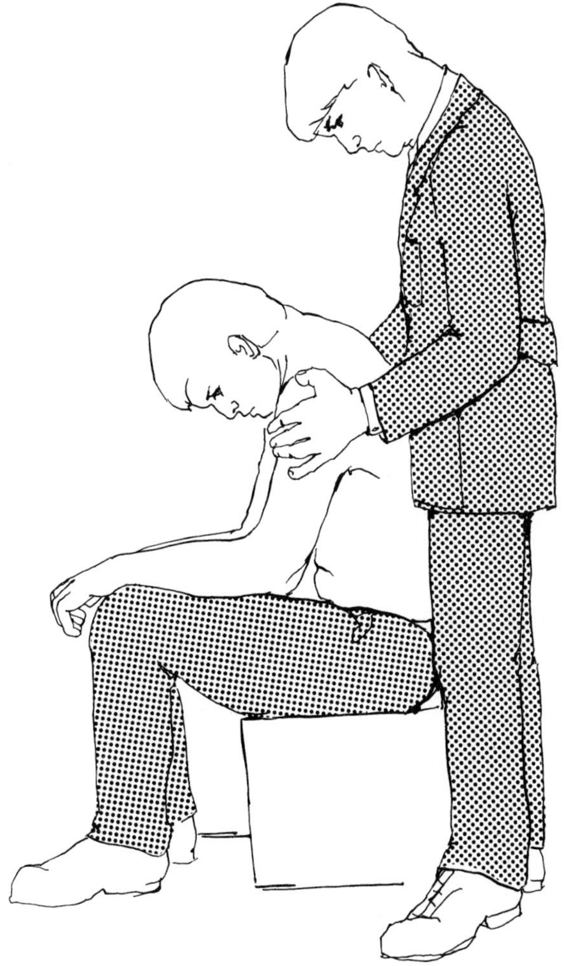

Fig. 17-6 Visualization of the anterior and posterior aspects of the shoulders may best be accomplished by having the patient sit on a low stool, with the therapist standing behind him. The injured shoulder may then be easily compared with the uninjured one. (From Rockwood CA, Green DP, editors: *Fractures*, ed 2, Philadelphia, 1984, Lippincott.)

acromion is apparent. Although a similar flat contour is also seen in patients with either wasted deltoid muscles or displaced surgical neck fractures, these latter patients score negative on the ruler test, since the humeral head is still in its normal position.[3] If the distance between the acromion process to the lateral humeral epicondyle on the involved side is not slightly greater than on the uninvolved side, a fracture of the proximal end of the humerus should be suspected.

13. What special tests are appropriate?

Crank, or apprehension, test (Fig. 17-7), sulcus test, and fulcrum test are for anterior instability; jerk test and posterior apprehension test (Fig. 17-8) are for posterior instability.[17]

Apprehension test With the patient sitting or standing, the examiner stands behind and raises the patient's arm to 90° of abduction and begins to rotate the shoulder externally. While one hand pulls back on the patient's wrist, the other is placed over the humeral head with the thumb pushing posteriorly for extra leverage. The other fingers are placed anteriorly to monitor any sudden instability that may occur.

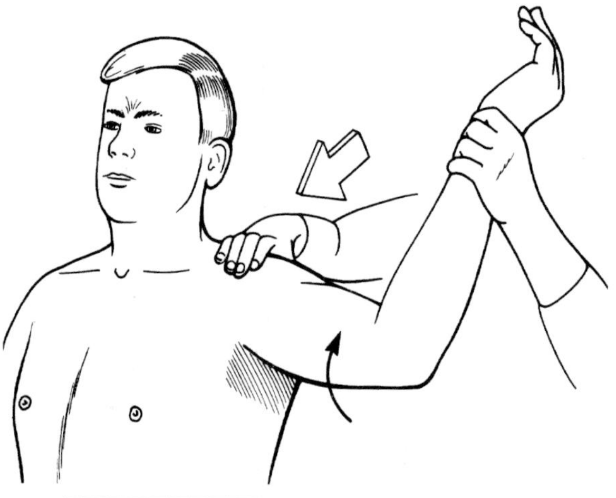

Fig. 17-7 Apprehension test for anterior dislocation.

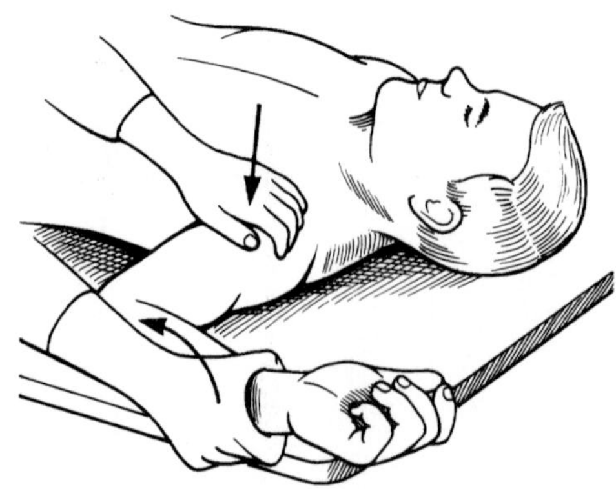

Fig. 17-8 Posterior apprehension test for posterior glenohumeral dislocation. The examiner abducts and medially rotates the patient's shoulder, followed by a posterior force applied on the proximal end of the patient's humerus. Resistance by the patient or apprehension observed on his or her face scores positive for this test.

Fulcrum test The fucrum test is a variation of the apprehension test that is performed with the patient supine for the purpose of using body weight to immobilize the scapula. Here the body acts as a counterweight. The table surface (or edge) or the examiner's hand under the glenohumeral joint acts as a fulcrum, and the patient's arm acts as a lever. With maintenance of gentle external rotation for 1 minute, the subscapularis is fatigued; apprehension will occur soon because the capsule then is challenged to maintain stability. This test isolates movement of the glenohumeral joint and allows a clear assessment of anterior translation. Also the range of external rotation causing apprehension will decrease as the patient recovers and therefore serves as an objective measure of improvement.

14. What are the three kinds of posterior dislocation?

Classification of posterior dislocation

- ***Subacromial (most common).*** Head lies behind the glenoid and beneath the acromion (Fig. 17-9).
- ***Subglenoid.*** Head behind and beneath the glenoid.
- ***Subspinous.*** Head medial to the acromion and beneath the scapular spine.[14]

15. What is the mechanism of posterior dislocation, and how is this managed?

Posterior dislocation tends to happen in the elderly.[16] The following are classic examples: when a purse is snatched from behind an owner who refuses to let go; from a blow to the front of the shoulder; or from a fall onto an outstretched upper extremity. Dislocation will occur from a combination of sudden forceful internal rotation, adduction, and flexion. Lesser tuberosity fractures are common and often cause the humeral head to become locked in the dislocated position. Reduction is accomplished by longitudinal

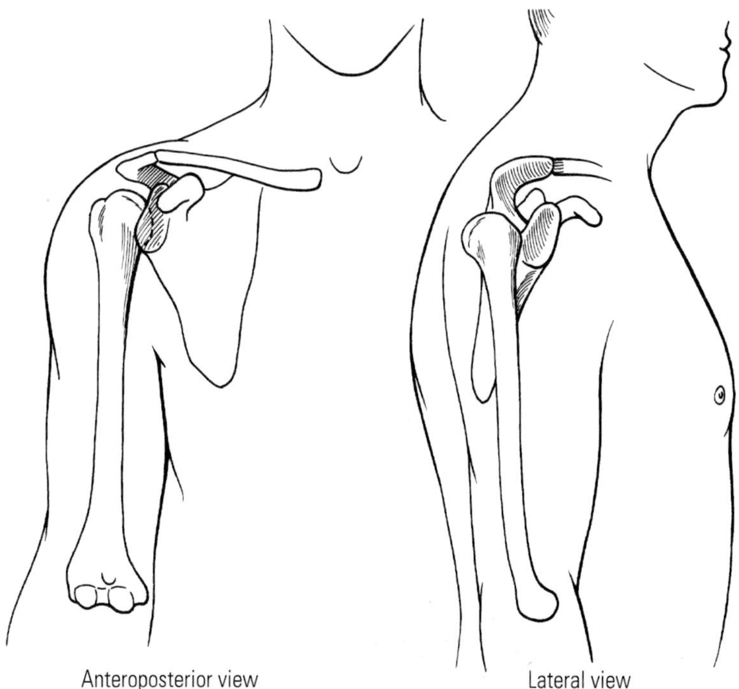

Fig. 17-9 Posterior (subacromial) dislocation.

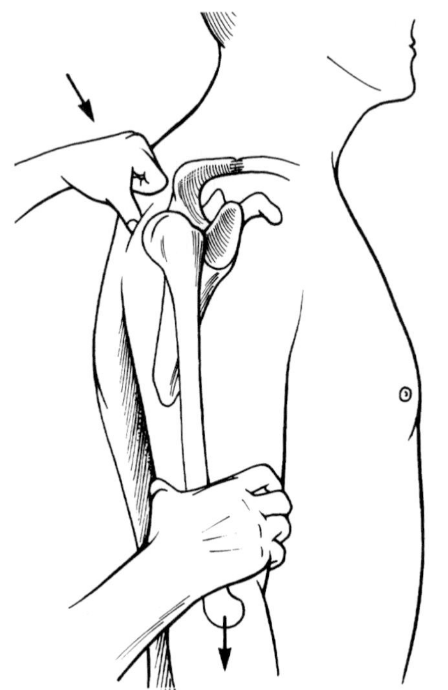

Fig. 17-10 Closed reduced of posterior glenohumeral joint dislocation.

forward traction on the arm with the elbow bent, accompanied by anterior pressure on the humeral head; the arm is then adducted, externally rotated, and then internally rotated to reduce the humeral head back into the glenoid cavity (Fig. 17-10). Immobilization in the elderly is only for 2 to 3 weeks in a handshake cast applied with the shoulder in neutral rotation and slight extension after confirmation of closed reduction by radiographs. Ice and nonsteroidal anti-inflammatory agents may bring relief. External rotation and posterior deltoid strengthening are emphasized during rehabilitation. Push-ups and bench-press exercises are to be avoided.[17]

16. Why is posterior dislocation more likely than anterior dislocation after electric shock?

Although convulsive seizures, accidental electric shock, or electric shock therapy may cause anterior dislocation, dislocation is usually posterior because the strong internal rotators simply overpower the relatively weaker external rotators. The reason is that the combined strength of the latissimus dorsi, pectoralis major, and subscapularis muscles overwhelms the infraspinatus and teres minor muscles by virtue of greater muscle bulk represented as a force vector of greater magnitude.[17]

17. What is the clinical presentation of posterior dislocation?

Recognition of posterior shoulder dislocation may be hampered by a lack of striking deformity as well as by the fact that any observed anomaly is masked by the shoulder being held in the traditional sling position of adduction and internal rotation.[17] Diagnosis may be missed because posterior dislocations are so rare (1%). In the initial interval before diagnosis of posterior dislocation is declared, the injury may be misdiagnosed as frozen shoulder, for which vigorous therapy may mistakenly be initiated in an attempt to restore range of motion.[11] A proper history is therefore absolutely necessary during the examination.

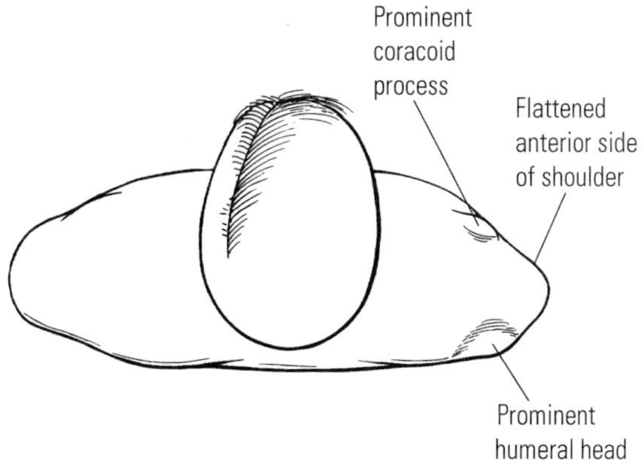

Fig. 17-11 Profile of posterior glenohumeral shoulder dislocation.

The classic clinical features of posterior dislocation include the following:

- Limited external rotation of the shoulder (often to less than 0°) and limited shoulder elevation (often to less than 90°) because of the humeral head becoming fixed or even impaled on the posterior glenoid rim by muscle forces. The shoulder appears fixed in abduction. Over time, the posterior rim of the glenoid may become further impacted into the fracture of the humeral head and produce a deep hatchet-like defect or V-shaped compression fracture of the lesser tuberosity, which engages the head and locks it even more securely in the position of posterior dislocation.
- Flattening of the anterior aspect of the shoulder and posterior prominence of the humeral head is best appreciated when one views the shoulders from above while standing behind the patient. The coracoid process may be prominent[17] (Fig. 17-11).

After confirmation of closed reduction by radiographs a handshake cast is applied in neutral shoulder rotation and slight extension for 3 weeks.

18. What radiographs are appropriate in detecting dislocation?

Anteroposterior views in the plane of the body are often deceptive and may lead the clinician into a diagnostic trap.[18] Rather, a series of radiographs in the plane of the scapula (that is, anteroposterior, scapular lateral, and axillary) are appropriate for all types of suspected dislocation.[17]

Humeral head defects confirming previous anterior dislocation in the case of posteromedial head defects and posterior dislocations in the event of anterolateral head defects are identified with special radiographic views.

19. What medical treatment is appropriate in the treatment of anterior dislocation?

Initial treatment includes the application of ice and the use of a sling. Although spasm occurs within a few minutes after dislocation, reduction should not be attempted until the shoulder is radiologically examined, regardless of how obvious the diagnosis may be. Reduction attempts are ill advised and may be dangerous if there is an associated fracture.[3] Acute GH joint dislocation should be reduced as quickly and gently as possible because early relocation quickly reduces stretch and compression of neurovascular structures, minimizes the degree of muscle spasm that must be overcome to reduce the joint, and prevents progressive enlargement of the humeral head defect in locked dislocations.[17]

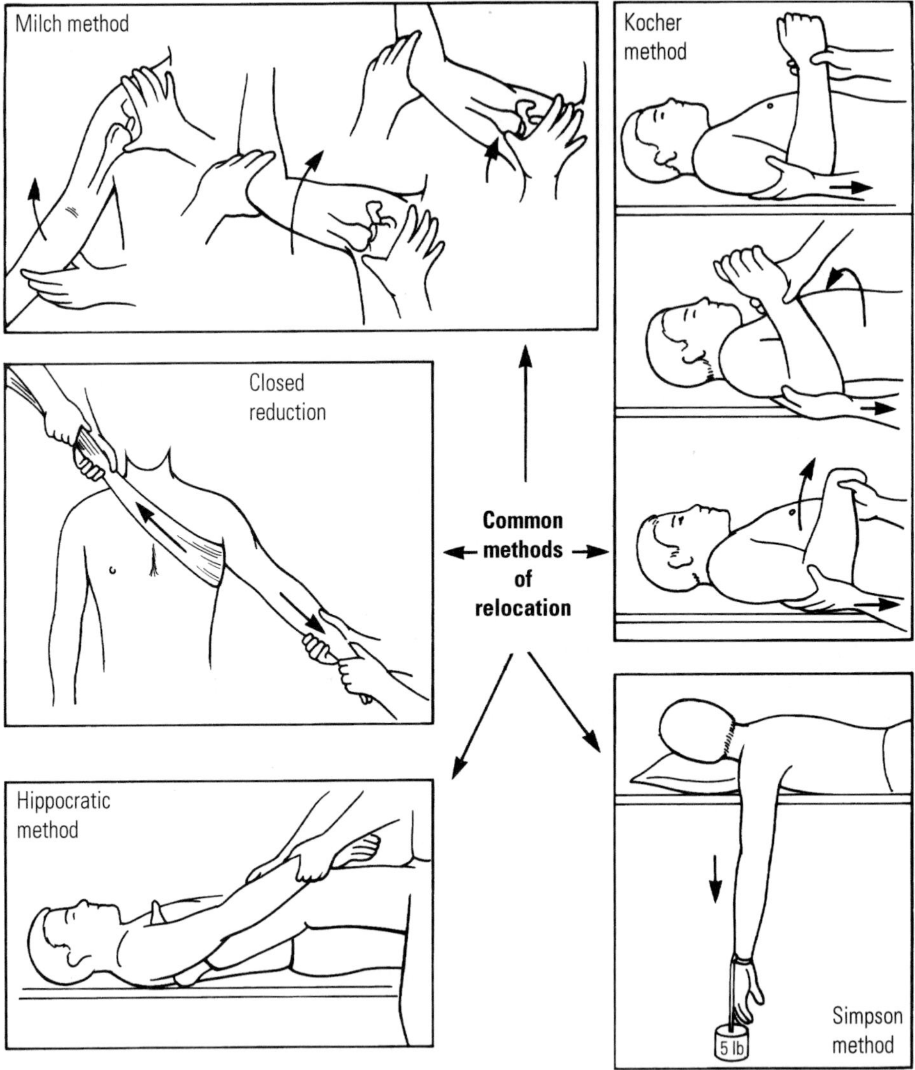

Fig. 17-12 Various methods of reduction of anterior shoulder dislocation.

20. What are some common forms of reduction?

There are two different principles used in the reduction (Fig. 17-12) of anterior shoulder dislocation: *traction* (or countertraction) and *leverage*. Leverage, however, involves the application of great force and may result in damage to the capsule, axillary vessels, or brachial plexus;[17] a simple and perhaps less painful reduction technique.

21. What is the postreduction management?

Postreduction treatment focuses on optimizing shoulder stability as well as muscle rehabilitation (that is, strengthening the rotator cuff and long biceps muscle) to impose a normal biomechanic pattern on a disrupted shoulder kinesiologic character.[17] Cryotherapy and nonsteroidal anti-inflammatory agents are appropriate when needed for either age group.

Controversy exists regarding the length of the immobilization period.[15] Because recurrent dislocation is common in patients less than 20 years old (90%) and may result from movements as trivial as raising one's hand behind the head, using the backstroke while swimming, or reaching into the back seat of a car, stability is essential to proper management. Thus, in young patients, immobilization should be approximately 3 weeks, while bearing in mind that young people are much less vulnerable to the effects of joint stiffness and the development of adhesions. However, once dislocation has occurred a second time in this age group, the chance of frequent recurrence is almost 100% and is therefore usually indication for open shoulder reconstruction.[10]

In patients older than 30 years of age, the chances of recurrence are lower because as one gets older the collagen composing the static shoulder restraints becomes stiffer and hence less elastic. In such patients, immobilization should not exceed approximately 1 week because the position of the immobilization sets the anteroinferior shoulder capsule in such a way that the capsular attachments may approximate and foreshorten (that is, adhesive capsulitis; Chapter 13).

22. What is the difficulty in managing chronic anterior traumatic dislocations?

A GH joint that has been dislocated for several days is a *chronic dislocation*. As the chronicity of dislocation persists, so do the complications of reduction. There are no established rules of management here because the age of the patient, length of time from dislocation, degree of symptoms, range of motion, radiographic findings, and general stability of the patient may vary greatly. When one encounters an elderly patient with shoulder pain and anterior dislocation on radiographs, a very careful history is mandatory to determine whether the injury occurred acutely or a week to several months earlier. The problem here is that by 2 to 3 weeks after dislocation the humeral head is so firmly impaled on the anterior glenoid and there is so much soft-tissue contracture and interposition that it is impossible to perform a gentle closed reduction.

If no more than 2 to 3 weeks have elapsed since the dislocation, a gentle closed reduction may be performed with minimal traction, without leverage, and with total muscle relaxation under general anesthesia. If this fails, a choice is made either to simply leave it alone, or to consider an open procedure. An open procedure can be very difficult because of the distorted anatomy of the axillary artery and nerves and because the structures are tight and "scarred" down.[17]

23. What accounts for the high incidence of recurrent dislocation?

In order to understand why it is that anterior shoulder dislocation is associated with a high incidence of recurrent dislocation, it is helpful to study Fig. 17-13.

In the normal shoulder, the motion of external rotation results in lateral rotation of the humeral head and stretching of the anterior capsule. In the absence of an intact anterior capsule glenoid labrum, as often occurs after anterior dislocation, there is a loss of balance of the static support of the glenoid rim. Subsequently, during attempted external shoulder rotation, arthrokinematic joint rotation is substituted by anteroinferior translation, resulting in redislocation. It is for this reason that chronic instability is obviated during external rotation of the shoulder. Instability is compounded when an indentation fracture is created by impaling of the humeral head on the anterior margin of the glenoid rim (Hill-Sachs lesion). A reverse lesion may occur on the anteromedial portion of the humeral head after posterior dislocation (reverse Hill-Sachs lesion).

24. What is the mechanism of recurrent dislocation?

In most cases of recurrent traumatic anterior instability, injury recurs from forced abduction and external shoulder rotation. This injury may occur from a fall onto an outstretched arm or after a blow delivered to

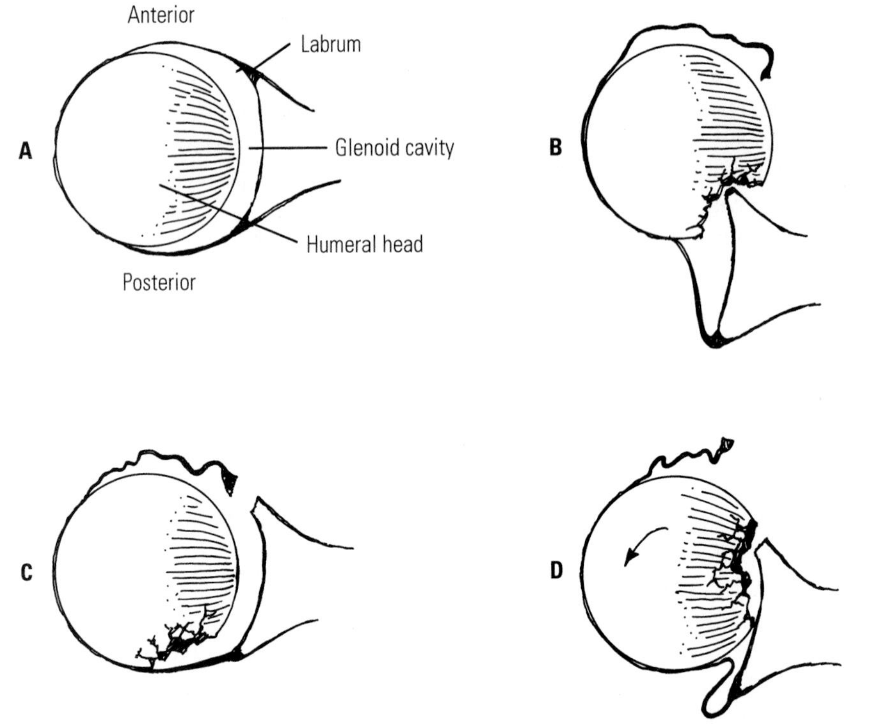

Fig. 17-13 Stages in the formation of a Hill-Sachs lesion with diagram of a left GH joint. **A,** Glenohumeral joint stability is enhanced by an intact labrum, a fibrous rim that deepens the glenoid cavity. **B,** Anterior dislocation with anterior glenoid rim indenting the posterolateral part of the humeral head. **C,** Reduction after anterior dislocation. **D,** After reduction there is chronic instability in external rotation, *arrow.* This tends to reinforce the head defect. (From Meals RA: *One hundred orthopaedic conditions every doctor should understand,* St. Louis, 1992, Quality Medical Publishing.)

the shoulder. A classic example is of a football player who tries to make an arm tackle on a ball carrier only to wind up having his own arm pulled back into extension, abduction, and external rotation. Similarly, a kayaker may have his arm pulled back over his head while bracing himself in white water, or a skier may fall onto an abducted arm. These movements yield a sharp and stabbing shoulder pain. Reduction may occur spontaneously or may require medical intervention. Subsequently the shoulder may demonstrate the "dead-arm syndrome,"[27] that is, recurrent dislocation,[25] or even frank dislocation when the arm assumes the positions of external rotation, abduction, and shoulder rotation.[17]

25. What is "apprehension shoulder"?

Apprehension shoulder is an overuse injury in swimmers, occurring most frequently during the backstroke, when the athlete enters the flip turn. At this instant the shoulder, in full abduction and external rotation, undergoes momentary anterior luxation onto the rim of the glenoid fossa as the swimmer's arm pushes off forcefully from the pool wall (Fig. 17-14).

26. What is recurrent instability with an atraumatic onset?

Recurrent instability may also have an atraumatic onset, that is, without a major injury the humeral head begins to slide out of its normal position. This instability may be anterior, posterior, inferior, or

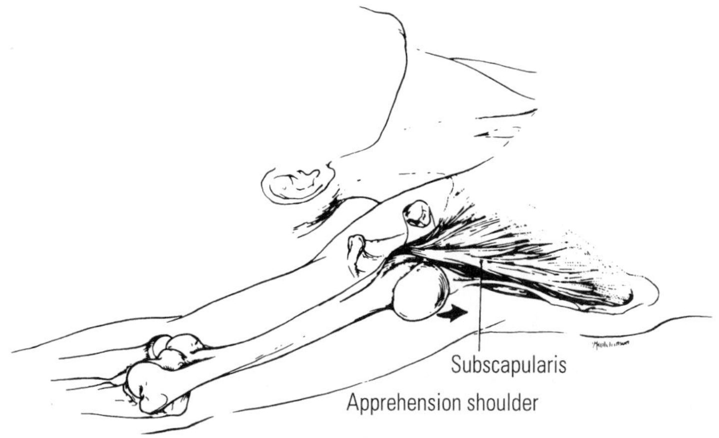

Fig. 17-14 Apprehension shoulder with vulnerable position of full abduction and external rotation as found in the backstroke turn. (From Kennedy JC, Hawkins R, Krissoff WB: *Am J Sports Med* 6:309, 1987.)

multidirectional. Careful questioning usually reveals that the original injury was minor in nature and occurred with actions such as lifting up a garage door, swinging a baseball bat, taking an overhead swing at a tennis ball, or having a minor fall on the shoulder. There are several important clues that hint at a diagnosis of atraumatic subluxation or dislocation: the original injury was minor and not usually associated with significant pain; the patient returned to his or her activities without much pain or difficulty; the subluxation or dislocation spontaneously reduced itself; or the patient has generalized ligamentous laxity.

In the event that one encounters a patient who can dislocate his or her shoulder voluntarily, the examiner must endeavor to determine whether voluntary instability, that is, the patient's desire to dislocate, is the underlying problem, in which case surgical stabilization is unlikely to succeed. However, surgery is appropriate if the patient's shoulder just happens to be able to be susceptible to dislocating itself. The patient with voluntary instability usually has no history of injury but has memories stretching back to childhood of the ability to slip one or both shoulders out of place with minimal discomfort. In the late teens or early twenties the patient may note how the shoulder begins to slip out of place when stress is placed on it.

27. How is recurrent instability categorized, and how is it managed?

It is helpful to categorize patients with recurrent shoulder instability into one of two groupings: the shoulder that goes out because it has suffered a major injury is different from one that goes out because it is constitutionally loose.[17]

The first of these categories, known as a *Bankart lesion,* is characterized by a history of definite trauma, as may occur to an 18-year-old skier whose recurrent anterior instability began with a fall on an abducted externally rotated arm. These shoulders have definite structural damage, particularly avulsion of the GH ligaments at their glenoid attachments, causing *unidirectional instability.* These shoulders frequently require surgery to reachieve stability.[17]

The second group of patients have no history of significant trauma, and instability hence is termed atraumatic. These patients are much more prone to *multidirectional instability.* Rehabilitation, particularly rotator cuff strengthening and flexibility exercises are the first line of management. In this situation the typical patient is a 16-year-old swimmer whose shoulders are becoming painful and on examination are found to be loose in all directions.[17]

28. What nonoperative management is appropriate after shoulder dislocation?

Although any form of GH joint instability may benefit from conservative rehabilitation, nonoperative management is particularly indicated in patients with atraumatic, multidirectional, bilateral instability.[17] Physical therapy is also appropriate for patients with voluntary instability or posterior GH joint instability and for those patients requiring a supranormal range of motion, such as baseball pitchers, swimmers, and gymnasts. These latter patients have looser GH joint capsules and a relatively greater dependence of the dynamic stabilizing mechanism and are not good candidates for surgical management because it does not permit return to a competitive level of function.

The mainstay of therapeutic rehabilitation for anterior GH joint instability is *strengthening* of the rotator cuff musculature. Both internal and external rotator strengthening contribute to anterior and posterior stability respectively, by serving as a buttress to hold the humerus in the glenoid and resist potentially displacing forces. Activation of the infraspinatus tendon and teres minor draw the humeral head posteriorly and thus unload stress on the damaged anterior capsule; an analogy may be made here to strengthening strategy of the hamstrings after anterior cruciate injury in the knee. A similar thesis may be advanced regarding the effects of internal rotation in the late treatment of posterior shoulder dislocation, similar to quadriceps strengthening after posterior cruciate knee injury.

Management of anterior dislocation

- *Rotator cuff strengthening* (see pp. 113-118) *exercises* are most effectively performed when one keeps the humerus close to the body in adduction and internally rotates the arm in the following progression: isometrics, isotonics, resistance, and eccentric strengthening. Strengthening of the internal rotators and adductors is appropriate, since increased tone in these antagonistic muscles serve to limit external rotation and abduction. Isolated external rotation is not an appropriate treatment modality at this early time. Additionally, contraction of the internal shoulder rotators causes the humeral head to migrate posteriorly, away from the anterior locus of instability.

  Pain-free isometrics are begun early on so as to prevent atrophy with avoidance of the combined motions of external rotation and abduction. At 2 to 4 weeks after injury, the patient may progress to isotonics and isokinetics as well as rubber tubing (resistive) exercises, spring exercises, or weights in the sidelying position as pain permits, while avoiding the aforementioned positions. Eccentric lengthening contractions are a velocity-decreasing strategy that slow things down during high-velocity movements; as such, they match the functional demands on these muscles when they are recruited to resist forced abducted and external rotation.

  At 4 to 6 weeks strengthening may be performed, if pain permits, with the shoulder no longer adducted to the patient's side. Only now may external rotation strengthening be added to facilitate centralization of the humeral head inside the glenoid fossa, which is possible only when all the cuff muscles are working harmoniously together. Abduction and adduction may now be performed to 90° of elevation while the shoulder is maintained in neutral rotation. Overhead flexion and shoulder extension is also permitted. This position is followed by the allowance of three different positions of internal and external rotation: 0° of abduction, 45° of abduction, and 90° of forward flexion. Strengthening of the scapular stabilizers is helpful and best performed if one begins with a modified push-up and progresses to standard push-ups. Push-ups should be performed with the arms somewhat adducted. Rubber Therabands and hand weights are to be used as part of a home exercise program, with emphasis on high repetition and low weight to improve endurance as well as low repetition and high weight to improve strength. Exercising the upper body in shoulder flexion and extension with an ergometer is appropriate at this phase of rehabilitation.[6]

- D_2 proprioceptive neuromuscular facilitation (PNF) muscle strengthening. D_1 extension is not recommended, since it involves posterior glenoid activity, hence anterior humeral head migration. (D, Diagonal pattern of movement.)
- Posterior GH joint *mobilization* to facilitate shoulder flexion that may have lessened during the 2- to 3-week period of immobilization in adduction and internal rotation.
- Use of single-channel electromyographic *biofeedback*, to centralize the humeral head, with emphasis on control rather than on strength and with electrode placement below the scapular spine for the purpose of learning to consciously contract and strengthen the rotator cuff musculature with the arm in neutral and slowly progressing through various levels and speeds of elevation. The basis of this treatment protocol derives from electromyographic studies showing the external rotators, particularly the infraspinatus, to be the primary dynamic shoulder stabilizers in abduction and overhead motion.[23] One performs this by tightening the rotator cuff muscles in the neutral position in order to glide and hold the humeral head posteriorly. Treatment should be performed for 10 sets of 10 repetitions before one progresses to active movement. By electronic monitoring and amplification of external rotation activity during an apprehensive motion, immediate visual and auditory feedback is provided to the patient. Performance is changed when muscle control is emphasized as an important adjunct to muscle strengthening. Movement progressions occur as the patient masters each level and include (1) forward flexion with a straight elbow, (2) forward flexion with increasing external rotation, (3) abduction with flexion, progressing to elbow extension, (4) abduction with elbow extension with increasing external rotation, (5) abduction from flexion, (6) abduction from flexion with increasing external rotation, and (7) reaching for objects behind the back or overhead. Electrode placement over the posterior deltoid is contraindicated because increased activity in this muscle drives the humeral head anteriorly.[28]
- Educate patients to avoid forced or high-velocity movement of external rotation, abduction, and hyperextension.
- Educate patients with voluntary shoulder instability by carefully explaining the importance of avoiding intentional GH joint subluxation and dislocation, stressing that each time they perform this maneuver they make their shoulder looser and more prone to unpredictable instability.
- Advise the patient to avoid following the standard Nautilus arm cross exercises on the double chest machine, regardless of position, latissimus pulldowns, behind the head military press, wide grip press, and lowering the bench press excessively into horizontal extension.

Management of posterior dislocation

Posterior dislocations are infrequent, but when they do occur, they are at risk for redislocating when the shoulder is internally rotated. Thus external shoulder rotation and posterior deltoid strengthening are emphasized during rehabilitation so as to limit internal rotation and adduction, with push-ups and bench press exercises being avoided. Initially, passive range of motion and pendulum exercises are started after several days of complete immobilization in a reverse sling or spica cast to hold the shoulder in external rotation. It is essentially to avoid excessive forward flexion and internal rotation during passive range of motion exercises. Later on, as dynamic strengthening ensues, it is important not to begin strengthening the external rotators in the position of full internal rotation. Similarly, as shoulder function improves, it is important to point out to the patient the importance of avoiding activities that would place the shoulder at the limits of shoulder flexion, internal rotation, or horizontal adduction so as not to redislocate.[6]

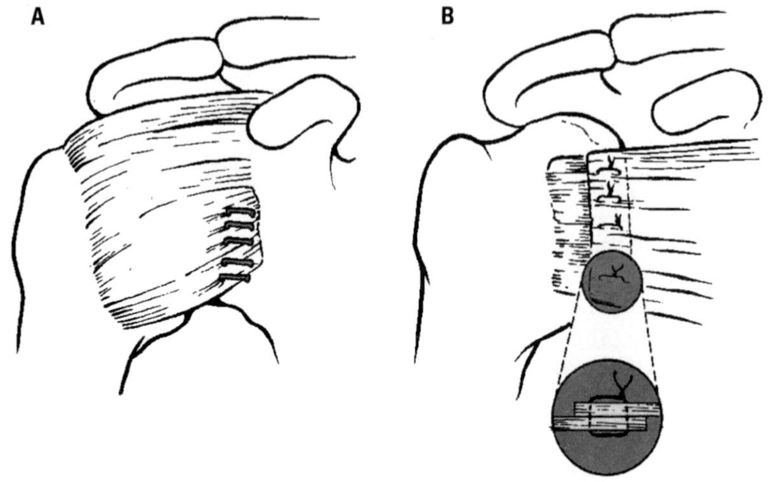

Fig. 17-15 Operations for recurrent anterior shoulder dislocation. **A,** Staple capsulorrhaphy involves reattachment of the inferior border of the capsule and labrum onto the glenoid using staples. **B,** Shortening of the subscapularis tendon. (From Dandy DJ: *Essential orthopaedics and trauma*, Edinburgh, 1989, Churchill Livingstone.)

29. What is surgical management in those patients for whom operative treatment is advisable?

The *Bankart procedure* involves suturing of the anterior capsule and labrum to the anterior glenoid rim. Many shoulder surgeons consider this the procedure of choice in management of traumatic unidirectional instability. This procedure requires a healthy capsule and most probably results in the best postoperative shoulder range of motion but is technically a more difficult operation to perform. Popularity of this procedure is attributable to the work of Bankart who first performed the operation in 1923 on one of his former house surgeons. Patients generally have their shoulder immobilized after surgery in the position of internal rotation and adduction by wearing a sling or a commercially available shoulder immobilizer. Immobilization is for 2 to 3 weeks after surgery and then only at night during the subsequent 3 to 6 weeks.[6]

With *staple capsulorrhaphy* (Fig. 17-15) the detached anterior capsule and labrum are secured back onto the glenoid by use of staples. This can be performed either as an open repair or arthroscopically. The advantage of this procedure is that range exercises, such as Codman's pendulum, may begin within the first week after surgery.

Putti-Platt procedure is an example of one of the subscapularis muscle procedures, first used by Sir Harry Platt of England and Vittorio Putti of Italy in the 1920s. Muscle transfers are considered to be *indirect repairs* and are designed to effect repair by altering the biomechanics extrinsic to the GH joint; this is to be distinguished from *direct repairs*, as are the Bankart and staple capsulorrhaphy procedures, which attempt to restore normal anatomy.

The results of surgery are often successful from the point of view of whether dislocation recurs. Clearly such dislocation does not recur. However this simply cannot be equated with an excellent result, since the patient now has 45° of external rotation and can no longer throw with that shoulder. The goal of postsurgical therapy is to ideally attempt ro regain as much external rotation and elevation as possible if one bears in mind that one inevitably falls short of meeting that goal. It is important to bear in mind that the patient must not place his or her shoulder at the limits of external rotation, abduction, or hyperextension during overenthusiastic exercise or activities of daily living because these ranges may potentially cause recurrence of dislocation. Patients need to have this explained to them.[17]

30. What postoperative therapeutic management is appropriate?

Surgery involving direct repairs may begin with submaximal isometrics during the first several weeks after the operation, since contractile tissues were not cut during surgery. With Bankart repairs, from 3 to 6 weeks after surgery, active abduction is permitted to 90°, whereas external rotation is limited to neutral. After these 6 weeks abduction and external rotation are slowly increased as pain and active motion permits. These exercises include progressive isometrics, isotonics, eccentric activities. A home program is instituted using rubber tubing and hand weights for isolated cuff, deltoid, and pectoralis strengthening and multiple plane strengthening, such as patterns of proprioceptive neuromuscular facilitation, to be later incorporated into a well-balanced program. Although attention is focused on the internal and external rotators and adductors, it is done at the expense of neglecting other prime movers of the GH joint. If motion is slow to return, more aggressive range of motion is initiated no earlier than 7 to 8 weeks after surgery. Functional activities may be performed from 8 to 12 weeks after surgery.[6]

With staple capsulorrhaphy, the patient is usually kept in a sling for 1 week, followed by active assistive range of motion permitted within pain tolerance during the second week. Progression to active range of motion then occurs at the beginning of week 3, as well as light resistance initiated from weeks 3 to 6. Rehabilitation of postsurgical Putti-Platt repairs differs in that the patient is usually kept wearing the sling for 2 to 4 weeks. Active range of motion to pain tolerance is encouraged for 3 to 6 weeks, at which time passive range of motion and strengthening exercises are initiated. Maximal internal rotation effort is usually delayed until 8 weeks after the operation, though some 10 to 15 repetitions may begin at 6 weeks.[8]

References

1. Blom S, Dahlback LO: Nerve injuries in dislocations of the shoulder joint and fractures of the neck of the humerus, *Acta Chir Scand* 136:461-466, 1970.

1a. Bracker MD: New treatment for dislocated shoulders. *The Physician and Sports Medicine.* vol 12, No 7, July 1984.

2. Cleland J: On the actions of muscles passing over more than one joint, *J Anat Physiol* 1:85-93, 1866.

3. Dandy DJ: *Essential orthopaedics and trauma*, Edinburgh, 1989, Churchill Livingstone.

4. Das SP, Roy GS, Saha AK: Observations on the tilt of the glenoid cavity of scapula, *J Anat Soc India* 15:114, 1966.

5. Duckworth T: *Lecture notes on orthopaedics and fractures*, ed 2, Oxford, 1984, Blackwell Scientific Publications.

6. Gould JA III: *Orthopaedic and sports physical therapy*, ed 2, St. Louis, 1990, Mosby.

7. Gowen I, Jobe F, Tibone J, et al: A comparative electromyographic analysis of the shoulder during pitching, *Am J Sports Med* 15:586-599, 1987.

8. Grana WA, Holder S, Schelberg-Karnes E: How I manage acute anterior shoulder dislocations, *Phys Sports Med* 15(4):88-93, 1987.

9. Grant JCB: *Grant's atlas of anatomy*, ed 6, Baltimore, 1972, Williams & Wilkins.

10. Henry JH: "How I manage dislocated shoulder," *The Physician and Sports Medicine* 12(9):66, 1984.

11. Hill NA, McLaughlin HL: Locked posterior dislocation simulating a "frozen shoulder," *J Trauma* 3:225-234, 1963.

12. Howell SM, Galinat BJ, Renzi AJ, Marone PJ: Normal and abnormal mechanics of the glenohumeral joint in the horizontal plane, *J Bone Joint Surg* 70A(2):227-232, 1988.

13. Jobe F, Tibone J, Perry J, et al: An EM analysis of the shoulder in throwing and pitching, *Am J Sports Med* 11:3-5, 1983.

14. Kumar VP, Balasubramaniam P: The role of atmospheric pressure in stabilising the shoulder: an experimental study, *J Bone Joint Surg* (Br) 67(5):719-721, 1985.

15. Lillegard WA, Rucker KS: *Handbook of sports medicine: a symptom-oriented approach*, Boston, 1993, Andover Medical Publishers.

16. Mallon B: *Orthopaedics for the house officer*, Baltimore, 1990, Williams & Wilkins.

17. Matsen FA, Thomas SC, Rockwood CA: Anterior glenohumeral joint instability. In Rockwood CA, Matsen FA: *The shoulder*, vol 1, Philadelphia, 1990, Saunders.

18. McLaughlin HL: Posterior dislocation of the shoulder, *J Bone Joint Surg* 34A:584, 1952.
19. Meals RA: *One hundred orthopaedic conditions every doctor should understand*, St. Louis, 1992, Quality Medical Publishing.
20. Moore KL: *Clinically oriented anatomy*, ed 2, Baltimore, 1985, Williams & Wilkins.
21. Moseley HF, Overgaard B: The anterior capsular mechanism in recurrent anterior dislocation of the shoulder, *J Bone Joint Surg* 44B:913-927, 1962.
22. Ovesen J, Nielson S: Stability of the shoulder joint: cadaver study and stabilizing structures, *Acta Orthop Scand* 56:149-151, 1985.
23. Perry J: Anatomy and biomechanics of the shoulder in throwing, swimming, gymnastics, and tennis, *Clin Sports Med* 2(2):247-270, 1983.
24. Poppen NK, Walker PS: Normal and abnormal motion of the shoulder, *J Bone Joint Surg* 58A:195, 1976.
25. Rockwood CA Jr, Burkhead WZ Jr, Brna J: Subluxation for the glenohumeral joint: response to rehabilitative exercise in traumatic vs. atraumatic instability. Presented at second open meeting of American Shoulder and Elbow Surgeons, New Orleans, 1986.
26. Roston JB, Haines RW: Cracking in the metacarpophalangeal joint, *J Anat* 81:165-173, 1947.
27. Rowe CR, Zarins B: Chronic unreduced dislocations of the shoulder, *J Bone Joint Surg* 64A:494-505, 1982.
28. Saboe L, Chepeha J, Reid D, et al: The unstable shoulder: electromyography: applications in physical therapy. Protocol from The Glen Suther Sports Medicine Clinic and Division of Orthopaedics at the University of Alberta, Thought Technology, Ltd, Edmonton, Alberta, 1990.
29. Saha AK: Dynamic stability of the glenohumeral joint, *Acta Orthop Scand* 42:491-505, 1971.
30. Saidoff DC: Diving accident results in acute pain and deformity in shoulder, *Advance for Physical Therapists* 3(9):12, 1992.
31. Salter RB: *Textbook of disorders and injuries of the musculoskeletal system*, ed 2, Baltimore, 1983, Williams & Wilkins.
32. Schwartz RR, O'Brien SJ, Patterson RF: Unrecognized dislocations of the shoulder, *J Trauma* 9: 1009-1023, 1969.
33. Simkin PA: Structure and function of joints. In Schumacher HR, editor: *Primer on the rheumatic diseases*, ed 9, Atlanta, Ga., 1988, Arthritis Foundation.
34. Symeonides PP: The significance of the subscapularis muscle in the pathogenesis of recurrent anterior dislocation of the shoulder, *J Bone Joint Surg* 54B:476-483, 1972.
35. Turkel SJ, Panio MW, Marshall JL, Girgis FG: Stabilizing mechanisms preventing anterior dislocation of the glenohumeral joint, *J Bone Joint Surg* 70A(2):227-232, 1988.
36. Unsworth A, Dowson D, Wright V: "Cracking joints": a bioengineering study of cavitation in the metacarpophalangeal joint, *Ann Rheum Dis* 30:348, 1971.

Recommended reading

Malone TR, McPoil T, Nitz A: *Orthopedic and sports physical therapy*, ed 3, St. Louis, 1997, Mosby.

Matsen FA, Thomas SC, Rockwood CA: Anterior glenohumeral joint instability. In Rockwood CA, Matsen FA, editors: *The shoulder*, vol 1, Philadelphia, 1990, Saunders.

Perry J: Anatomy and biomechanics of the shoulder in throwing, swimming, gymnastics, and tennis, *Clin Sports Med* 2(2):247-270, 1983.

Part Four

Brachial Plexus, Thoracic Outlet, and Shoulder Girdle

Pain, Dysesthesia, and Paresthesia in Ulnar Three Digits Caused by Proximal Lesion

18

A 41-year-old violin virtuoso belonging to the Metropolitan Opera orchestra complains to you of numbness, paresthesia, dysesthesia, pain, and clumsiness in his right ulnar three digits toward the end of long operas that significantly compromise his performance. He occasionally complains of nocturnal pain that abates if he sits up in bed. His pain coincides with the three nights per week during which he follows a disciplined regimen of weight lifting to stay in shape and strengthen his shoulder girdle. Symptoms also appear when he blowdries his hair. The gentleman, a bachelor, spends his time reading despite his severe myopia and admits to being a long-time heavy smoker. Upon calling the referring physician you learn that recent apical chest radiographs are clear and there is no evidence of the presence of a cervical rib or abnormally long C7 transverse process. Nor is there any sign of cervical spine disease. Electrolytes are at normal levels. An electromyogram and a nerve conduction velocity test proved negative. The patient denies any color changes, hyperhidrosis, swelling, trauma, joint pain, dry eyes, dry mouth, or photophobia. His past medical history is normal, as is his family history.

OBSERVATION Forward neck posture with rounded shoulders; minor atrophy of right interossei and thenar and hypothenar eminences, and proximal and middle portions of the medial forearm. There is apparent hypertrophy of pectoralis major, pectoralis minor, and all the anterolateral neck muscles, which seem to stand out strongly. There is noted hypertrophy of bilateral scalene muscles. Upon observing the patient's breathing pattern, you notice that his chest moves up and down with each breath without any apparent accompanying diaphragmatic component.

PALPATION No point tenderness over neck or upper extremity; there is no redness of warmth anywhere.

RANGE OF MOTION Full painless range present in bilateral upper extremities.

MUSCLE STRENGTH Normal to bilateral upper extremities.

SELECTIVE TENSION Resistive testing at midrange demonstrates no pathologic condition.

JOINT PLAY Hypermobility is noted in the lower cervical spine, and hypomobility is present in the sterno-clavicular joint, particularly anterior and inferior glide.

A. Sternocostovertebral space

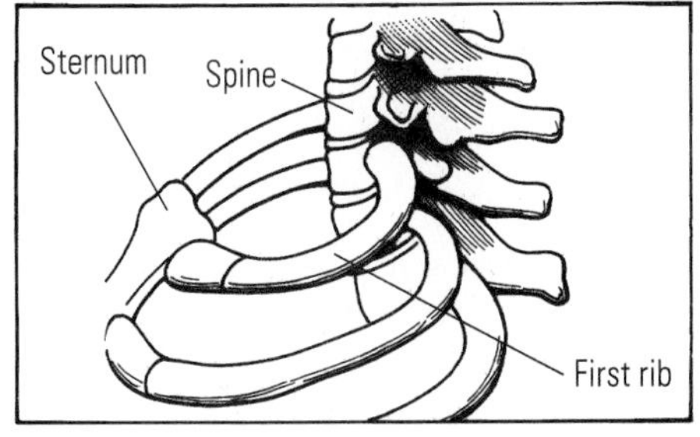

B. Scalene triangle

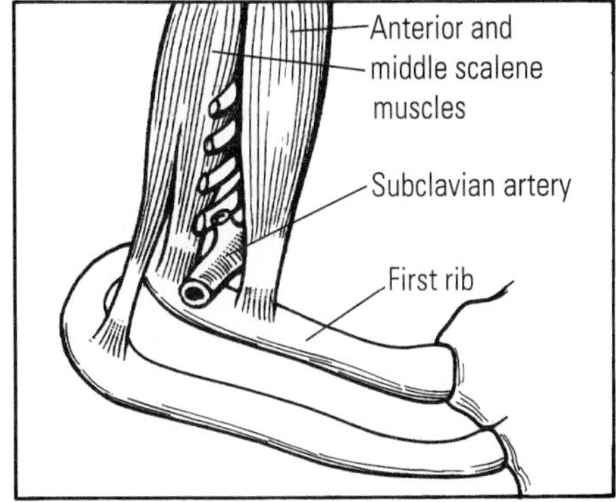

C. Costoclavicular space

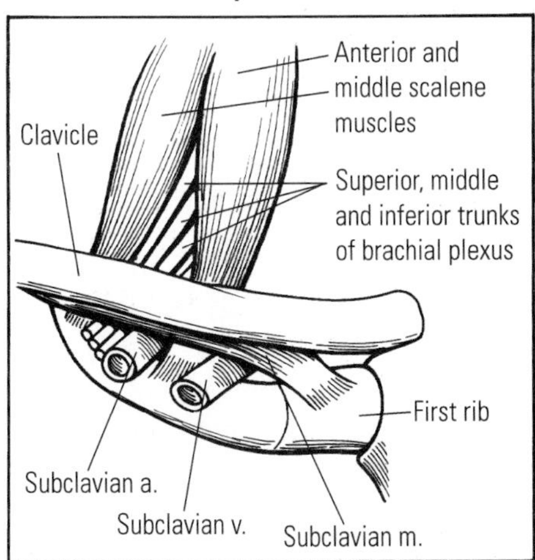

D. Coracopectoral space

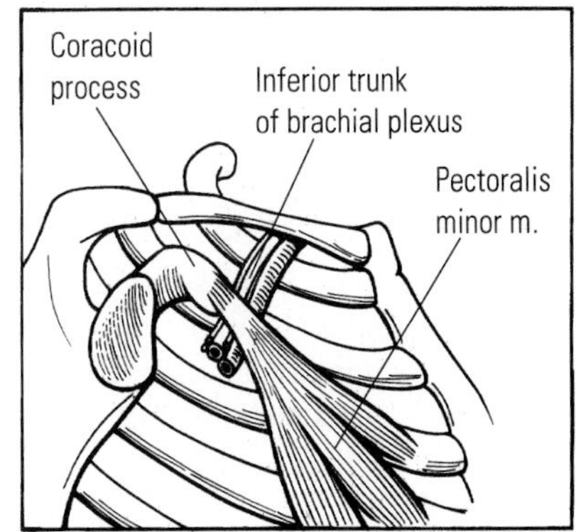

Fig. 18-1 The thoracic outlet has four sections. **A,** *Sternocostovertebral space.* Pancoast tumors present at this locale. **B,** The *scalene triangle* is narrower in many patients with thoracic outlet syndrome resulting in emergence of the neurovascular bundle from the apex of that triangle.* This may cause excessive rubbing of the neurovascular bundle against adjacent structures. Additionally, nerve adhesion to muscle may occur at this site. **C,** The *costoclavicular space* contains all the structures of the scalene triangle and the subclavian vein. **D,** The *coracopectoral space* contains the inferior trunk of the brachial plexus.

*Sanders RJ, Roos DB: The surgical anatomy of the scalene triangle. *Contemporary Surgery,* 1989, 35:11-16.

SENSATION Decreased to light touch to proximal and middle portions of the medial area of the forearm.

REFLEXES C5, C6, and C7 are normal.

VITAL SIGNS Normal, with clear breath sounds.

SPECIAL TESTS Negative compression and distraction of the cervical spine; negative Tinel sign at the ulnar groove adjacent to the medial epicondyle; negative Adson's maneuver, negative costoclavicular maneuver; positive hyperabduction test though no bruit is auscultated over the supraclavicular fossa; radial pulse pressure is less pronounced with contralateral neck flexion and rotation.

1. **What disorder is most likely the cause of this man's symptoms?**
2. **What relevant anatomy is requisite to understanding this disorder?**
3. **What are the three categories of risk factors in the development of thoracic outlet syndrome (TOS)?**
4. **What congenital factors directly cause or predispose for TOS?**
5. **How do forms of local and distal trauma alter the *local* anatomy of the thoracic outlet?**
6. **What is the relationship between posture and TOS?**
7. **What anatomic sex differences might account for a higher incidence of TOS in certain females?**
8. **What is the relationship between affective depression and the thoracic outlet?**
9. **What is the typical presentation of the postural variety of TOS?**
10. **What are the clinical signs and symptoms?**
11. **What is the differential diagnosis?**
12. **How common is vascular compromise in TOS?**
13. **What problems are there with many of the time-honored clinical tests used to diagnose TOS?**
14. **Describe the Hunter's test and Elvey's upper extremity tension test.**
15. **Are electrodiagnostic tests helpful in confirming the presence of TOS?**
16. **What rehabilitative therapy is appropriate in the treatment of TOS?**
17. **What is the prognosis of TOS?**
18. **What surgical options are available after a failed conservative regimen of treatment?**

1. What disorder is most likely the cause of this man's symptoms?

The *thoracic outlet syndrome* (TOS) complex refers to a series of neurovascular compression syndromes in the shoulder region. The plethora of specific nomenclature for this pathologic condition include cervical rib syndrome, scalenus anticus syndrome, subcoracoid pectoralis minor syndrome, costoclavicular compression syndrome,[17] scalenus medius syndrome, first thoracic rib syndrome, hyperabduction syndrome, Paget-Schroetter syndrome, and droopy shoulder syndrome.[25] Each syndrome name may be said to reflect a shift in thinking as to the origin of the disorder in question. Over time, disenchantment of given nomenclature gave way to a new theory and treatment of the symptoms and that in turn fell into disfavor because treatment of that entity did not conclusively cause abatement of symptoms. Today, TOS is recognized as an entrapment compression vasculopathy of the subclavian vessels but more commonly involving the lower trunk or medial cord of the brachial plexus at any one of four sites[20] (Fig. 18-1).

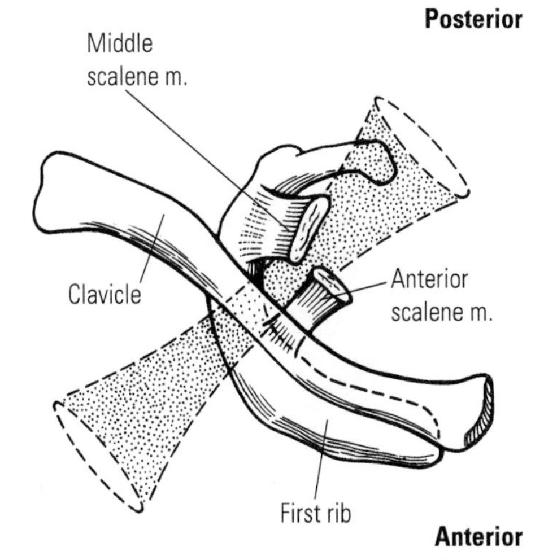

Fig. 18-2 Superior view of the dimensions of the thoracic outlet.

2. What relevant anatomy is requisite to understanding this disorder?

The thoracic outlet is bounded by the anterior scalene muscle anteriorly, medial scalene muscle posteriorly, clavicle superiorly, and first rib inferiorly[25] (Fig. 18-2). The uniting of the ventral primary rami of the 5 cervical through the first thoracic roots to form the superior, middle, and inferior trunks of the brachial plexus occurs supraclavicularly in that part of the neck known as the posterior triangle.[14] The brachial plexus travels away from the spinal cord by passing between the cleft of the scalenus anticus and medius muscles into the supraclavicular region.[14] Here the ventral primary rami unite to form the superior, middle, and inferior trunks.[14] The ventral rami of C8 and T1 unite to form the inferior trunk, which exits the neck to enter the axilla by crossing between the first rib[14] and the clavicle (costoclavicular space)[20] on its way to the upper extremity. After leaving the costoclavicular space those nerve fibers composing the inferior trunk pass infraclavicularly underneath the muscular fibers of pectoralis minor en route to their distal destination by way of the coracopectoral space. Upper plexus involvement may occur after spasm of the scalenus muscles, whereas lower plexus involvement may occur in the costoclavicular space or underneath the pectoralis minor.[20]

The thoracic outlet has four sections: (1) The *sternocostovertebral space.* Pancoast tumors present themselves here. (2) The *scalene triangle* is narrower in many patients with TOS resulting in the emergence and rubbing of the neurovascular bundle against the apex of this triangle. Additionally, nerve adhesion to muscle may occur at this site. (3) The *costoclavicular space* contains all the structures of the scalene triangle plus the subclavian vein. (4) The *coracopectoral space* containing the inferior trunk of the brachial plexus (see Fig. 18-1).

3. What are the three categories of risk factors in the development of thoracic outlet syndrome (TOS)?

- Congenital-structural anomaly
- Traumatic-structural alterations in the size of the thoracic outlet
- Postural alteration in the size of the thoracic outlet.[25]

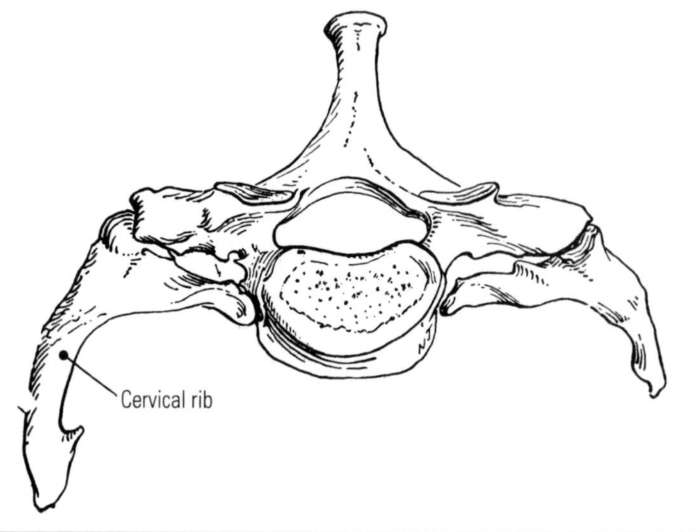

Fig. 18-3 Cervical rib. (From Moore KL: *Clinically oriented anatomy*, ed 2, Baltimore, 1985, Williams & Wilkins.)

4. What congenital factors directly cause or predispose for TOS?

Anatomic anomalies include the presence of a *cervical rib* (Fig. 18-3), unusually *long transverse processes* of the seventh cervical vertebrae, or soft tissue in the form of an *anomalous fibrous band*. This band is located near the cervical rib and may cause as much trouble as a bony rib though it is radiographically undetected because it is not ossified.[4] The presence of this band is suggested when the seventh cervical transverse process projects as far as the thoracic rib instead of being 1 cm shorter.[4] Cervical ribs, which articulate with the seventh cervical vertebra (Fig. 18-4), are present in 1% of the population, where they extend into the neck where their anterior end may either be free or attach to the first rib or sternum.[14] Although the presence of these variations may cause little or no trouble under normal circumstances, after injury and loss of normal posture they represent a risk factor in the development of TOS.[25]

5. How do forms of local and distant trauma alter the *local* anatomy of the thoracic outlet?

Posttraumatic alterations of local anatomy may be caused by a malunited clavicle fracture resulting in exuberant callus formation and significantly diminishing the space between the clavicle and the first rib.[25] Another common example of local trauma is whiplash tears to the scalene muscle, which often result in protective spasm. Increased scalene muscle tone will excessively elevate the first rib and reduce the thoracic outlet aperture.[25] A delayed onset of local trauma would be whiplash-caused tears of the scalene muscle. The resultant tear fills in with scar tissue that, over time, undergoes contractures and fibrosis,[25] strangling that portion of the plexus that travels through its substance. Compression within the interscalene space may occur after reflex muscle spasm of the scalenes, cervical spondylosis because of facet joint inflammation attributable to degenerative disk disease or cervical radiculopathy, overhead work postures, or heavy lifting.[1]

Distant trauma refers to painful lesions of the upper extremity that occur distal to the thoracic outlet. For example, a painful lesion of the hand, such as a neuroma, results in an involuntary guarding posture of the entire upper extremity. Although an abnormal posture protects the injured part from potential mechanical stimulation, it does so at the expense of altering the carriage of the shoulder girdle and

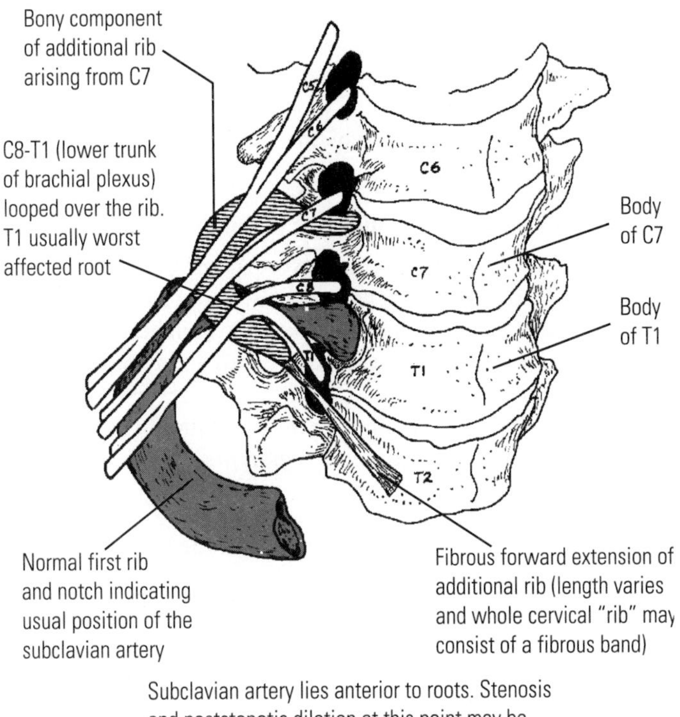

Fig. 18-4 Relation of the cervical rib to its surrounding structures. (From Patten J: *Neurological differential diagnosis,* ed 2, London, 1996, Springer-Verlag.)

hence potentially decreasing the size of the thoracic outlet. This decreased size may cause direct compression of the brachial plexus, especially in the presence of extra ribs or aberrant fibrous bands. The latter is an example of how postural abnormality can exacerbate a previously asymptomatic congenital factor. The involuntary maintenance of an abnormal posture causes compression, which is worsened by a vicious cycle of muscle spasm.[25]

6. What is the relationship between posture and TOS?

Loss of correct posture of the shoulder girdle is highly significant in the development of thoracic outlet syndrome and is explained in the following manner. During embryologic development, the forelimb buds must rotate 270° to produce the human upper extremity. Rotation occurs at the thoracic outlet level, and the nerves of the brachial plexus are twisted (circumducted) and positioned precariously at the center of rotation between the clavicle anterosuperiorly and the first rib posteroinferiorly.[25] Thus the descending neurovascular bundle exits the upper thorax by way of a bony aperture with limited diameter. This outlet may be thought of as a dynamic tunnel that changes diameter as a direct function of postural alteration. What we have here is the creation of a unique situation in which the diameter of aperture of this tunnel-like outlet is maintained by soft tissue attaching onto the scapula.*

*Wearing a backpack or scuba tank may result in an acute postural alteration that may precipitate neurovascular compression at the thoracic outlet.

Descent, or *ptosis*, of the scapula[13] manifests with age, especially with the advent of middle age,[4] because of gravity. As such, TOS is yet another example of a malady caused by forcing an anatomy designed for the quadruped position to tolerate the erect posture. In light of the above, we may state that alteration of the scapular posture will alter the thoracic outlet and may cause symptoms of TOS.[13] Nearly all humans may experience compromise of the thoracic outlet since the human shoulder is itself a risk factor.[25]

7. What anatomic sex differences might account for a higher incidence of TOS in certain females?

The upper margin of the sternum is level with the lower part of the second dorsal vertebra in males and on the lower part of the third dorsal vertebra in females. In the female, the medial third of the clavicle is lower than that in the male and thereby decreases the available space between the clavicle and the first rib (costoclavicular space). In addition, scapular ptosis may be greater in females with large breasts. Attaching to the pectoralis major muscle, the breasts exert a downward pull of the superior proximal attachment off the sternal half of the clavicle and thus further reduce the thoracic outlet aperture. This problem, referred to as *droopy shoulder syndrome*, may be accelerated by increased pressure from a narrow brassiere strap.

8. What is the relationship between affective depression and the thoracic outlet?

The distal attachment of the upper fibers of the trapezius insert onto the lateral third of the superior border of the clavicle and unilaterally act as a dynamic sling. The normal tone of these upper fibers elevates the clavicle while simultaneously preventing the shoulder girdle from sagging down on the chest. The individual who feels defeated by life will not hold his or her head up high because of "loss of face." Instead there are slumped shoulders in the absence of this normally acting dynamic sling. Thus, emotional depression may be physically expressed as scapular ptosis.[13]

9. What is the typical presentation of the postural variety of TOS?

The patient, nearly always a middle-aged woman, succumbs to inferior trunk compression by day resulting from stooped posture, which often accompanies middle age. Complaining of waking up anytime at night from severe "pins and needles" in one or both hands, the patient finds relief by letting her arms hang over the edge of the bed or by sitting or standing up. She then falls back asleep only to be awakened several hours later with recurrence of symptoms, or she may sleep uninterrupted until morning. On waking, the hands may feel numb for half an hour and exhibit clumsiness during small motions such as turning on the light or holding a toothbrush. The nocturnal symptoms may be a release phenomenon representing ischemic recovery of the nerve trunk, manifesting during sleep when the day's constant downward strain is relieved by the recumbent position. Thus the lower brachial plexus trunk moves upward and out of contact with the first rib in the gravity-eliminated, recumbent position. By day the patient is little troubled unless he or she wears a heavy overcoat, carries a heavy weight, or simply holds the arm in a dependent position for any length of time. The patient may eventually come to realize that the more she exerts herself physically by day the more pain she is likely to experience that night. Moreover, nocturnal symptoms may entirely abate after a bout of influenza causing the patient to remain essentially bed bound for several days or even after a "lazy holiday."[4]

10. What are the clinical signs and symptoms?

Thoracic outlet syndrome is an affectation of the brachial plexus and not of the cervical nerve roots. Consequently the patient will not experience symptoms at the base of the neck (supraclavicular fossa) where the lesion lies but rather distally along the upper limb.[4] The cutaneous distributions affected are those of the ulnar nerve and the medial cutaneous nerve of the forearm corresponding to the ulnar distribution in the hand and medial aspect of the forearm.[7,12] These two nerves represent the last two adjacent branches off the medial cord of the brachial plexus before that cord joins with the lateral cord to form the median nerve.

Paresthesias may later be accompanied by aching pain that is either poorly localized or over the whole arm. Paresthesia is often confined to the medial area of the forearm as well as hypothenar region of the hand. Either symptom may be exacerbated by such use of the arm as lifting and carrying heavy objects such as a container of milk or a suitcase or just standing about or walking. The patient may aggravate symptoms by merely reading[30] (think posture!), and the clinician may observe unequal shoulder heights and guarded posture.[25]

Motor deficits are not usually pronounced with TOS[25] and, when present, consist of a sense of weakness and clumsiness in the fingers. The patient may state that his or her grip or pinch strength is reduced. Atrophy, reflective of long-term TOS, will affect all the intrinsic hand muscles, since the involved plexus fibers are derived from the C8 and T1 roots, which furnish intrinsic hand innervation. Atrophy may also manifest in either the thenar[5] hypothenar eminences.[25] Tendon reflexes remain normal.[5]

11. What is the differential diagnosis?

The major problem of diagnosis stems from the lack of a good definitive objective test to confirm the presence of TOS.[25] Because of this the diagnosis is a clinical one that is largely reached by exclusion.[20]

- *Ulnar nerve entrapment* is also suggested by nocturnal numbness, but these patients never have sensory loss in the proximal or middle portions of the forearm.[5] In addition, patients with ulnar nerve entrapment should have no atrophy of the intrinsic muscles innervated by the median nerve in the thenar eminence.[5]
- *Carpal tunnel syndrome* may also cause thenar atrophy, but the sensory loss, if present, manifests in the first two digits. The former is additionally differentiated from TOS by electrophysiologic studies indicating distal and not proximal compression.
- In *C8 cervical radiculopathy* there is compression with an almost identical pattern of T1 nerve fibers as in TOS. However, TOS may also involve the subtraction of some T1 and even C8 fibers that do not travel in the medial cord of the plexus. Cervical spondylosis rarely involves the C8 root emerging from the C7 to T1 interspace but should be suspected if there is obvious involvement of several other roots as well. Neck pain, triceps weakness, reduced triceps reflex, and weakness of finger extensors furnish a clue toward involvement of the C8 nerve root.[5]
- *Intramedullary* or *extramedullary spinal cord processes* such as syringomyelia, glioma of the spinal cord, extramedullary cervical tumor, infarction of the spinal cord, or meningioma in the foramen magnum may mimic TOS. The following signs direct attention away from the thoracic outlet: long tract signs such as brisk reflexes or extensor plantar response, loss of tendon reflexes in the arms, Horner's syndrome, or weakness of the upper arm or shoulder.[5]
- *Pancoast tumor*, also known as pulmonary superior sulcus tumor, is accompanied by rapid and severe weakness of all the small muscles of the hand and, in advanced cases, results in radiographically visible cancerous erosion of the first and second ribs, as well as possible hoarseness attributable to paralysis of one vocal cord.[4] A regular anteroposterior radiograph may yield a false-negative result, whereas apical views or computerized tomography is more definitive.[20] The apical lung tumors ought to be especially suspect in patients who have a history of smoking.[13]
- *Pronator teres syndrome* (see pp. 25-27 and Fig. 4-3) shares many of the same symptoms as TOS. In TOS pain generally arises in the shoulder and the proximal area of the arm with radiation into the ulnar aspect of the hand with numbness experienced in the fifth digit and along the ulnar aspect of

the forearm. With pronator teres syndrome symptoms are primarily at the elbow with radiation into the radial aspect of the hand and numbness that extends into the median nerve distribution. With the passage of time, atrophy of the thenar musculature will occur. The different provocative maneuvers eliciting the symptoms of each respective disorder as well as the absence or presence of Tinel's sign should additionally help differentiate the two conditions.[5]

12. How common is vascular compromise in TOS?

Most patients with TOS do not have vascular symptoms and therefore do not require arteriography. When symptoms do occur, they include distal edema,[3] coldness, muscle ache, and loss of strength on continued use, which are more typical of vascular compromise than of neural compression.[17] The patient may notice that his or her hand grip gives out while carrying a heavy suitcase. In addition, the hand may turn pale and cyanotic similar to Raynaud's phenomenon though most authorities agree that the full set of changes typical to Raynaud's phenomenon are not a component of TOS. Gangrene of the fingertips or trophic skin and nail changes may occur secondary to arterial insufficiency.[5] When evidence of vascular insufficiency presents, arteriography should be done and the lesion promptly repaired, since the lesion is progressive and delay will only exacerbate it.[5]

13. What problems are there with many of the time-honored clinical tests used to diagnose TOS?

The Adson, hyperabduction, and costoclavicular maneuvers are provocative movements and postures that attempt to reproduce pain, paresthesias, a change in radial pulse, or a supraclavicular bruit. The reliability of these tests has never been established, and it is now apparent that positive findings occur in many normal people who have no arm symptoms whatsoever.[24] Nevertheless, judgment of the clinical significance of a positive result may be made when one considers the speed of onset and the severity of symptoms during examination.[25] Cyriax advocates lifting the lower trunk of the brachial plexus off the first rib by having the patient lie supine with the arm passively resting over the head for 10 minutes, resulting in a positive sign of relief and abatement of symptoms. All this, against the backdrop of suggestive history and differential exclusion, enable a firm diagnosis to be made.[4]

14. Describe Hunter's test and Elvey's upper extremity tension test.

Hunter test The test is begun with the shoulder abducted to 90° and the elbow flexed to 90°. The arm is then straightened. A positive sign results in a painful shooting sensation down the arm in the distribution of the involved nerves presumably from sudden traction of the tethered medial cord of the brachial plexus.[25] Similar tension tests may be performed to stretch the ulnar and radial nerve tracts. The appropriate limb postures may be extrapolated when one studies Fig. 24-20 and positions the various joints of the upper extremity so as to stretch each tract by considering its relation to the axis of the joints it crosses. A proximal-to-distal sequence of medial shoulder rotation and depression, forearm pronation, elbow extension, wrist flexion, and ulnar deviation may isolate the radial nerve. An ulnar-nerve stretch bias may be performed by wrist extension and radial deviation, forearm supination, elbow flexion, shoulder depression, and abduction.[2]

Upper extremity tension test Elvey's upper extremity tension test (UETT) determines the mobility of the brachial plexus and nerve root, particularly the median nerve. Similar to the straight leg raise test in the lower extremities, this test may determine if any restrictions of the nerve roots or plexus have occurred in those structures stretched by a sequence of upper extremity movements. The three superimposed component movements include (1) shoulder abduction, lateral rotation, and extension behind the coronal plane; (2) forearm supination and elbow extension; and (3) wrist and finger extension[6,11] (Fig. 18-5).

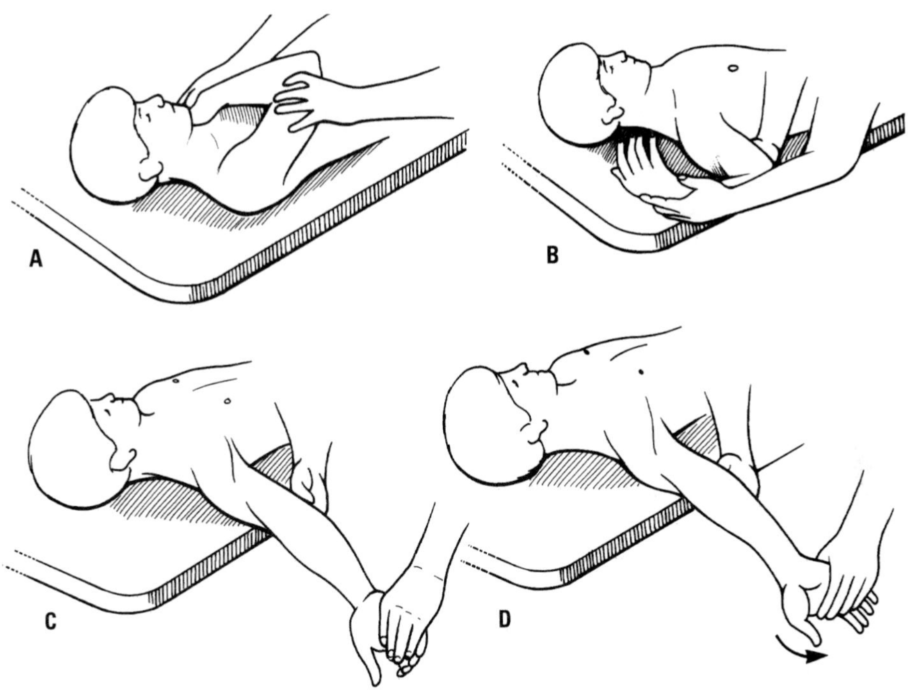

Fig. 18-5 Elvey's upper extremity tension test is a provocative sequence of motions that determines mobility (that is, gliding) of the nerve tract including the brachial plexus and nerve root. This particular test biases the *median nerve* and the anterior interosseous nerve for tension by way of mechanical stretch. **A,** First the arm and scapula are placed in a resting position. **B,** Next the arm is placed in the position of 90° shoulder abduction, lateral rotation, and elbow flexion with the forearm pronated. **C,** The elbow and forearm are then extended and supinated. **D,** The wrist is then extended to reproduce symptoms. Cervical lateral flexion to the left or right may then be added. It is essential for the examiner to maintain each posture before superimposing the next position in this sequence.

Similar tension tests may be performed to stretch the ulnar and radial nerves. Provocative upper limb postures may be extrapolated from a study of Fig. 24-20. Limb postures that tension-bias certain nerves may be inferred by reflecting upon the course of given nerve in relation to axis of the joint it crosses. A proximodistal sequence of imposed upper limb postures in the following order tenses the *radial nerve:* shoulder depression and medial rotation, elbow extension, forearem pronation, wrist flexion, and ulnardeviation. An *ulnar nerve* bias is provoked by the following sequence: shoulder depression and abduction, elbow flexion, forearm supination, wrist extension, and radial deviation.[2]

15. Are electrodiagnostic tests helpful in confirming the presence of TOS?

Electrophysiologic testing for TOS is controversial[5] because consistent electromyographic (EMG) criteria are often not met, thus calling into question the existence of the diagnosis or even of the syndrome itself.[25] Nevertheless, testing should include EMG and measurement of ulnar nerve sensory action potential as well as ulnar motor conduction at the elbow, the latter to rule out an elbow (ulnar nerve) lesion.[5] A ruled-out ulnar nerve lesion may suggest a proximal compromise of the thoracic outlet. Characteristic electrodiagnostic changes include but are not limited to prolonged latency of the ulnar F wave and reduced amplitude of the ulnar sensory evoked amplitude.

16. What rehabilitative therapy is appropriate in the treatment of TOS?

Rehabilitative therapy

- The treatment strategy is to facilitate more balance in the shoulder girdle so as to effect permanent lifting of the lower trunk of the brachial plexus off the first rib or to reduce pressure from the pectoralis over the nerve or nerves coursing beneath. This strategy is accomplished by a threefold approach of (1) postural reeducation, (2) selective muscle strengthening, and (3) selective soft-tissue stretching. This program must be introduced gently so as to avoid provocation of symptoms.[18] The therapist must be in close contact with the patient so that the program may be closely monitored. If a particular exercise causes pain, it must be modified or eliminated. Simply admonishing a patient to "stand straight like a West Pointer and get the shoulders back" is likely to result in frustration rather than relief. The time limit for this program should be 3 to 4 months.[13]

  The goals of therapy include (1) control of symptoms, (2) restoration of foreshortened tissues to normal length, (3) restoration of muscle balance, (4) improvement in posture, (5) development of stress-management techniques, and (6) prevention of recurrence of symptoms.[8]
- The use of *modalities* such as heat, cold, ultrasound, electrical stimulation (of high-frequency), diathermy, laser, and electroacupuncture have been used in providing temporary pain relief.[1]
- Careful *positioning* of the upper extremity such that the brachial plexus is neither compressed nor stretched (Fig. 18-6). This rest position is with the scapula in abduction and elevation and the shoulder in internal rotation and adduction (that is, the hand is placed on the contralateral shoulder). The patient must be warned, however, that maintaining this position for long periods will only inhibit progress, since the plexus will tend to become adhered to the underlying tissue and further motion may be lost.[1]
- *Stretching* of tightened soft tissue such as the levator scapula,[3] pectoralis major (see Fig. 10-2) and pectoralis minor, and all neck musculature.[19] Cervical spine exercises restore normal muscle length to the scalenes. Exercises include cervical retraction (Fig. 18-7), side flexions, and cervical flexion and extension. Patients should begin from either the position of minimal or absent pain, and proceed to the point

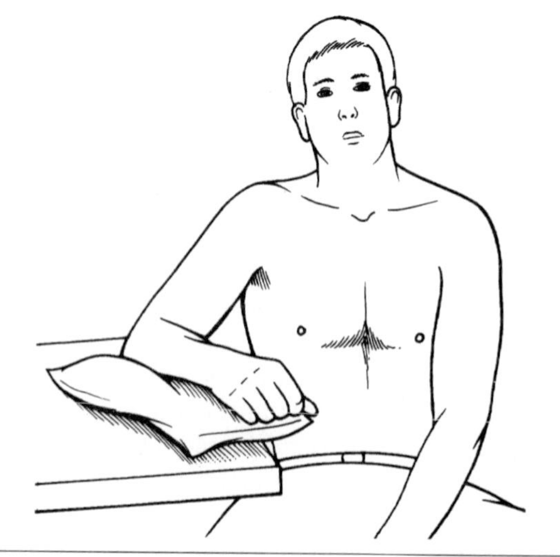

Fig. 18-6 Sitting rest position using a pillow to support the arm.

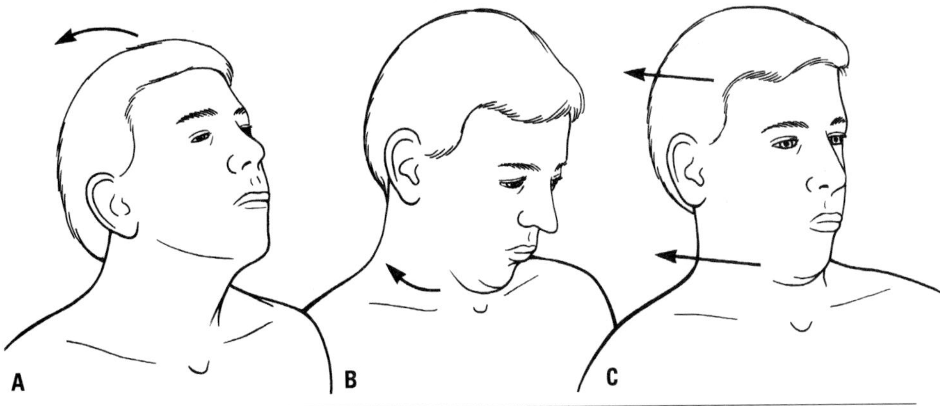

Fig. 18-7 Cervical retraction exercises. **A,** Poor technique—elevated chin. **B,** Poor technique—depressed chin. **C,** Good technique.

of discomfort or strain without pushing through their pain. If there is no pain or strain felt, the patient or therapist may apply gentle overpressure.[1] Targeting tight structures is a major facet of the evaluation and treatment of this condition. Restoration of normal length of adaptively shortened tissue is paramount to successful treatment. Foreshortened tissue may either compress or prevent normal movement of the brachial plexus. Lengthening of such tissue, provided that inflammation has receded, is imperative to a successful treatment regimen. Pain-reducing modalities may need to be used before or during lengthening to offset the inflammatory response.[1] Slow leaning into a corner with both hands on each wall at shoulder level, inhaling as the body leans forward, and exhaling as the body leans back is a particularly good stretch.[18]

- A self-stretching program of 5 to 10 repetitions every 2 to 4 hours throughout the day. Each repetition ought to be performed from a position of rest or neutral to the point where pain or strain is felt. The patient is warned not to push through the pain because doing so may lead to more inflammation and hinder progress. As treatment progresses, the point at which pain or strain is perceived is progressed further into that range. Between exercises, the patient may use the arm within tolerable limits or maintain the arm in the rest position.[1]
- Gentle *brachial plexus gliding exercises* (Fig. 18-8) to maintain free excursion of the plexus within the upper extremity. Free excursion is necessary, since inflammation of the plexus may cause adhesive binding of the plexus to surrounding tissue. Gliding may be accomplished by use of the UETT as an exercise. Each repetition should proceed from an area of minimal or no discomfort to the point at which discomfort starts and back to the rest position. As the restriction diminishes, more shoulder abduction and external rotation may be incorporated into the exercise. During the later stages of treatment, wrist extension and contralateral cervical side flexion may be added to produce further stretch. These gliding exercises are not appropriate to the acutely inflamed thoracic outlet condition.[1]
- *Strengthening* of muscles antagonistic to tightened muscle groups.[18] An appropriate strengthening and stretching strategy focuses on strengthening the protractors and scapula elevators (serratus anterior and upper trapezius) while stretching the scapula retractors and depressors (rhomboids and middle and lower trapezius).
- *Postural reeducation* is a major facet of conservative treatment.[13] Exercises to make the trapezius repeatedly contract and relax altogether miss the point, since these muscles are already strong in most people.

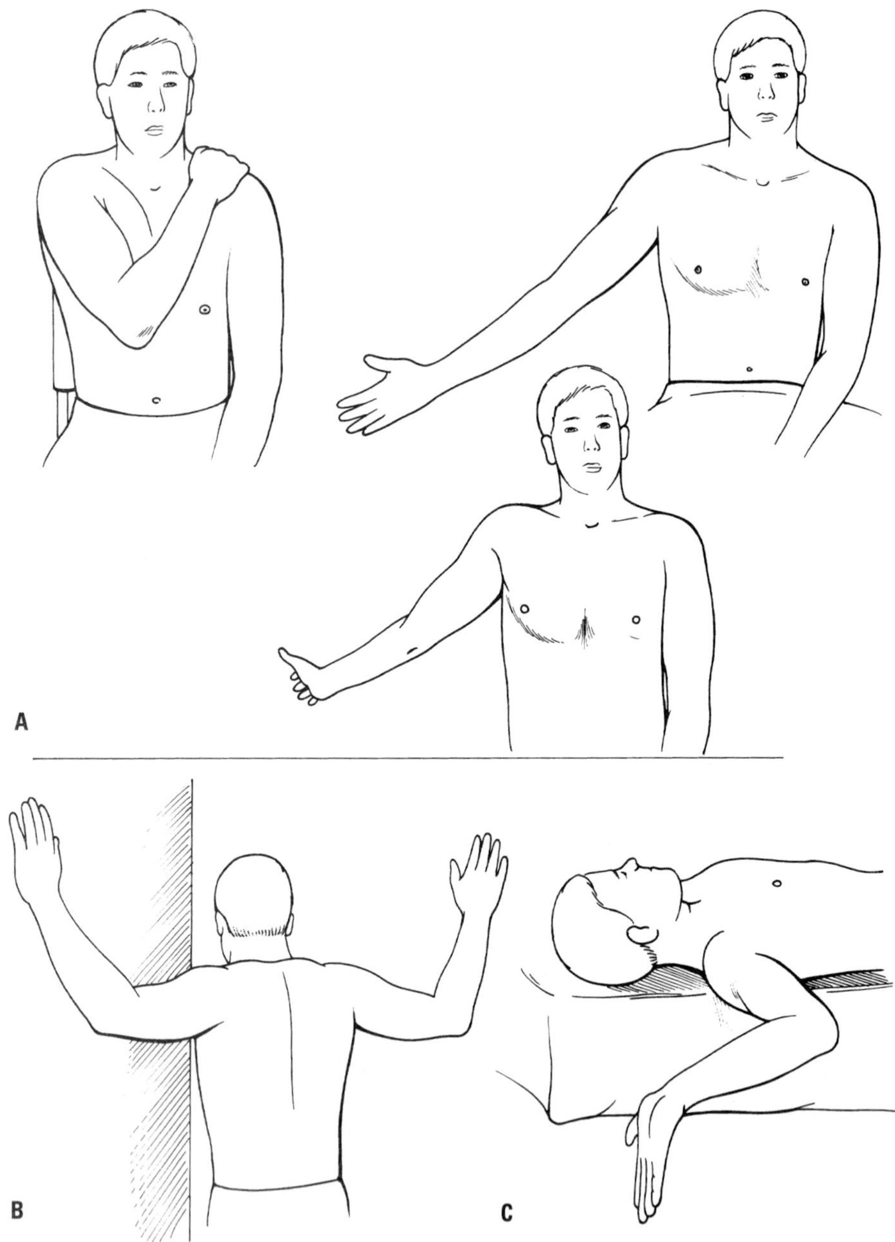

Fig. 18-8 Brachial plexus gliding exercises mobilize the nerves and may help prevent adhesions. **A,** Brachial plexus stretch while sitting. **B,** Brachial plexus stretch while leaning into a corner. **C,** Brachial plexus stretch in supine position using wrist extension and external rotation at 90° of abduction.

The patient must learn to keep his or her shoulders very slightly shrugged most of the time, that is, to maintain a slight constant postural tone in the trapezii because this habit can be inculcated.[4]

- Use of a figure-of-eight *harness strap* to pull the shoulders back out of their forward round-shoulder posture.
- *Joint mobilization* of the sternoclavicular joint[19] emphasizing anterior and inferior glide as well as scapular mobilization.[18] Mobilization of the first and second rib articulations are indicated to facilitate increased thoracic cage flexibility.
- Emphasize *diaphragmatic breathing*. When the patient works with his hands at or above chest level, as in the case of a violin player, the scalene and sternomastoid muscles, secondary respiratory muscles, are recruited and may eventually hypertrophy because of continued use. The diaphragm actively contracts and descends during normal quiet breathing. Ascent against gravity occurs during exhalation and is synergistically assisted by the recoiling properties of the lung and expiratory chest muscles. During quiet breathing diaphragmatic mobility is about 1 to 3 cm and is responsible for approximately two thirds of pulmonary ventilation, with the remaining third accomplished by other respiratory muscles. Breathing facilitated by the use of secondary respiratory muscles may gradually result in a weakened diaphragm and alter this 1:3 respiratory muscle ratio. The diaphragm may be strengthened by abdominal breathing (Fig. 18-9) exercises. The patient lies on his or her back with the legs drawn up with one hand on the chest and the thumb of the other just below the navel. During inhalation the chest remains stationary while the abdomen protrudes. Instruct the patient to exhale through pursed lips while manually assisting the abdomen to draw inward. The exercise may be performed for 3 minutes for two or three times per day and may be done without the use of hands once mastery is achieved. Abdominal weight exercises (Fig. 18-10) are performed with the foot of the bed raised approximately 16 inches and use of a one-pound weight (that is, a sandbag, book, or hot water bottle). Breathing is performed as during the latter exercise though the patient lies supine. This may be performed for 5 to 10 minutes twice per day and with addition of one-half pound every third day to a total of 5 pounds. This exercise may be prolonged up to 10 minutes as the patient progresses. Teach the patient to make use of primary respiratory muscles so that a therapist placing his hands over the patient's chest will move out and inward.[19]

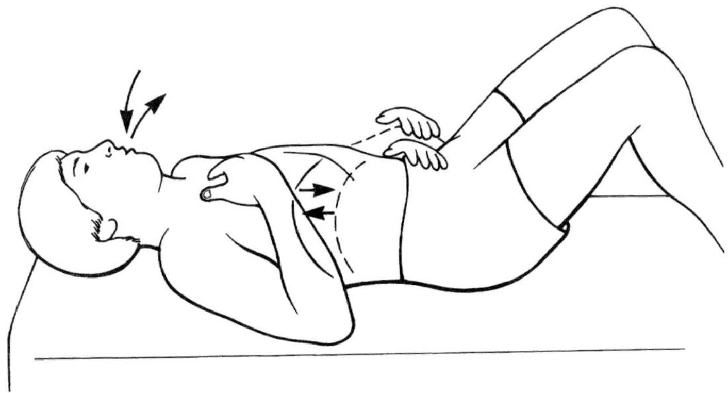

Fig. 18-9 Abdominal breathing exercises.

- *Weight reduction* when the patient is obese.[13] The use of an underwire brassiere with wider straps may be helpful.
- Emotional depression may negatively affect TOS because it can be physically expressed in scapular ptosis and should be appropriately dealt with either by the help of a mental health professional or by the use of antidepressants.[13]
- Scrutinize daily living activities as well as the patient's work conditions so that appropriate adjustments may be made.[13]
- Avoid wearing a heavy coat. Down coats are preferable. Avoid carrying heavy weights.
- Patients with nocturnal pain should sleep with their affected arm supported and in a neutral position. The pillow should not lift the shoulders off the bed[19] (Fig. 18-11).
- While one is sitting, arm supports such as those provided by an armchair are a must[19] because they unload the weight of the upper limb through the forearms so that the scapula is supported without effort. Use of a lumbar support during sitting may be helpful.
- Sitting each evening for one-half hour in an armchair before one goes to bed allows the nerve trunk to recover, as evidenced by the reappearance of familiar symptoms during sitting and eventual abatement after several minutes. The patient may then sleep, free from fear of being awakened.[4]
- Relaxation exercises to relax the upper thorax.[3]
- Massage of the trapezius and surrounding musculature.

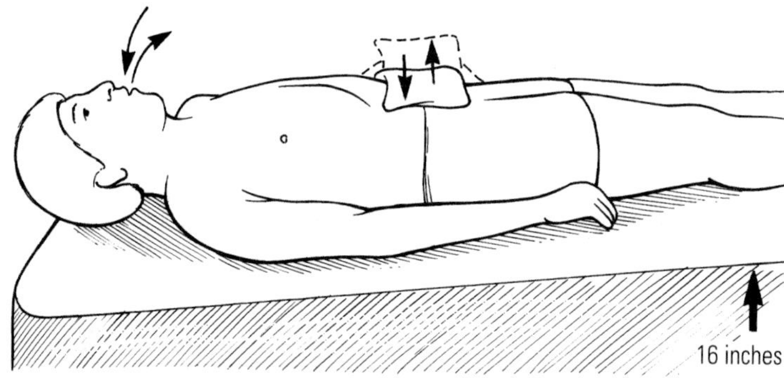

Fig. 18-10 Abdominal weight exercises.

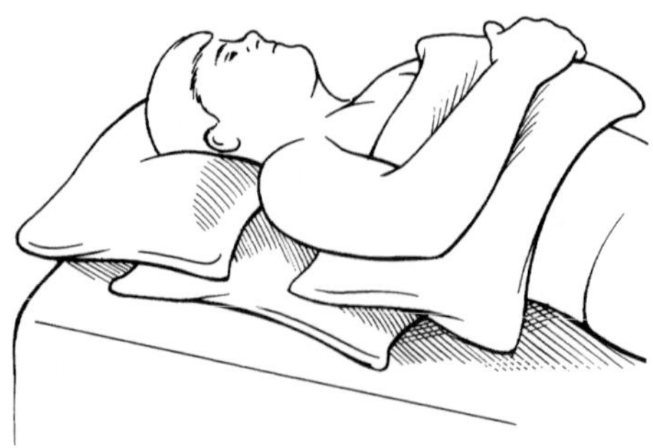

Fig. 18-11 Rest position in supine. Pillows or use of a triangle foam wedge should be used to support the thoracic spine, scapula, and arm.

17. What is the prognosis of TOS?

Fifty to ninety percent of sufferers of TOS respond rapidly and favorably to a conservative treatment program[3,9] and regain normal pain-free function of the upper extremity. The remainder may require surgery or a more extensive program that requires psychologic counseling as well as more involved rehabilitative intervention. Patients who do not respond to either conservative or surgical intervention often suffer from a host of physical and psychologic problems and should be referred to chronic pain centers, which are designed to address these problems.[10]

18. What surgical options are available after a failed conservative regimen of treatment?

The criteria for surgical treatment that demonstrate failure of conservative treatment include (1) signs of muscle wasting, (2) intermittent paresthesias being replaced by sensory loss, and (3) pain becoming incapacitating.[16] Surgery not performed by most shoulder surgeons[13] includes depression of the scalene muscles and resetting of the first rib, removal of the cervical rib if present, removal of the clavicle, severing of the pectoralis minor muscle, and trisection of the subclavius muscle above the coracoid ligament.[19] Eighty percent of surgical candidates respond favorably after surgery, and a period of rehabilitation emphasizing maintenance of full range of motion so as to reduce adhesions of the brachial plexus by scar tissue as well as postural correction is indicated.[21]

References

1. Barabis J: Therapist's management of thoracic outlet syndrome. In Hunter JM, Schneider LH, Mackin EJ, Callahan AB, editors: *Rehabilitation of the hand: surgery and therapy*, ed 3, St. Louis, 1990, Mosby.
2. Butler D: *Mobilisation of the nervous system*, Melbourne, 1991, Churchill Livingstone.
3. Kisner C, Colby LA: *Therapeutic exercise: foundations and techniques*, ed 2, Philadelphia, 1990, FA Davis.
4. Cyriax J: *Textbook of orthopaedic medicine*, vol 1: *Diagnosis of soft tissue lesions*, ed 8, London, 1982, Bailliere-Tindall.
5. Dawson DM, Hallet M, Millender LH: *Entrapment neuropathies*, ed 2, Boston, 1990, Little, Brown & Co.
6. Elvey R: Brachial plexus tension tests and the pathoanatomical origin of arm pain. In Glascon E, et al, editors: *Aspects of manipulative therapy*, ed 2, New York, 1985, Churchill Livingstone.
7. Gilliatt RW, LeQuesne PM, Ligue V, et al: Wasting of the hand associated with a cervical rib or band, *J Neurol Neurosurg Psychiatry* 33:615, 1970.
8. Hawkes C: Neurosurgical considerations in thoracic outlet syndrome, *Clin Orthop* 207:24, 1980.
9. Hoffman J: Electrodiagnostic techniques for and conservative treatment of thoracic outlet syndrome, *Clin Orthop* 207:21, 1986.
10. Jaeger S, Read R, Smullens SM, Breme P: Thoracic outlet diagnosis and treatment. In Hunter JM, Schneider LH, Mackin EJ, Callahan AD, editors: *Rehabilitation of the hand*, St. Louis, 1984, Mosby.
11. Kenneally M, et al: The upper arm tension test: the SLR of the arm. In Grant R, editor: *Physical therapy of the cervical and thoracic spine*, New York, 1988, Churchill Livingstone.
12. Lascelled RG, Mohr PD, Neary D, Bloon K: The thoracic outlet syndrome, *Brain* 100:501, 1977.
13. Leffert RD: Neurological problems. In Rockwood CA, Matsen FA, editors: *The shoulder*, vol 1, Philadelphia, 1990, Saunders.
14. Moore KL: *Clinically oriented anatomy*, ed 2, Baltimore, 1983, Williams & Wilkins.
15. Netter FH: *The CIBA collection of medical illustrations*, vol 7: *Respiratory system*, Ardsley, N.Y., 1980, CIBA-Geigy Corp.
16. Pang D, Wessel H: Thoracic outlet syndrome, *Neurosurgery* 22:105, 1988.
17. Peet RM, Hendriksen JD, Anderson TP, Martin GM: Thoracic outlet syndrome: evaluation of a therapeutic exercise program, *Staff Meet Mayo Clin* 31:281, 1956.
18. Peet RM, Hendriksen JD, Anderson TP, Martin GM: Thoracic-outlet syndrome: evaluation of a therapeutic exercise program, *Proc Mayo Clin* 3:265, 1956.
19. Pronsati MP: Treatment of thoracic outlet syndrome comes under scrutiny, *Advance for Physical Therapists*, p 14-15, Sept 9, 1991.
20. Schumacher HR, Bomalski JS: *Case studies in rheumatology for the house officer*, Baltimore, 1990, Williams & Wilkins.

21. Sunderland S: *Nerves and nerve injuries*, ed 2, London, 1978, Churchill Livingstone.
22. Swift TR, Nichols FT: The droopy shoulder syndrome, *Neurology* 34:212, 1984.
23. Swift TR, Roos DB: TOS or just droopy shoulders, *Aches Pains* 6:813, 1984.
24. Telford ED, Mottershead S: Pressure at the cervico-brachial junction: an operative and anatomical study, *J Bone Joint Surg* 30:2490, 1948.
25. Whitenack SH, Hunter JM, Jaeger SH, Read RL: Thoracic outlet syndrome complex: diagnoses and treatment. In Hunter JM, Schneider LH, Mackin EJ, Callahan AD, editors: *Rehabilitation of the hand: surgery and therapy*, ed 3, St. Louis, 1990, Mosby.

Recommended reading

Barbis J: Therapist's management of thoracic outlet syndrome. In Hunter JM, Schneider LH, Mackin EJ, Callahan AD, editors: *Rehabilitation of the hand: surgery and therapy*, ed 3, St. Louis, 1990, Mosby.

Butler D: *Mobilisation of the nervous system*, Melbourne, 1991, Churchill Livingstone.

Peet RM, et al: Thoracic outlet syndrome: evaluation of a therapeutic exercise program, *Staff Meetings Mayo Clin*, p 281, 1956.

Sanders RJ, Haug CE: *Thoracic outlet syndrome: A common sequelae of neck injuries.* J.B. Lippincott, Philadelphia, 1991.

Whitenack SH, Hunter JM, Jaeger SH, Read RL: Thoracic outlet syndrome complex: diagnosis and treatment. In Hunter JM, Schneider LH, Mackin EJ, Callahan AD, editors: *Rehabilitation of the hand: surgery and therapy*, ed 3, St. Louis, 1990, Mosby.

Large and Broad-Shouldered Infant with Monoparetic Arm after Breech Delivery

19

While working at the community hospital outpatient clinic 3 days a week, you are referred a case in the neonatal nursery. The infant, only 2 days old, presented with a breech delivery and appears to limply hang her left lower extremity adducted to her side with the forearm held in pronation. The baby weighed 9 pounds at birth, scored 6 on the Apgar test initially and then 7 five minutes later, and appears to have well-defined, almost broad shoulders. The infant is a first born. Radiographs have ruled out any clavicle or shoulder fracture.

CLUE:

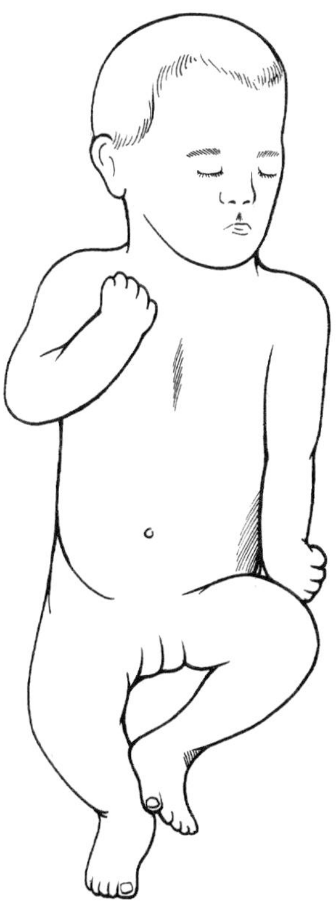

1. **What is most likely afflicting the infant?**
2. **What is the mechanism involved in brachial plexus injury?**
3. **How does brachial plexus injury most commonly occur in the neonate?**
4. **How does brachial plexus injury most commonly occur in the adult?**
5. **What is the anatomy of the brachial plexus?**
6. **How does architectural design of the brachial plexus serve as a force distributor?**
7. **What are the clinically observed patterns of injury?**
8. **What is the range of severity of injury?**
9. **What other conditions are associated with brachial plexus injury after birth trauma?**
10. **What abnormal respiratory function may occur with Erb's palsy?**
11. **What primary soft-tissue deformities occur after upper root paralysis?**
12. **What secondary contractures and osseous deformity occur after upper plexus injury?**
13. **What osseous deformities occur over time after upper root paralysis?**
14. **What radiographic changes eventually occur in the newborn after upper brachial plexus injury?**
15. **What is the difference between a preganglionic and a postganglionic nerve lesion?**
16. **Describe avulsion pain after preganglionic root avulsions.**
17. **What electrodiagnostic tests are appropriate?**
18. **What is the differential diagnosis of Erb's palsy?**
19. **What is the prognosis for recovery?**
20. **What is the prognosis after root avulsions?**
21. **How do evaluations of motor function differ when one is assessing a flail arm?**
22. **What operative management is appropriate in adults after brachial plexus injury?**
23. **What surgery is appropriate to improving elbow biomechanics?**
24. **What operative management is appropriate in infants or children after brachial plexus injury?**
25. **What are the goals of nonoperative management after brachial plexus injury?**
26. **How is the passive range of motion modality best administered?**
27. **How is the active range of motion modality best administered?**
28. **What is the role of electromyography in rehabilitative management?**
29. **How is the modality of stretching exercises most appropriately administered?**
30. **What positioning is appropriate in the infant after brachial plexus injury?**
31. **What is the role of electrical stimulation in the conservative treatment of plexus injury?**
32. **How is pain managed?**
33. **Is splinting appropriate in the management of brachial plexus injury?**
34. **What is a flail arm splint?**

1. What is most likely afflicting the infant?

Upper brachial plexus injury known as Erb's palsy.

2. What is the mechanism involved in brachial plexus injury?

After the elimination of poliomyelitis as a serious cause of paralysis in the industrial world, brachial plexus injury has become the most common cause of shoulder paralysis. The brachial plexus is attached by fascia to the first rib medially and to the coracoid process laterally, so that lateral head movement with simultaneous shoulder depression will both stretch the upper plexus and compress it against the first rib. This upper brachial plexus injury, known as *Erb's palsy,* is the most common type of shoulder paralysis and

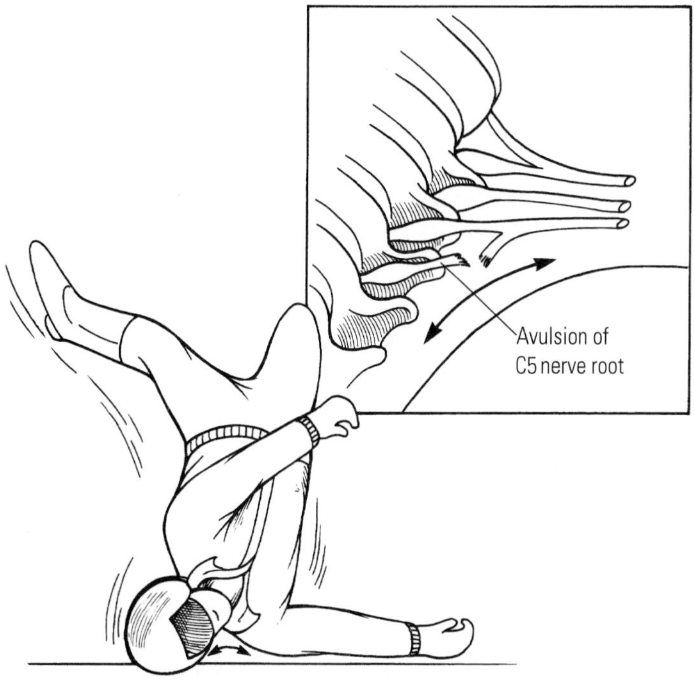

Fig. 19-1 Avulsion of C5 nerve root after a motorcycle accident.

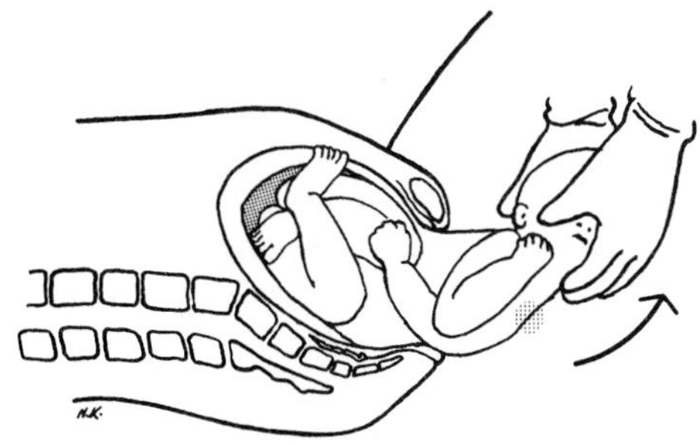

Fig. 19-2 Mechanism of upper brachial plexus birth injury. Excessive traction and lateral flexion of head and neck during delivery. (From Moore KL: *Clinically oriented anatomy*, ed 2, Baltimore, 1985, Williams & Wilkins.)

occurs after violent excessive separation of the shoulder from the neck (Fig. 19-1). Lower brachial plexus injury occurs from excessive, often violent hyperabduction of the shoulder attributable to upward arm traction causing stretch to the lower plexus and simultaneous compression by the underside of the coracoid process.[20]

3. How does brachial plexus injury most commonly occur in the neonate?

Obstetrical Erb's palsy commonly occurs during the last phase of vaginal delivery, especially when the infant has disproportionately large shoulders (fetal dystocia) in which the obstetrician facilitates delivery by way of traction and lateral flexion (Fig. 19-2); this is complicated by the presence of a narrow (that is, android) maternal pelvis. Other birth risk factors include midforceps delivery, vacuum extraction, and low forceps delivery in decreasing order of incidence. Other significant factors, regardless of method of delivery, include high birth weight (macrosomia), that is, greater than 3500 g, pregnant mothers succumbing to glucose intolerance (gestational diabetes), use of oxytocin, vertex and breech deliveries, occipitoposterior or transverse presentations, rotation of the head in cephalic presentation, and first pregnancies. Additionally, infants with such injury often have lower Apgar scores and are more commonly delivered after spinal or epidural anesthesia after a prolonged second stage of labor.[8,14,16,18]

Overall incidence of brachial plexus injury has shown epidemiologic variation according to the quality of prenatal care and neonatal care during delivery. The incidence is approximately one in 1000 births.[16] Although the likelihood of such injury after cesarean delivery is extremely unlikely, it may occasionally occur because of either a failed attempt at forceful vaginal delivery or an imperfect extraction during cesarean surgery.[18]

William Heinrich Erb, a professor at the University of Heidelberg and the first neurologist to utilize a reflex hammer,[17] demonstrated with electrical studies (1874) that pressure at the junction of the fifth and sixth brachial nerve roots, that is, *Erb's point,* located 2 to 3 cm above the clavicle and just behind the posterior edge of the sternomastoid muscle,[18] yields the characteristic type of muscle paresis.

In 1884, Augusta Dejerine-Klumpke described a paralytic lesion of the lower brachial plexus that was subsequently named after her. Erb-Duchenne-Klumpke's palsy (C5-T1) represents the second most common brachial plexus injury. Pure Klumpke's palsy (C5-T1) represents the second most common brachial plexus injury. Pure Klumpke's palsy (C8-T1) occurs very infrequently.[22]

4. How does brachial plexus injury most commonly occur in the adult?

The majority of upper brachial plexus injuries in the adult population result from high-velocity motorcycle accidents during which the driver is thrown forward and lands on the point of the shoulder, resulting in excessive separation of the neck and shoulder. This may also occur after a bicycle injury, after a pedestrian is struck and thrown by an automobile, or after a hard blow to the lateral area of the head, as by a baseball bat while the ipsilateral shoulder is simultaneously depressed. Patients are usually young males in their late teens or early twenties, often unskilled or beginning manual occupations.[12]

A common mechanism of lower brachial plexus injury is that of *excessive hyperabduction* as may occur after free fall in which an individual attempts to break his fall by attempting to grasp an object such as a tree limb[15] (Fig. 19-3). In the newborn, injury may have been incurred during attempted extraction of the upper limb by way of hyperabduction. (Fig. 19-4). The plexus may also suffer injury from heroin injection, delayed reaction to radiation treatment, serum injection, apical lung tumors (such as Pancoast's tumor), or during an operation on the axilla; the last two may cause lower brachial plexus injury.

Postanesthetic upper brachial plexus palsy may occur from malposition of the head, neck, or arm during general anesthesia and surgery. This is not permanent, and the prognosis for full recovery is excellent.[12]

5. What is the anatomy of the brachial plexus?

That interlacing of nerve fibers composing the brachial plexus (Fig. 19-5) is fascinating, complex, and yet frustrating because although one might memorize a textbook diagram of the plexus it would not be adequate for application to a significant number of clinical situations because of the significant variations in plexuses. Generally the "classic" brachial plexus is composed of the distal distribution of the anterior primary rami of C5 to T1 *spinal roots* (or nerves). The brachial plexus has contributions from C4 (cervical plexus) in a significant number of patients and is said to be "prefixed." Similarly, T2 contributions, occurring in a very small proportion of the population, lend the designation of "postfixed plexus."

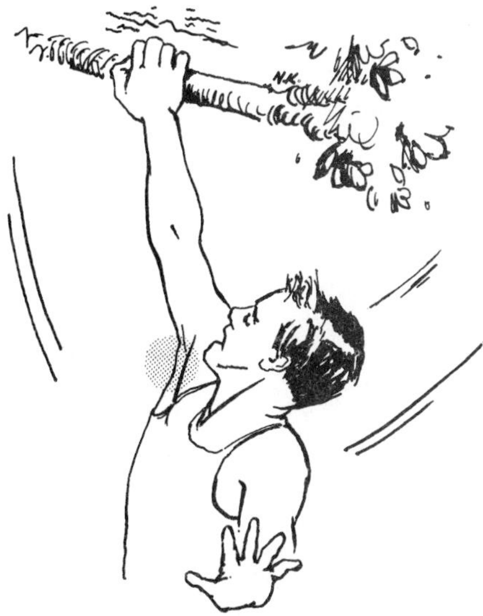

Fig. 19-3 Mechanism of injury in lower brachial plexus injury involves excessive, sudden, and forceful hyperabduction of the upper extremity. (From Moore KL: *Clinically oriented anatomy*, ed 2, Baltimore, 1985, Williams & Wilkins.)

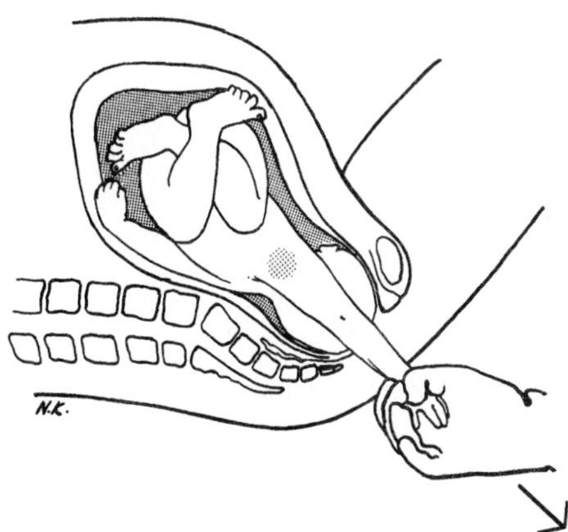

Fig. 19-4 Mechanism of lower brachial plexus injury incurred during birth. Forceful pull of the upper limb during birth into hyperabduction. (From Moore KL: *Clinically oriented anatomy*, ed 2, Baltimore, 1985, Williams & Wilkins.)

The roots continue distally to form *trunks*. The fifth and sixth cervical roots merge into the *upper trunk*, the seventh root continues to become the *middle trunk*, whereas the eighth cervical and first thoracic roots form the *lower trunk*. Each trunk then separates into anterior and posterior divisions (relative to the axillary artery). The anterior divisions of the upper and middle trunks unite to form the *lateral cord*, whereas the anterior division of the lower trunk forms the *medial cord*. The posterior divisions of each trunk unite and together form the *posterior cord* of the plexus. Although individual nerves such as the dorsal scapular nerve to the rhomboids and levator scapulae muscles come directly off the fifth cervical root before the upper trunk is formed, the aforementioned cords give off the largest number of terminal nerves. There is then a further sub-

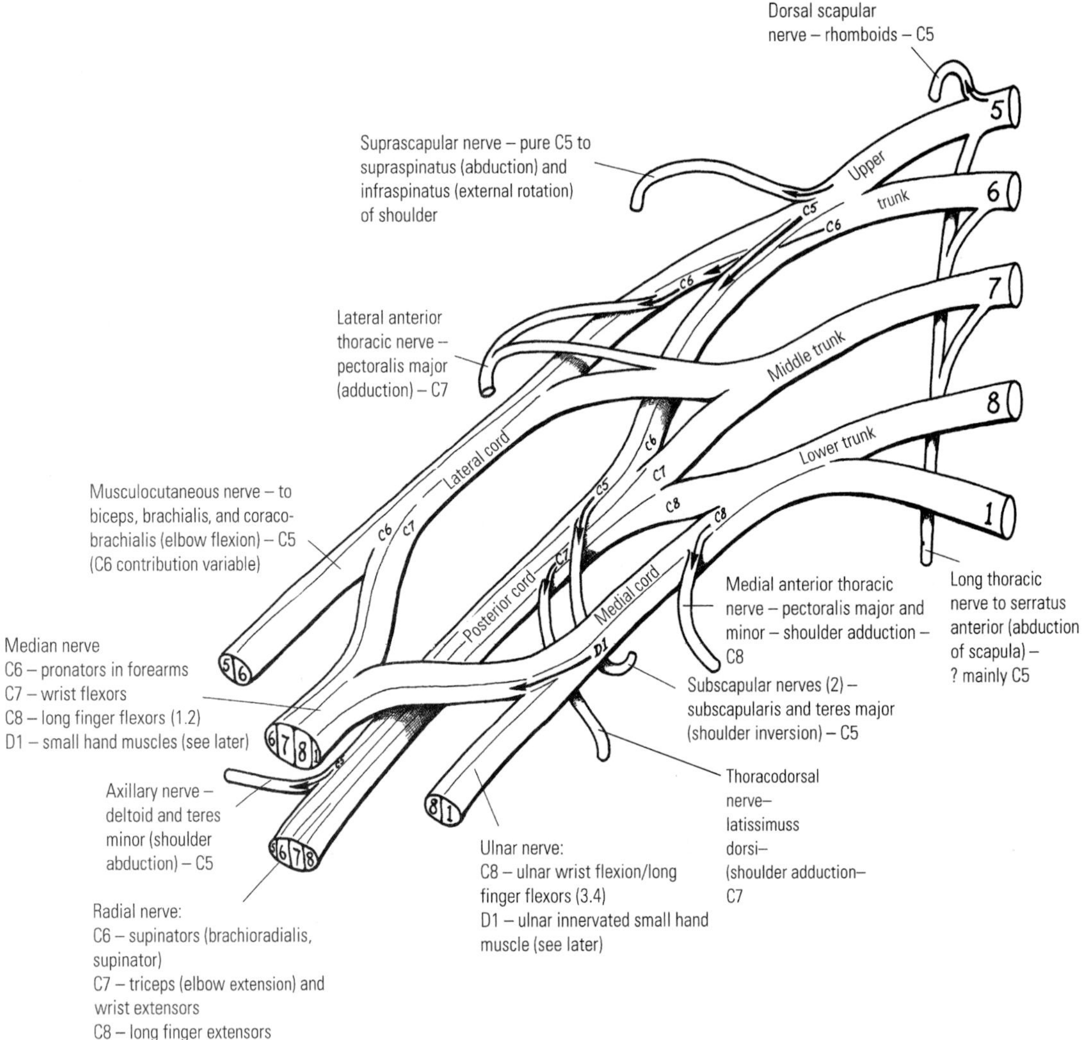

Fig. 19-5 Diagram of the brachial plexus. Contributions from each root are shown in the cross section of each cord as well as the median, ulnar, radial, and musculocutaneous nerves. (From Patten J: *Neurological differential diagnosis*, ed 2,London, 1996, Springer-Verlag.)

division in which the lateral and medial cords subdivide into branches, two of which fuse to become the median nerve. The remaining branches of the medial and lateral cords continue distally and respectively give rise to the medial cutaneous nerve to the upper arm, forearm, and the musculocutaneous nerve; the latter is the physical continuation of the lateral cord. Additionally the medial and lateral pectoral nerves derive from the medial and lateral cords respectively.

6. How does architectural design of the brachial plexus serve as a force distributor?

In the course of phylogenetic changes of the human upper extremity from closed kinetic chain (weight-bearing) function to that of open kinetic chain function, there occurred changes in plexus design to reflect

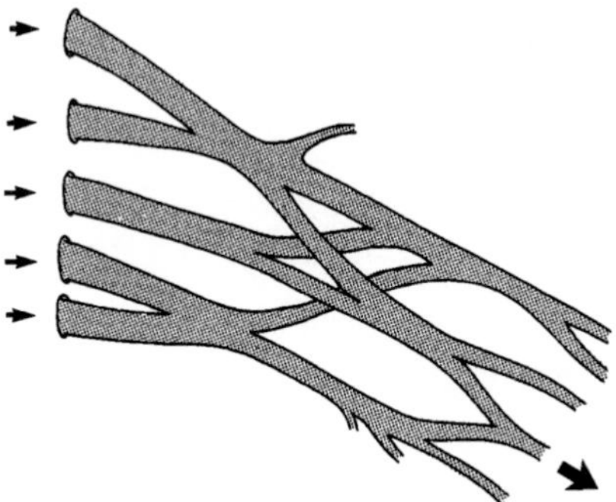

Fig. 19-6 The brachial plexus as a force distributor. Tension on one trunk will be distributed throughout the entire plexus. The angulation inherent to this design strategy enhances rather than minimizes the plexus reaction to the disruptive stretch by means of elongation and distribution of stress. (From Butler D: *Mobilisation of the nervous system,* Melbourne, 1991, Churchill Livingstone.)

this divergence of function. The architectural zigzag mesh composing the brachial plexus (Fig. 19-6), by virtue of design, is more capable of dissipating force by means of elongation, so that tension delivered to one trunk is distributed throughout the whole plexus.[22]

This force-distributing strategy is absent in the lumbosacral plexus, since destabilizing traction to the lower extremity is less likely, given the relatively greater stability present at the hip joint. Again we appreciate the price paid in terms of increased likelihood of upper extremity disorder in lieu of stability exchanged for mobility as mankind evolved from the quadruped to the biped posture. It is significant to note that the brachial nerves have spiral bands enabling them to stretch a full 16% without damage; this accommodating elasticity is absent in the lumbosacral plexus[2] (Fig. 19-7).

7. What are the clinically observed patterns of injury?

Patterns of muscle disfunction include the following:

C5-C6 lesion

Muscle weakness and paralysis manifest in the rhomboids, levator scapulae, serratus anterior (that is, the scapular movers), supraspinatus and infraspinatus (lateral humeral rotators), the deltoid muscle, biceps brachii, brachioradialis, and supinator (the elbow flexors and forearm supinators), which accounts for the forearm becoming contracted in pronation. The wrist extensors may or may not be paralyzed, and, if they are, patients may still be able to dorsiflex the wrist if the finger extensors are preserved. Functional deficits include an inability to control shoulder movement, which can neither be forward flexed nor abducted. Although the elbow may be extended, it cannot be actively flexed. Active hand motion is infrequently affected. Sensory loss, which is difficult to distinguish, is often absent and when present may show variable deficits along the outer surface of the upper arm, forearm, thumb, and index finger.

The upper extremity will assume a characteristic *waiter's tip posture*[15] (Fig. 19-8) with the shoulder held in internal rotation and adduction next to the trunk. The elbow is extended, the forearm pronated, and the hand held in flexion. This is the posture, conceivably, that one would assume while accepting a tip or bribe without letting the giver have the satisfaction of seeing the receiver's face, while scouting the periphery to ensure that no one was looking. After brachial plexus injury, this posture is accounted for when one considers how the normal magnitude of tonal output is shunted to the remnant undamaged nerves and hence expressed as excess tone in the antagonistic muscles: the adjacent C7-C8-T1 level muscles. This clinical presentation makes the diagnosis obvious. Whether accompanied with a history of injury in the adult patient,

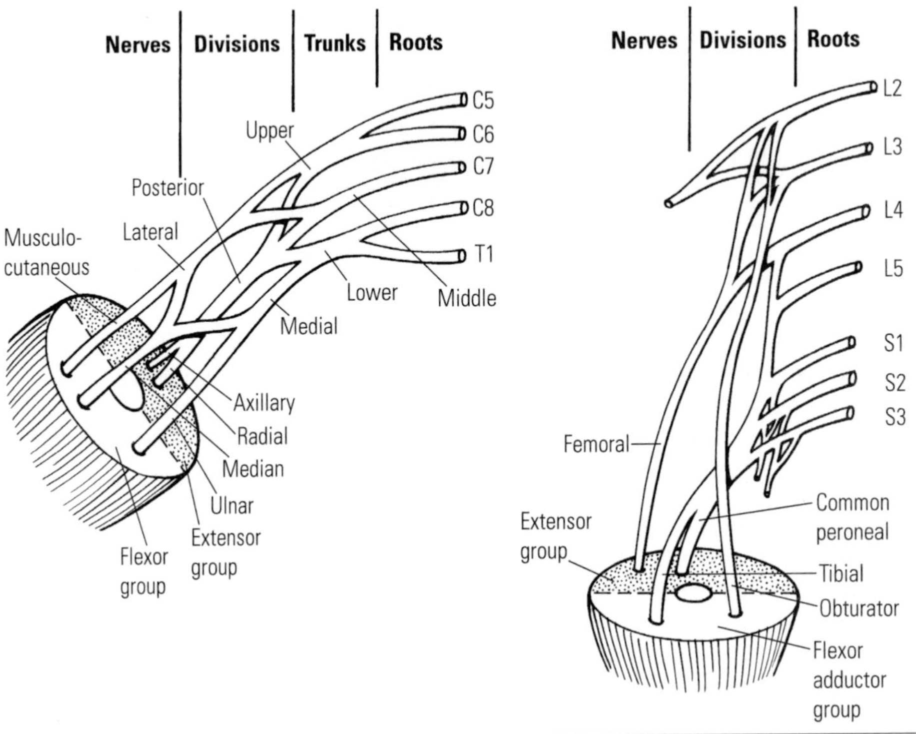

Fig. 19-7 Comparative architechture of plexus design. Although the brachial plexus is suited to dissipate tension by means of distribution of force throughout the plexus, the lumbosacral plexus lacks this design method.

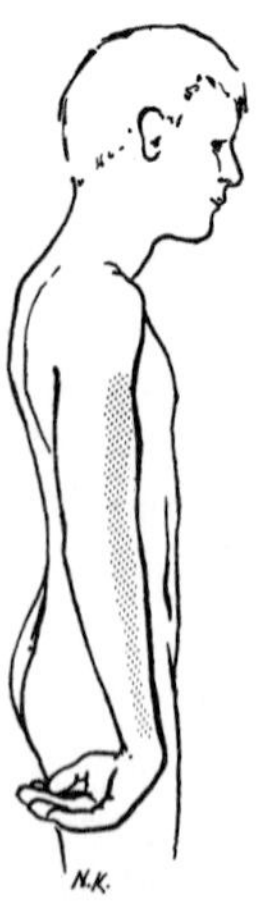

Fig. 19-8 Characteristic waiter's tip posture associated with upper brachial plexus injury. (From Moore KL: *Clinically oriented anatomy*, ed 2, Baltimore, 1985, Williams & Wilkins.)

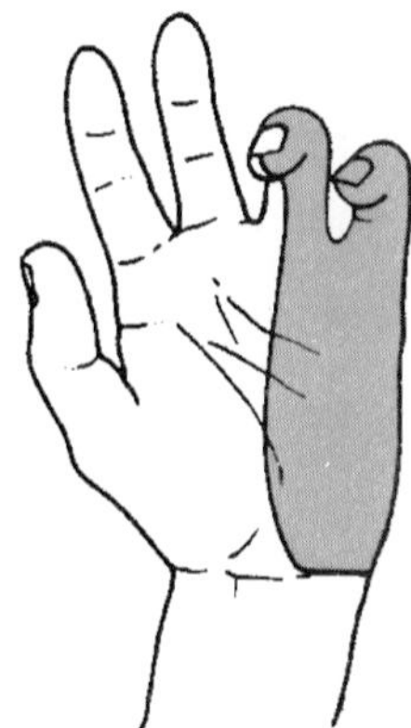

Fig. 19-9 Ulnar nerve palsy resulting in *main en griffe,* or clawhand. (From Ellis H: *Clinical anatomy,* ed 7, Oxford, 1983, Blackwell Scientific Publications.)

or after birth trauma in an infant, the patient essentially fails to move the shoulder, which is held limp against the trunk with only some active wrist and finger flexion. In the neonate, an asymmetric Moro reflex[16] confirms the diagnosis. Erb's palsy is commonly diagnosed within 24 hours after birth.[17]

C5-C6-C7 lesion

The C5 to C7 lesion includes all the deficits of the previous group with the addition of loss of active elbow, wrist, and finger extension. It is as if a radial nerve palsy were superimposed upon a C5-C6 lesion. As a result, there is a slightly wider area of sensory loss, that is, one involving the middle finger.

C7-C8-T1 lesion

The uncommon C7 to T1 lesion essentially presents as a combined median and ulnar nerve palsy of the hand as well as some radial nerve deficit manifesting as partial weakness in wrist extension, since the radial nerve receives some fibers from C8 and T1. Denervation of flexor muscles in the wrist and hand manifests as loss of active finger flexion and extension and as loss of all intrinsic hand function without producing a clawhand deformity[12] in some patients. A *clawhand* deformity (Fig. 19-9) occurs from loss of intrinsic hand function and from overpull of the extrinsic extensor muscles (that is, innervated by the radial nerve) of the proximal phalanx of the fingers. Thus the metacarpophalangeal joints become hyperextended while the proximal and distal interphalangeal joints become flexed. Therefore, if radial innervation is preserved, a clawhand deformity will manifest; otherwise it will not.

Sensory loss is usually confined to the little and ring fingers as well as to the ulnar border of the hand and inner forearm; however, if C7 dermatome is involved, the middle finger will lose sensation as well. The former two fingers are hyperextended at the metacarpophalangeal joints because the medial two lumbricale muscles are paralyzed and the extensor digitorum is unopposed.[15] Proximal function of the upper arm and shoulder are preserved with this lesion, though triceps function may be compromised. Horner's syndrome may be present because of involvement of sympathetic nerve fibers from T1. In the neonate, an absent grasp reflex is the most prominent clinical feature.[16] Infants and children may unwittingly, because of sensory loss, traumatize their fingertips even to the point of occasionally losing a fingertip.

C5 to T1 lesion

Trauma to the entire plexus is unfortunately the second most common type of brachial plexus injury.[12] This disastrous injury is accompanied by profound motor weakness and total loss of sensation resulting in flail-anesthetic limb. Prognosis for spontaneous recovery is extremely poor.

8. What is the range of severity of injury?

Stretching of the nerve roots or trunks of the plexus beyond the elastic limit of that nerve may result in one of several types of injuries. The range of injuries includes (1) minimal stretch causing mild edema, which may in turn damage more myelin with subsequent blocking of nerve impulses, (2) hemorrhage and subsequent scar formation within the nerve, (3) axonal rupture (tearing) of the nerve with or without wide separation of segments[4] or, at the very worst, (4) intraspinal root avulsion off the spinal cord. Considerable variation also exists in the number of levels affected, ranging from the mildest stretch and subsequent edema of only one or two roots to avulsion of the entire plexus.

9. What other conditions are associated with brachial plexus injury after birth trauma?

The most commonly associated condition of obstetrical brachial plexus injury is *facial nerve paralysis* resulting from difficult delivery that necessitated forceps use. There is also significant occurrence of ipsilateral idiopathic infantile muscular *torticollis* in breech-presentation infants. *Spasticity* occurs in those neonates afflicted with more severely involved root avulsions, since this results in focal hemorrhage up and down as well as in the vicinity of the cervical and thoracic spinal cord. *Fractures* of the clavicle, proximal humerus, and humeral shaft occur in that order of decreasing frequency. Other nerve injuries may include sympathetic nerve function associated with the first thoracic root producing ipsilateral *Horner's syndrome.* Additionally, involvement of the fourth cervical root may produce phrenic nerve injury[18] and subsequent paralysis of the diaphragm.

10. What abnormal respiratory function may occur with Erb's palsy?

More commonly occurring in those individuals with a prefixed plexus, injury to the upper brachial plexus may be accompanied by phrenic nerve disruption and hence hemidiaphragmatic paralysis. This is often observed by asymmetric thoracic and abdominal movement upon unilateral diaphragmatic observation. Phrenic nerve paralysis may result in respiratory distress and cyanosis and may mimic diaphragmatic hernia.[19] Examination of diaphragmatic function by electromyograph and fluoroscopy is not routinely carried out for infants with upper or whole types of paralysis, since ultrasound may yield accurate information in a noninvasive fashion. If the lesion is only a temporary neurapraxia, it is important to prevent respiratory problems such as atelectasis until recovery occurs. Positioning with the paralyzed side underneath is to be avoided. Prevention of secretion retention in relatively immobile portions of lungs is facilitated by postural drainage in the prone position at a 45° angle in the home several times a day. Respiration may be aided by oxygen and continuous positive airway pressure or continuous negative pressure[22] in severe cases.

11. What primary soft-tissue deformities occur after upper root paralysis?

After upper brachial plexus injury and resultant paresis or paralysis of the shoulder abductors and flexors as well as the scapular protractors and retractors, excess tone expressed to the intact neuromuscular junctions postures the shoulder in adduction, internal rotation, and slight forward flexion (Fig. 19-10). The summation of these unbalanced forces disturbs the synchronized and exquisitely balanced force couples that maintain normal kinesiologic function. Proximal muscle imbalance favors the shoulder adductors and medial rotators with soft-tissue contractures into the extremes of these latter ranges because those muscles adaptively foreshorten.

The scapula too is affected because both the serratus anterior and the rhomboids are weakened or nonfunctional. As a result, those muscles linking the humerus to the scapula (subscapularis, teres minor, latissimus dorsi) now cause the scapula to adhere to the humerus. This in turn upsets the normal 6:1 scapular-humeral rhythm during the first 30° of movement, and so any shoulder elevation, if any, is accompanied by a 1:1 ratio instead.[22]

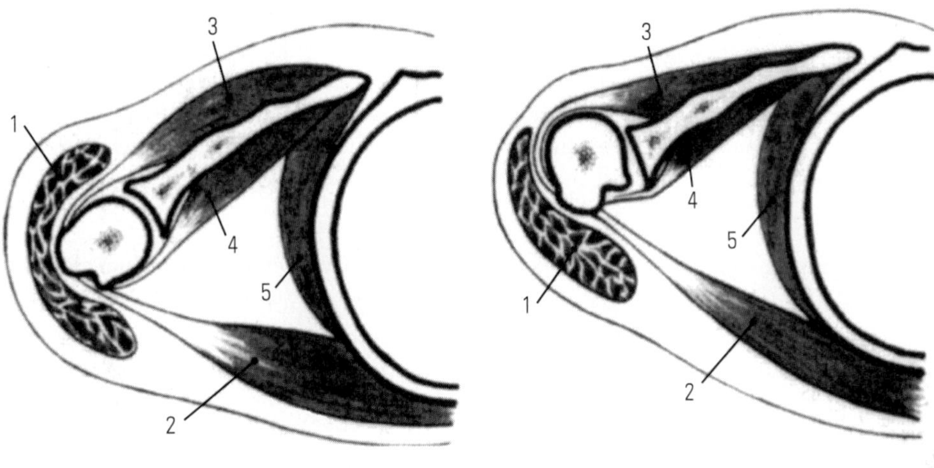

Fig. 19-10 Resulting muscle imbalance after upper brachial plexus injury results in shoulder deformity. Horizontal section comparing the normal shoulder *(left)* with the shoulder affected with an upper root lesion *(right)*. *1,* Deltoid; *2,* pectoralis major; *3,* infraspinatus; *4,* subscapularis; *5,* serratus anterior. Such imbalance postures the shoulder in adduction, internal rotation, and slight forward flexion. (From Scaglietti O: *Surg Gynecol Obstet* 66:868-877, 1938.)

The functional result of muscle imbalance is abnormal movement or abnormal combinations of movement that most commonly manifest as compensatory shoulder abduction with elbow flexion while one is attempting to reach out. This apparent disorganization of movement is actually the patient's attempt to reach in the most biomechanically advantageous manner, given the preservation of some muscle group as well as newly adapted muscle length. This substitution pattern, termed *Erb's engram,*[10] is a reasonably effective attempt at reaching, given the unfortunate state of affairs. A *visuokinesthetic motor engram*[8a] is a movement formula for the organization and execution of action.[13] When this movement substitution is practiced by the infant, it becomes learned to the extent of becoming "engrammed" on the motor cortex and eventually becomes automatic and dominant despite apparent substantial recovery.

At the elbow joint, the elbow flexors and anterior capsule become contractured over time because of weakness of the biceps brachialis and supinator. This also accounts for the forearm becoming contracted in pronation.[21] There may be only partial weakness of the triceps because that muscle receives most of its innervation from the C7 dermatome.

12. What secondary contractures and osseous deformity occur after upper plexus injury?

Secondary soft-tissue contractures include atrophy of the posterior deltoid, contracture of the subscapularis as well as the pectoralis major, and lengthening and atrophy of the infraspinatus contributing to posterior capsular insufficiency. Because of incessant and unbalanced internal shoulder rotation, the humeral head eventually suffers posterior subluxation. Additionally the anterior shoulder joint capsule becomes tight while the posterior capsule stretches. Secondary bony changes may also occur in the acromion, which bends forward and downward to hook over the front of the posteriorly subluxed humeral head. This hooking increases with age and varies directly with the degree of posterior subluxation. The coracoid process may become greatly elongated because of the pull of the now contractured coracobrachialis muscle. The clavicle becomes shorter because of its becoming slowly curved more acutely than on the opposite side secondary to the unopposed weight of the upper extremity and from the vector sum of unbalanced muscular forces.

13. What osseous deformities occur over time after upper root paralysis?

Because of muscle imbalance in favor of those muscles (that is, the middle and lower root levels) antagonistic to a given level of injury, accompanying bony deformities will eventually occur. Over time the humeral head will become retroverted, and persistent unbalanced internal shoulder rotation will cause flattening of the medial aspect of the humeral head. Additionally the glenoid fossa will in turn become hypoplastic and sclerotic and may even form a "saddle" type of joint with the depressed humeral head.[6]

14. What radiographic changes eventually occur in the newborn after upper brachial plexus injury?

Radiographic changes include the following: In the newborn the proximal humerus will lie more distant to the glenoid, and development of the proximal epiphyseal ossification center is retarded. This epiphyseal center is lateral to that of the greater tuberosity as ossification occurs because of the internally rotated humerus. The humeral head succumbs to posterior subluxation, the coracoid process becomes elongated, and the acromion is elongated, hooked, and flared on its end. The clavicle and glenoid are undeveloped. The diaphragm may be elevated if there is phrenic nerve paralysis.[7]

15. What is the difference between a preganglionic and a postganglionic nerve lesion?

Preganglionic lesions (that is, root avulsions) are characterized by the following signs, symptoms, and history: (1) a high-speed impact injury, (2) a period of loss of consciousness, (3) associated injuries such as multiple fractures, (3) a head injury, (4) vascular injury, (5) positive Horner's sign, (6) presence of sensory action potentials, (7) presence of meningoceles on a myelogram (which indicates avulsion), and (8) pain in the anesthetic limb.

Postganglionic lesions (that is, distal ruptures) are characterized by the following signs, symptoms, and history: (1) slow-speed impact injury, (2) no loss of consciousness, (3) no associated injuries, (4) negative Horner sign, (5) negative sensory action potentials, (6) normal myelogram, (7) positive Tinel's, or neuroma, sign, and (8) no pain[5] (Fig. 19-11).

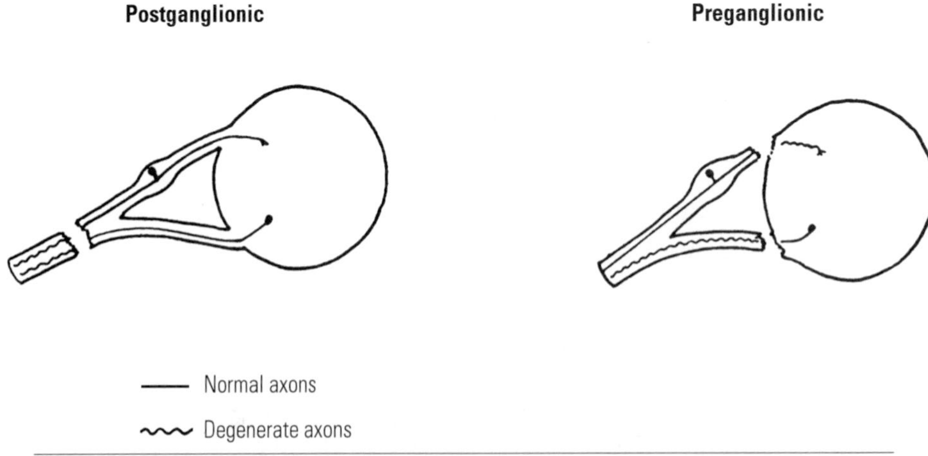

Fig. 19-11 Site of lesion may be preganglionic or postganglionic, each of which manifests a different clinical presentation. (From Bonney G: *Brain* 77: 588-609, 1954.)

16. Describe avulsion pain after preganglionic root avulsions.

Preganglionic avulsion pain is not usually immediate but occurs 2 to 3 weeks after injury. Patients describe the pain as a constant, burning, or crushing sensation akin to the hand being crushed in a vice. Pain may manifest as sudden, sharp, electric, or shooting paroxysms of pain that crescendo for several seconds to 1 minute and gradually recede to a constant burning. The pain may be so intense that the patient may stop talking as pain literally takes his breath away as he grips his arm during the peak of discomfort. The pain does not vary with external stimuli. Patients may experience difficulty falling asleep but, once asleep, are not usually awakened by pain. This incessant pain is accounted for by a lack of central inhibition and hence unsuppressed firing of the cells of the dorsal horn.[24] This lack of central inhibition originates in sudden deafferentation of the spinal cord at the time of injury. Pain is frequently felt in the dermatome of the root that has been avulsed. This is curious, since no pathways remain between that dermatome in the arm and the spinal cord.

Preganglionic and postganglionic lesions respectively score positive and negative to histamine and cold vasodilatation response.[1] These data are useful in evaluating preoperative nerve repair in adults with accidental brachial plexus injury.[18]

17. What electrodiagnostic tests are appropriate?

Needle electromyograph of the paraspinal muscles is appropriate in determining whether root avulsion has occurred (Fig. 19-12). The reason is that the posterior cervical musculature is serially innervated by

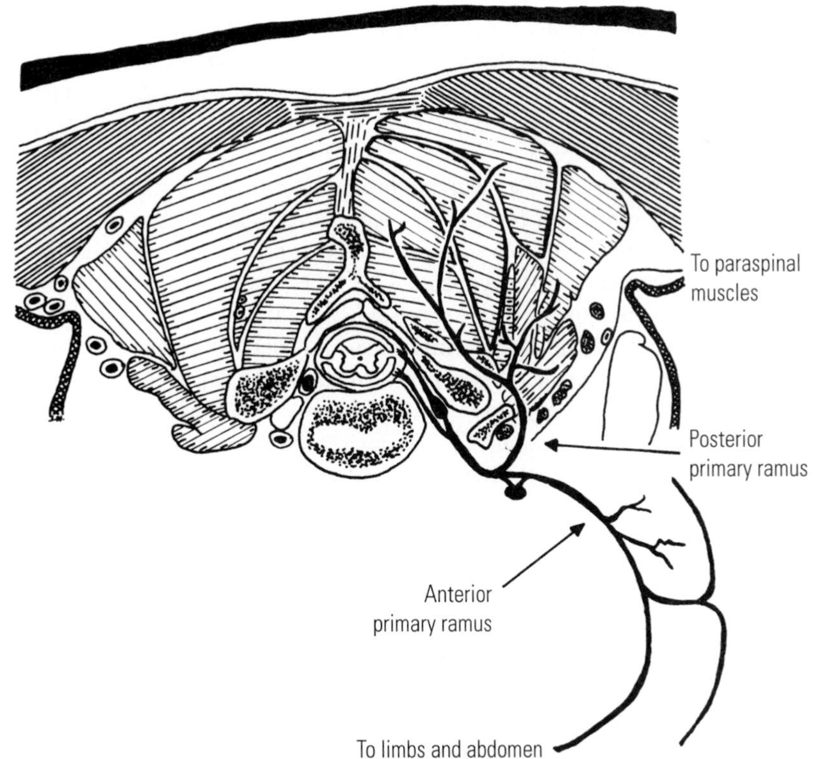

Fig. 19-12 Anterior and posterior primary rami. (From Hunter JM, Schneider LH, Mackin EJ, Callahan AD, editors: *Rehabilitation of the hand: surgery and therapy,* ed 3, St. Louis, 1990, Mosby.)

the posterior primary rami of the same-level spinal nerves innervating the anterior primary rami that make up the plexus. For example, if the limb musculature is denervated but the erector spinae muscles corresponding to that level are functioning normally, we have confirmation that the posterior rami at that level are intact. We may then make the following deduction: given that the posterior primary rami are given off immediately after the spinal nerves as they exit the intervertebral foramen, the lesion must be farther distally (that is, postganglionic rupture) somewhere along the course of the trunk, cord, or nerve branch and not proximally (that is, preganglionic avulsion). If, on the other hand, both sets of muscles are denervated, we may assume that an avulsion has occurred. Furthermore, the site of lesion can often be defined from the distribution of fibrillation activity.[12] Absence of fibrillation activity several weeks after nerve insult is suggesive of a good prognosis, since most of the axons are probably intact.

Nerve conduction velocity (NCV) studies can also distinguish between distal ruptures and root avulsions. The latter will manifest as preservation of sensory conduction only, without a value recorded for motor conduction velocity, since the axon is separated from the anterior horn cell in the spinal cord. Sensory conduction is preserved however, since the dorsal root ganglion remains in continuity with the axon or dendrite.[12]

Electromyographic studies (EMGs) are very difficult to perform with small infants. Rather than determining the site of lesion, they are more useful in determining the extent of injury and the presence or absence of recovery.[18]

18. What is the differential diagnosis of Erb's palsy?

Fractures of the humerus or clavicle are differentiated from brachial plexus injury by voluntary elbow motion elicited by forearm or hand stimulation. With spastic hemiplegia, the ipsilateral lower extremity is involuted as well and may be accompanied by persistent Babinski's sign and sustained ankle clonus.

19. What is the prognosis for recovery?

Most cases of brachial nerve injury have a favorable prognosis.[23] If only a small segment of the axon is stretched but not ruptured, quick self-repair and recovery are likely. Temporary blockage of nerve impulses from swelling will resolve as edema subsides as long as no axon damage has occurred. However, if the axon is interrupted, reinnervation may take a long time, if one considers the slow rate of axonal growth in the peripheral nervous system (about 1 mm a day).[16] Although Erb's palsy is generally reported as having the best prognosis of all types of brachial plexus injuries, if no deltoid or biceps recovery has occurred by the third month, the result is often poor. Prognosis for full recovery is poor in Klumpke's palsy, and complete axon rupture is unlikely to recover regardless of level of injury. Similarly, a whole-plexus type of injury has an extremely poor prognosis for recovery. If recovery occurs, reinnervation will generally be complete in 4 to 5 months with Erb's palsy and anywhere between 7 months to 2 years in total plexus injury.[4]

20. What is the prognosis after root avulsions?

For plexus lesions determined to be of the root avulsion type, prognosis for spontaneous recovery is very poor. Given our present level of technology it is impossible to replant a spinal nerve that has been avulsed from the cord. However, if there is sufficient nerve length available distal to the intervertebral foramen, surgical repair may be attempted.[12] The results are often unsatisfactory.

21. How do evaluations of motor function differ when one is assessing a flail arm?

Motor functional assessment of a flail arm is approached differently from that of ordinary muscle testing. The examiner attempts to identify flickers of movement (as in the rhomboids) that would indicate sparing of the C5 nerve root from rupture. Bear in mind that a trace muscle grade of the upper pectoralis major (that is, clavicular) fibers implies sparing or recovery of the mainly upper trunk, whereas such a grade or greater observed in the lower pectoralis major fibers (sternal fibers) would indicate lower trunk recovery. A muscle gradation of trace flicker (that is, grade 1) means that there is evidence of slight contractility on observation or palpation, without observable joint motion.[5]

22. What operative management is appropriate in adults after brachial plexus injury?

In adults with brachial plexus injury, surgery is most often considered only when no evidence of either electromyographic or clinical recovery has occurred within the first 6 months after injury, since the outlook for spontaneous recovery is poor. The time in which surgery holds most promise for reinnervation is within the first 6 to 9 months after injury. A lapse of more than 1 year makes it hardly worthwhile considering. Neural reconstruction by microsurgery is accomplished by use of an autograft, usually the sural nerve and occasionally the medial cutaneous nerve of the forearm.[12] Surgery is considered successful if the interval between surgical repair and onset of observable recovery of elbow flexion is between 1 year and 18 months.[12] Results of repair for elbow restitution are significantly better than that for shoulder function, and about three forths of these patients regain the ability to flex the elbow against gravity and resistance. With regard to the shoulder, success is often no better than the ability to shrug one's shoulder or overcome inferior shoulder joint subluxation. In all cases it is absolutely vital that the suprascapular nerve be repaired or else the all-important lateral rotary stability will be lacking. Most patients will not be able to raise their arms overhead after surgical reinnervation of shoulder musculature. Repair is rarely performed in the lower trunk of the plexus, since intrinsic muscle fibrosis will have occurred in the hand by the time nerve growth is complete.

It is because of the often poor functional result of neural reconstruction that many authorities consider secondary peripheral reconstruction the mainstay of surgical intervention. Surgery attempts correction of secondary osseous and soft-tissue deformities that have developed as a result of muscle imbalance. Reinforcement of weak or paralyzed muscles may be addressed by the use of tendon transplants, whereas osseous deformities may be addressed by humeral derotation osteotomy or shoulder arthrodesis. With the latter procedures, it is imperative that the trapezius and the serratus anterior function normally, since this is the minimal operating muscle pattern that will allow good postoperative function. In the event of flail glenohumeral joint, arthrodesis overcomes painful joint subluxation and will permit the patient to utilize the upper limb functionally. Limitation of abduction and rotation make it impossible to move the involved arm passively with the healthy hand in some activities of daily life such as dressing and combing one's hair.[3]

23. What surgery is appropriate to improving elbow biomechanics?

After brachial plexus injury, lack of full elbow flexion is not considered to be a significant disability, whereas the latter coupled with a fixed supination deformity is considered significant because this permits only limited hand function. Hand function is limited because this forearm deformity places the palm of the hand in a position useless for anything more than carrying objects. A weakened hand is much more useful if the forearm is partially pronated, since the functional portion of the hand faces the working surface of a desk or table. Correction is most simply performed by forearm osteotomy[18] or by correcting the excessive internal rotation at the shoulder (Fig. 19-13). Although effective, elbow flexorplasty, such as pectoralis major or latissimus dorsi transfer, may result in a conspicuous scar. Procedures to improve hand and wrist use are often individualized according to the given pattern of dysfunction.

24. What operative management is appropriate in infants or children after brachial plexus injury?

Microsurgery is generally not performed during infancy and is indicated only in the event of (1) a completely flail arm with Horner's syndrome after 1 month or (2) absence of biceps function after 3 months.

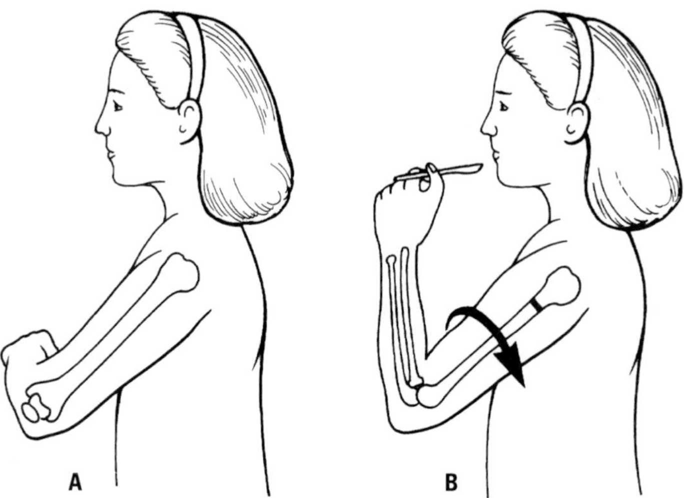

Fig. 19-13 Rotational osteotomy at the shoulder may improve function. (Redrawn from Rockwood FA, Matsen CA, editors: *The shoulder,* vol 2, ed 2, Philadelphia, 1990, Saunders.)

Postoperative immobilization involves a body jacket for 3 weeks. The prognosis for recovery after pediatric surgery is more favorable than surgery in the adult brachial plexus injury. In the older child (such as 5 or 6 years of age) surgery to stabilize the joints, tendon transplant, and soft-tissue elongation may be performed because patients may benefit from regained improvement in function.[12]

25. What are the goals of nonoperative management after brachial plexus injury?

The cornerstone of initial treatment in all cases of brachial plexus injury is nonoperative management.[9] Unfortunately, in some instances ignorance, inexperience, or lack of financial resources stymies success of an early nonoperative treatment approach. Goals of management include prevention of (1) soft-tissue contracture, (2) neglect, (3) substitution patterns, (4) injury to insensate parts, (4) and prevention of subluxation. Of paramount importance is appropriate psychologic support to control anxiety and fears of the future, address the injury to the patient's body schema, and discuss issues of vocation and depression.

26. How is the passive range of motion modality best administered?

Passive range of motion (PROM). Initially the infant is passively supported in a swing or swathe together with a collar or cuff to support the shoulder so as to prevent subluxation. No passive range of motion is to be performed for the first several days so as to permit early traumatic neuritis to subside.[18] This also avoids tension on the irritated plexus and allows resolution of hemorrhage and edema.[22] PROM of the shoulder girdle should then commence in those planes in which loss of active muscle contraction occurs in external shoulder rotation and abduction, forearm supination, wrist extension, finger extension, and thumb abduction. These exercises serve to stretch the weakened or paralyzed muscles. All movements must be performed gently so as not to damage the shoulder. The infant should not cry as a result of these movements. Additionally the normal scapulohumeral relationship should be manually mimicked during shoulder joint elevation. The scapula should not be manually restrained once the humerus rises above the 30°[20] elevation mark. The reason is that elevation unaccompanied by scapular rotation (or lateral humeral rotation) results in potential impingement within the subacromial arch beyond 30°. Particular effort should be taken to teach the infant's parents how to perform passive movements appropiately. An overzealous parent can severely injure an infant's arm and must be carefully impressed with the importance of keeping within the normal range.

In the adult, the hand often tends to conform to the contour of the abdomen against which it rests, resulting in eventual ankylosis of the metacarpophalangeal joints in full extension, with the thumb in the plane of the hand and therefore useless even if motor control returns. PROM taught to the adult ought to be simple and few in quantity because the more complex and numerous, the less likely the patient is to perform them regularly.[12]

27. How is the active range of motion modality best administered?

Active range of motion (AROM). The therapist must not simply stimulate movement. Rather he or she must perform *motor training,* that is, stimulation of movement while minimizing and preventing disorganized limb movement, that is, habituated substitution patterns. To facilitate this, the therapist uses manual guidance of the limb during elevation together with verbal praise to the infant, such as appropriate cooing and wooing, to ensure that the infant moves as normally as possible. Abnormal tone dominates the limb, and, given the sheer limits or practicality, the infant's nervous system may, despite well-intentioned therapy, engram a substitution movement pattern. It is for this reason that motor training must involve *intense* training of the limb in specific planes of movement. For example, in training the deltoid and external rotators to contract and elevate the shoulder, the exercise is first done on the child's side where gravity is eliminated. The therapist then slowly progresses the child to gravity-resisted movements in the supine position while simultaneously deemphasizing unwanted substitutions. Objects of grasp used to stimulate should be irresistible in form and color so as to motivate the child. Verbal feedback and positive reinforcement in the form of tone and smile are a must, and part and parcel of the repertoire of skills the therapist cultivates while treating such children. Additionally, the object of attraction (such as a bright fishing lure without its hook) is best kept 5 to 7 inches away from the child's face because this range includes the infant's acute field of vision.[22] Objects will also be more easily detected if they move rather than if they are simply held stationary. AROM is performed, at the very least, with each diaper change.

When the child is old enough to interact with adults and to obey simple commands, play activities are initiated. The therapist must be very imaginative, so that games are performed and nursery rhymes may be sung with each exercise so as to stretch contracted muscles or strengthen weakened muscles.

28. What is the role of electromyography in rehabilitative management?

Serial electromyographic (EMG) studies ought to be begun within the first few weeks after birth and repeated at 6- to 8-week intervals for as long as indicated. EMG signs of return such as decreased denervation potentials and the appearance of reinnervation potentials often predate clinically apparent return by several weeks. Potential recovery is maximized when the appearance of these EMG findings is immediately followed by intense therapy to stimulate activity in affiliated muscle groups. Although excessive fatigue is to be avoided, specific motor training at this juncture may be crucial to actualizing potential neural recovery. Thus EMG is used as a guide to the motor training program.[20,22]

29. How is the modality of stretching exercises most appropriately administered?

Stretching activities of the active musculature are appropriate, since the excess tone delivered to the unopposed muscles causes them to shorten more quickly. Muscles that require regular stretching include wrist and finger flexors, elbow extensors, forearm pronators, shoulder adductors, and internal rotators.

30. What positioning is appropriate in the infant after brachial plexus injury?

Positioning. When placed in supine or prone positions, infants should have their arm placed with the shoulder in midrange of abduction and external rotation and with the elbow in flexion. This position somewhat approximates a natural neonate posture, avoids excessive joint stretch, and reinforces the goals of range of motion exercises. Propped and sidelying on the sound side is a position that permits the involved arm to be free for play and permits encouragement of midline orientation as well as hand-to-hand or hand-to-mouth activity; however, the affected arm is relatively nonfunctional secondary to paralysis. Occasional sidelying on the affected side is permitted with appropriate protection from undue compression achieved by propping of the infant in a well-supported position, with the trunk slightly rolled back toward supine to reduce body weight on the arm. A small pillow or folded baby blanket is tucked under the infant's head so as to achieve a neutral alignment of the neck along the body axis. This position allows the baby to play with the sound arm, which is less influenced by gravity.[20]

31. What is the role of electrical stimulation in the conservative treatment of plexus injury?

Electrical stimulation is appropriate in most kinds of brachial plexus injury, including those in infants. The goal of electrical stimulation is to prevent muscle atrophy and fibrosis from setting into denervated muscle.[13] Here, the reference electrode is placed on the baby's ipsilateral forearm or leg while the active electrode is attached to the dorsum of the therapist's hand. In this fashion the therapist feels everything that the infant does and can thus monitor the magnitude of stimulation directly. Pinpoint stimulation is then provided by way of the therapist's fingers, for example, by placement of the tip of each finger on the motor points of shoulder force-coupled muscles. Treatment should be minimized in the pediatric population to no longer than several minutes at a time.[11]

32. How is pain managed?

Pain treatment. A significantly high percentage of patients with traction injuries to the brachial plexus suffer pain that may initially be very severe; this is particularly true after an avulsion of the nerve root. Fortunately, discomfort usually diminishes with time. In the interim, however, pain may be managed with transcutaneous electric stimulation (TENS) or acupuncture. The deafferentation of the spinal cord after an avulsion injury leads to changes in the firing of the dorsal horn cells in the spinal cord. One might argue that TENS artificially restores the afferent input to the spinal cord by allowing completion of the disrupted circuit. Thus, if TENS is to work by this mechanism, electrodes ought to be placed proximally to the level of the lesion (Fig. 19-14). Single-channel units are usually adequate, though large pads are preferable so as to facilitate as large an afferent input as possible.

Electrode placement involves one large pad placed over the appropriate damaged dermatome (providing that there is some residual afferent input), whereas the other pad is placed over the nerve trunk of the appropriate root level of damage. Electrodes may be placed more distally in the event of some residual arm sensation. Pads may also be applied over the impaired area of sensation, provided that the area is not anesthetic, since this arrangement would provide no afferent pathway along which the electrical stimulus could pass to the spinal cord. A minimum duration of treatment of 8 hours a day for 3 weeks is recommended.[5] TENS treatment is contraindicated in infants.

The treatment of pain with narcotics on a long-term basis is contraindicated, since this is chronic, "benign" pain. Once the patient is started on the use of narcotic medication by well-meaning physicians, the result is often considerable difficulty in weaning patients from these drugs. Cordotomy, rhizotomy, or sympathectomy as sources of pain relief are not considered appropriate by some authorities. Indeed, the problem of pain occurring after brachial plexus injury continues to be a difficult one for which no clearly dependable solution exists.[12]

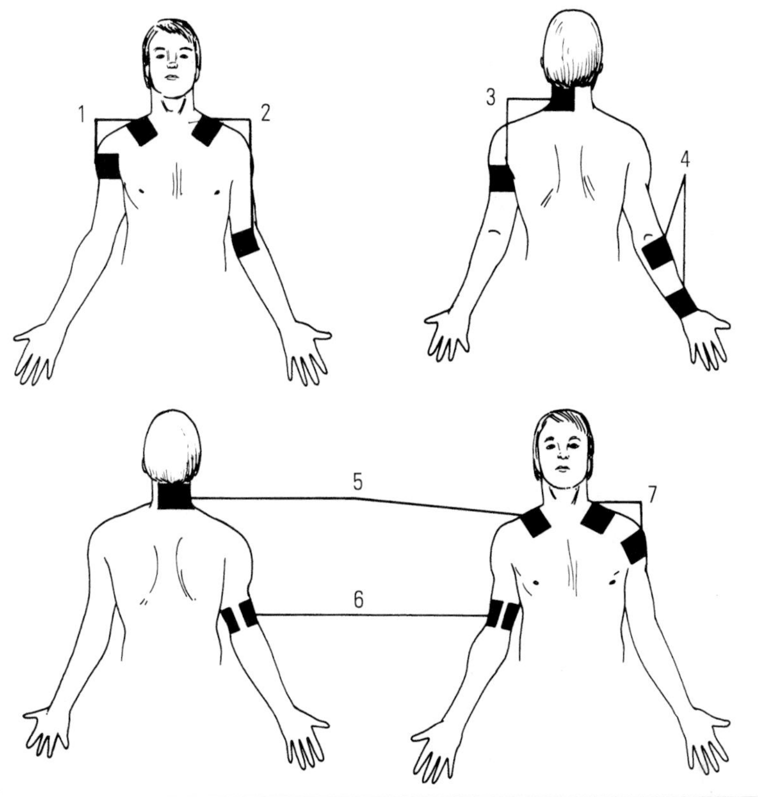

Fig. 19-14 Transcutaneous electric stimulation (TENS) electrode placements *1* to *7* for brachial plexus patients with avulsion pain. (From Hunter JM, Schneider LH, Mackin EJ, Callahan AD, editors: *Rehabilitation of the hand: surgery and therapy*, ed 3, St. Louis, 1990, Mosby.)

33. Is splinting appropriate in the management of brachial plexus injury?

Continuous *splinting* of the extremity after a brachial plexus injury is a controversial topic and is no longer routinely employed as a treatment modality. A once commonly used splint is the "Statue of Liberty" position designed to immobilize the shoulder in the corrected position, but it may eventually cause hypermobility and even anterior glenohumeral dislocation. Pinning the sleeve to a pillow or mattress with the shoulder in 90° abduction and external rotation essentially does the same thing and is inappropriate. Intermittent positional splinting is appropriate during those times when active intervention with the infant is not possible, provided that it is not substituted for regular active range of motion activities. Elbow splints have also been known to cause a pathologic condition such as elbow flexion contracture, dislocation and flattening of the radial head, and bowing of the proximal end of the ulna.

Resting hand splints are often appropriate to prevent flexion contractures of the fingers and to stabilize the thumb and fingers in good functional alignment. Dynamic splints to reinforce and reeducate wrist and finger extensors have been used with infants sustaining C7 injury.[20]

34. What is a flail arm splint?

Flail anesthetic limb is defined as total loss of limb sensitivity compounded with profound motor weakness; it has an extremely poor prognosis for spontaneous recovery. The adult with a flail arm should never

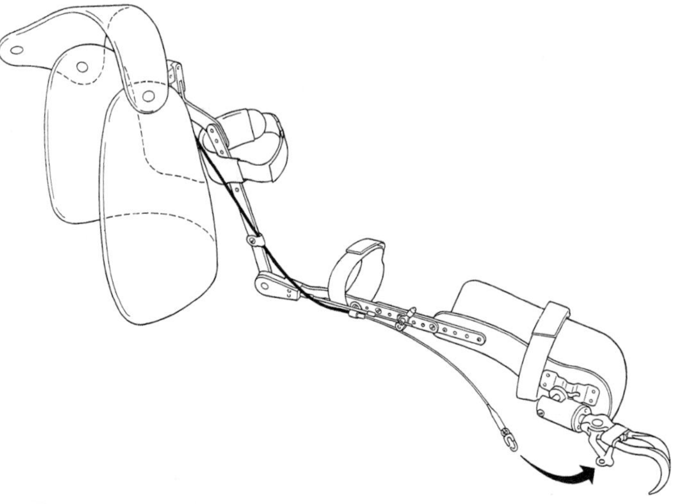

Fig. 19-15 Flail arm splint. (From Robinson C: *Br J Occup Ther* 49(10):1986.)

be splinted because of the rapidity with which contractures set in. However, wearing a functional *flail arm splint* is appropriate in providing the patient with bilateral upper extremity function while he or she waits for recovery to occur. It is up to the rehabilitation team or the patient's therapist to discern whether a given patient is appropriate for this splint. The reason is that the patient who is not truly motivated or suitable for a flail arm splint may well cause a lot of time to be wasted by both therapist and patient.

The flail arm splint (Fig. 19-15) is a lightweight modular splint that is actually a skeleton of an upper limb prosthesis that fits over the paralyzed arm. This orthosis provides the necessary shoulder support to allow for some shoulder abduction while preventing subluxation. An elbow lock device permits alternative positions for elbow flexion as well as being a forearm-to-wrist support trough having a platform on the volar aspect, onto which standard artificial limb appliances may be fitted. The splint is operated in the same manner as a prosthesis, that is, by a cable running from the terminal appliance to a shoulder strap on the opposite shoulder. The flail arm splint can be fitted in 1½ to 2 hours, functions as a tool for use at work as well as for hobbies, and can be taken off when not in use. When compared to an upper extremity prosthetic, its advantage over a prosthetic is a cosmetic one that allows the patient to retain his or her limb after and hence the psychologic benefit of maintaining his or her sense of body schema, which is lost after amputation. Amputation is uncommon because paralysis of the shoulder girdle muscles in most brachial plexus injuries precludes good operation of the artificial limb.[5]

References

1. Bonney G: The value of axon responses in determining the site of lesion in traction injuries of the brachial plexus, *Brain* 77:588-609, 1954.
2. Bonney G: Prognosis in traction lesions of the brachial plexus, *J Bone Joint Surg* 41B:4, 1959.

2a. Butler D: *Mobilisation of the nervous system*, Melbourne, 1991, Churchill Livingstone.

3. Comtet JJ, Sedel L, Fredenucci JF, Herzberg G: Duchenne-Erb palsy: experience with direct surgery, *Clin Orthop Rel Res* (237):17-23, Dec 1988.
4. Eng GD, Koch B, Smokvina MD: Brachial plexus palsy in neonates and children, *Arch Phys Med Rehabil* 59:458, 1978.

5. Frampton YM: Therapist's management of brachial plexus injuries. In Hunter JM, Schneider LH, Mackin EJ, Callahan AD, editors: *Rehabilitation of the hand: surgery and therapy*, ed 3, St. Louis, 1990, Mosby.
6. Goddard NJ, Fixsen JA: Rotation osteotomy of the humerus for birth injuries of the brachial plexus, *J Bone Joint Surg* 66B:257-259, 1984.
7. Gorden M, Rich F, Deutschberger J, et al: The immediate and long term outcome of obstetric birth trauma. 1. Brachial plexus paralysis, *Am J Gynecol* 117:5-56, 1973.
8. Griffen PP: *Orthopedics in the newborn: neonatology, pathophysiology and management of the newborn*, ed 2, edited by GB Avery, Philadelphia, 1981, Lippincott.
8a. Heilman KM, Rothi LJG: Apraxia. In Heilman KM, Valenstein E, editors: *Clinical neuropsychology*, ed 2, Oxford, 1985, Oxford University Press.
9. Jackson ST, Hoffer MM, Parrish N: Brachial plexus palsy in the newborn, *J Bone Joint Surg* 70A(8):1217-1220, 1988.
10. Johnson EW, Alexander MA, Koenig WE: Infantile Erb's palsy (Smellie's palsy), *Arch Phys Med Rehabil* 58:175, 1977.
11. Kahn J: *Principles and practice of electrotherapy*, ed 2, New York, 1991, Churchill Livingstone.
12. Leffert RD: Rehabilitation of the patient with an injury to the brachial plexus. In Hunter JM, Schneider LH, Mackin EJ, Callahan AD, editors: *Rehabilitation of the hand: surgery and therapy*, ed 3, St. Louis, 1990, Mosby.
13. Liberson WT, Terzis JK: Some novel techniques of clinical electrophysiology applied to the management of brachial plexus palsy, *Electromyogr Clin Neurophysiol* 27:371, 1987.
13a. Leipmann H: *Drei Aufsätze aus dem Apraxiegibiet*, Berlin, 1908, Karger.
14. McFarland LV, Raskin M, Daling JR, Benedetti TJ: Erb/Duchenne's palsy: a consequence of fetal macrosomia and method of delivery, *Obstet Gyneco* 68(6): 784-788, 1986.
15. Moore KL: *Clinically oriented anatomy*, ed 2, Baltimore, 1985, Williams & Wilkins.
16. Netter FH: *The CIBA collection of medical illustrations*, vol 1: *Nervous system*, Part 2, Summit, N.J., 1986, CIBA-Geigy Corp.
17. *Phys Ther Forum* 1x(12):1, 1990.
18. Rockwood CA, Matsen FA, editors: *The shoulder*, vol 2, Philadelphia, 1990, Saunders.
19. Rose FC, editor: *Paediatric neurology*, Oxford, 1979, Blackwell Scientific Publishers.
20. Semmer CJ, Hunter JG: *Early occupation therapy intervention: neonates to three years*, Gaithersburg, Md., 1990, Aspen Publications.
21. Sever JW: Obstetric paralysis: a report of 470 cases, *Am J Dis Child* 12:541-578, 1916.
22. Shepherd RB, Campbell SK: Brachial plexus injury. In Campbell, SK, editor: *Pediatric neurologic physical therapy*, ed 2, New York, 1991, Churchill Livingstone.
23. Sjöberg I, Erichs K, Bjerre I: Cause and effect of obstetric (neonatal) brachial plexus palsy, *Acta Paediatr Scand* 77:357, 1988.
24. Wells PE, Frampton VM, Bawsher D: *Pain management in physical therapy*, vol 1, East Norwalk, Conn., 1988, Appleton & Lange.

Recommended reading

Frampton YM: Therapist's management of brachial plexus injuries. In Hunter JM, Schneider LH, Mackin EJ, Callahan AD, editors: *Rehabilitation of the hand: surgery and therapy*, ed 3, St. Louis, 1990, Mosby.

Leffert RD: Rehabilitation of the patient with an injury to the brachial plexus. In Hunter JM, Schneider LH, Mackin EJ, Callahan AD, editors: *Rehabilitation of the hand: surgery and therapy*, ed 3, St. Louis, 1990, Mosby.

Shepherd RB: Brachial plexus injury. In Campbell SK, editor: *Clinics in physical therapy: Pediatric neurologic physical therapy*, ed 2, New York, 1991, Churchill Livingstone.

Semmer CJ, Hunter JG: *Early occupation therapy intervention: neonates to three years*, Gaithersburg, Md., 1990, Aspen Publications, p 86.

20

Exquisite Pinpoint Muscle Pain and Taut Bands within Muscle Substance and Remote Referral to a Locale within the Same Myotome

A 38-year-old fireman fell through the roof of a burning building and sustained a superficial laceration of the right dorsal wrist and right dorsoproximal forearm. Several weeks later he was referred for physical therapy because of persistent paresthesia along the ulnar aspect of the right hand. He has been unable to return to work.

PALPATION Elicited stabbing wrist pains on ulnar or radial deviation as well as dorsal numbness in digits four and five of his right hand.

MOTION AND STRENGTH ARE DECREASED AS SHOWN:

	Left	Right
Wrist flexion:	85°	75°
Wrist extension:	62°	30°
Radial deviation:	20°	20°
Ulnar deviation:	45°	15°
Grip strength:	31 kg	6 kg
Lateral pinch:	5.8 kg	4 kg
Pulp pinch:	6.2 kg	5 kg

SENSATION There is decreased sensation to touch and pinprick along the ulnar distribution of the hand.

SPECIAL TESTS The patient tested negative for all clinical neurologic and electrodiagnostic testing.

1. **What is myofascial pain syndrome (MFP)?**
2. **What historical overview is necessary to an understanding of the development of MFP?**
3. **What is a trigger point?**
4. **What triggers a muscle to develop an active trigger point?**
5. **Is there a relationship between loss of range of motion and the presence of trigger points?**
6. **What is the cause of trigger points?**

7. **What is the relationship between the trigger point and the referred pain?**
8. **How are trigger points quantitatively measured?**
9. **What steps are involved in an MFP evaluation?**
10. **What palpation technique is employed when one is searching a length of muscle for trigger points?**
11. **What is the rationale for the referral of pain several segmental levels caudad or cephalad?**
12. **With MFP, is the precipitating injury chronic or acute?**
13. **What therapeutic intervention is appropriate in the treatment of MFP?**
14. **What is the spray and stretch treatment?**
15. **What is injection treatment, and is there a less invasive alternative in the treatment of MFP?**
16. **What forms of electrotherapy are appropriate in the treatment of MFP?**
17. **What connective-tissue techniques are appropriate in the treatment of MFP?**
18. **What is the ischemic-pressure technique in the treatment of MFP?**
19. **What cold modalities may be used in the treatment of MFP?**
20. **What role does static splinting play in the treatment of MFP?**
21. **What exercises are helpful in the treatment of MFP?**
22. **Describe a hypothetical treatment sequence for the injured fireman's hand.**

1. What is myofascial pain syndrome (MFP)?

Myofascial pain (MFP) is defined as a local irritation mainly in muscle and possibly fascia, tendon, or ligament that exhibits local tenderness, specific pain patterns, and autonomic symptoms that are easily reproducible and specific to that tissue. Myofascial pain is essentially a single-muscle syndrome that may combine to form single myotome or dermatome patterns of involvement. Detection and management of this condition follow established parameters.Terms such as *trigger point, referred pain,* and *locus of pain* are concepts characteristic of MFP symptoms.

2. What historical overview is necessary to an understanding of the development of MFP?

Myofascial pain is not a new concept but is rather an evolving clarification that slowly emerged after a legacy of confusion regarding this disorder.

A confusing series of names has alternately been used in describing MFP and include muscular rheumatism, nonarticular rheumatism, myalgia spots, idiopathic myalgia, fibrositis, rheumatic myalgia, and rheumatic myopathy. The nomenclature describing myofascial pain is understood in the historical context of the evolution of this condition. In the early twentieth century the term *muscular rheumatism* was commonly employed to describe generalized musculoskeletal pain of unknown cause. With time, this appellation was criticized as serving as a diagnostic scrap box for painful ailments that could not be otherwise classified. In response, Sir William Gowers, the English neurologist, in 1904 renamed this condition *fibrositis* and thus implied a proposed cause of inflammation of fibrous or connective tissue.[9]

Half a century and many scientific books and papers later, Janet Travell, M.D., began in 1952 to promote the terminology *myofascial pain* and *myofascial syndrome.* Travell was the first female physician for the White House, serving as President Kennedy's personal physician and friend. She treated Kennedy's trigger points in his back and prescribed his famous rocking chair as part of his treatment program.[24]

Notwithstanding, MFP continued to be a controversial topic and was considered to be a wastebasket term in need of redefinition. It was not until the 1986 Symposium on Fibrositis/Fibromyalgia debate that MFP came into its own with the understanding and clarification of clinical presentation and management.

3. What is a trigger point?

Central to an understanding of MFP is the idea of the trigger point. *Trigger points* are described as small hypersensitive areas in muscle, ligament, or fascia, which, when stimulated, give rise to referred pain.[25] This is a consistent feature of the trigger point. Trigger points are classified as either *latent* or *active.*

Latent trigger points evoke pain and tenderness in those same locales as active trigger points do, and they can be made to refer pain remotely by palpation. Additionally, latent trigger points may be present in individuals without a diagnosis of MFP and are differentiated from active trigger points by the following circumstance: When the individual is asked whether he or she has ever felt this pain at any time other than palpation of the given area, the answer is no; in other words, the latent trigger point is only painful when provoked.[17] Without perpetuating factors, an active trigger point tends to revert to and persist as a latent trigger point.[21]

An acute strain caused by sudden overload of muscle can produce an active trigger point that causes referred pain. Chronic repetitive strain of a muscle may also yield an active trigger point. If the demands of the muscle are reduced, the referred pain may spontaneously subside within several days or weeks. However, in the event that the provoking stimulus continues incessantly, an acute MFP syndrome may persist or even become chronic. With time, MFP may even propagate to other muscles within the same or nearby myotomes as secondary and satellite trigger points.[21]

Interestingly, studies have shown that up to 71% of trigger points have been found to have identical locations with acupuncture points.[16] This, however, could be coincidental, since there are some 1000 acupuncture points identified in the literature on that topic.[22]

4. What triggers a muscle to develop an active trigger point?

A variety of situations can incite a muscle to develop a trigger point. These include direct trauma, stress, overuse, fatigue, posture, stressful sleeping, and work postures. Two common findings characteristic of trigger points are (1) the local twitch response elicited by snapping palpation of the trigger point and (2) reproduction of the patient's pain by sustained pressure applied to that area.

5. Is there a relationship between loss of range of motion and the presence of trigger points?

The shoulder musculature frequently contains an abundance of trigger points, though the diagnosis is often mistaken as a bursitis or tendinitis. Typically, when the patient fails to respond to conventional treatment, he or she is told to simply "live with it." However, on closer examination the clinician will often discover a limitation of joint motion produced by adaptive or reflexive shortening of the structure containing the trigger point that crosses that joint.[2,18,23] Similarly the involved muscle may produce pain when stretched. For example, if the trigger point is found to be located in the substance of the infraspinatus muscle, the resultant limitation of motion will be at the glenohumeral joint in external rotation and horizontal abduction.[17]

6. What is the cause of trigger points?

Various attempts to explain the existence of trigger points in physiologic, anatomic, or neurophysiologic terms have proved frustrating. Proposed causes include inflammatory, anatomic, ischemic, neurophysiologic; altered autonomic nervous system; and connective tissue irritation. Interestingly, when viewed under the electron microscope, trigger points have a moth-eaten ragged appearance similar to that of overused muscle.[2]

Trigger points develop most commonly in antigravity muscles such as trapezius, the erector spinae, or gastrocnemius because of the unrelenting burden of contraction these muscles experience in the erect posture. For example, the trapezius, along with other muscles, bears the task of supporting the head in normal posture. This burden possibly taxes the ability of muscles to disburse concentrations of lactic acid,

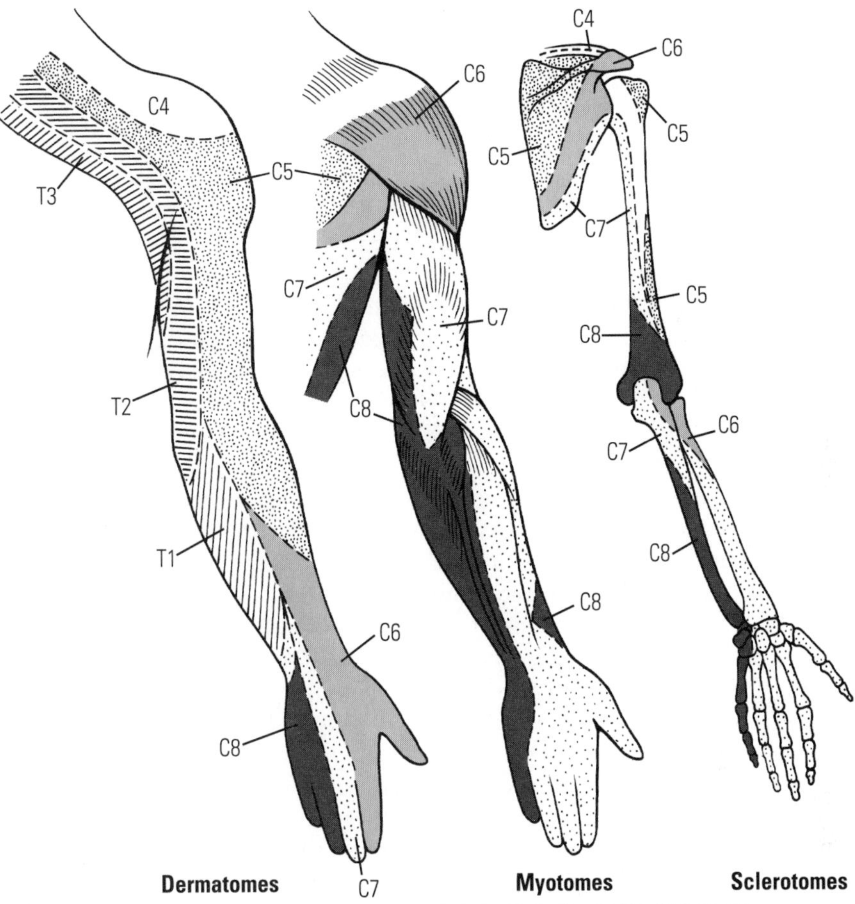

Fig. 20-1 Dermatomes, myotomes, and sclerotomes of the upper extremity.

which aggregates at specific areas known as trigger points. Having developed trigger points, a muscle is more likely to become fatigued. Hence a vicious cycle is established in which continued contraction sustains and perhaps fortifies the cycle.

7. What is the relationship between the trigger point and the referred pain?

Trigger points often *refer* pain remotely but consistently to specific areas, such as the interosseous muscles of the hand. So consistent are these remote referrals of pain that mappings demonstrate a relationship that appears remarkably consistent with dermatome or myotome patterns[10] (Fig. 20-1).

Thus the *locus of pain* refers to the origin of pain resulting in remote and often distal, referral sites. This relationship between the trigger point and the reference area of pain emphasizes the following emergent principle of management: patients with MFP must be treated according to the locus of their pain and not necessarily the presentation site.

8. How are trigger points quantitatively measured?

The tissue compliance meter (TCM) is a hand-held instrument that, unlike other devices that measure the presence of trigger points, offers the advantage of being objective, since measurements are not dependent on a patient's reaction or cooperation. This device offers an immediate and simple reading of the depth of penetration of a rubber disk at a known pressure, the relation of which expresses tissue compliance. The TCM objectively documents compliance for trigger points, taut bands, scar tissue, fibrositic nodules, edema, and spasm and thus provides an early objective indication of either healing or resolution in the soft-tissue disorder.

The universal clinical dynamometer is a pocket-sized, hand-held device that is used in quantitative measurement of muscle strength. Thermography documents trigger points that appear as areas that are discoid. Thermography also measures the presence of muscle spasm.[6]

9. What steps are involved in an MFP evaluation?

Once all conventional pathologic conditions have been ruled out, the clinician explores the possibility of the myofascial component as the source of pain. MFP is a diagnosis of exclusion, and laboratory and imaging studies are helpful only to rule out other diseases. The MFP evaluation follows a sequence of gathering information regarding the patient's subjective complaints as well as objective measurements taken before one searches for the source of pain. Diagnosis is accomplished when one takes a history and a physical examination.

The patient's history may reveal a direct or indirect trauma precipitating the pain. The chief complaint may be local, referred, or both, and may be colored in by the patient on a body chart. The diagram is then reviewed with the patient, who goes over additional factors such as the date on onset, nature of the pain (that is, dull, sharp, or a deep ache), and precipitating factors. The patient may initially have a limitation in the range of motion, experience autonomic changes, and frequently complain of weakness and stiffness. Pain intensity is preferably recorded on an analog pain scale. If the patient complains of numbness, as many do, then Semmes-Weinstein monofilaments and a vibrometer may be used.[17]

The "hands-on" portion of the evaluation commences with the clinician seeking a myofascial component in the form of positively identified trigger points that reproduce the patient's pain. Two findings that greatly help to make the diagnosis are the presence of exquisite spot tenderness at the trigger point and a palpable band of taut muscle fibers running through the trigger point. Once the source of pain is discovered, it is confirmed by pain on active contraction or passive stretching of the structure. It is important to note that palpation of the entire length of the identified muscle ought to be performed by the therapist. In the event that no source is found, an investigation of the muscles innervated by, at the very least, one spinal segment above or below should commence. A successful MFP evaluation cannot be limited to examining the muscles innervated by the same level of the pain presentation.

Remotely referred pain is most often perceived distally to the source of pain and is mapped out carefully with the therapist screening for a pattern following a dermatomal or myotomal distribution. However, Travell and Simons identified the following muscles in the upper quadrant that typically refer pain proximally: sternocleidomastoid, biceps brachii, the long head of triceps, supinator, brachioradialis, and adductor pollicis. Palpation continues so as to identify any pain elicited in muscles innervated by the same level of dermatome or myotome of the pain presentation.[17]

10. What palpation technique is employed when one is searching a length of muscle for trigger points?

Palpation of muscle for the presence of trigger points is similar to the palpation for tendinitis. The purpose of evaluation is twofold: (1) reproduction of pain and (2) tissue turgor.

The examiner applies firm pressure with the pulp of the thumb across the entire span of the muscle, from origin to insertion. The patient is asked to inform the therapist if he or she feels pain and, if so, whether the pain is his or her pain. At times the patient may literally jump and exclaim, "That is my pain," in what is known as a *positive jump sign.*[7]

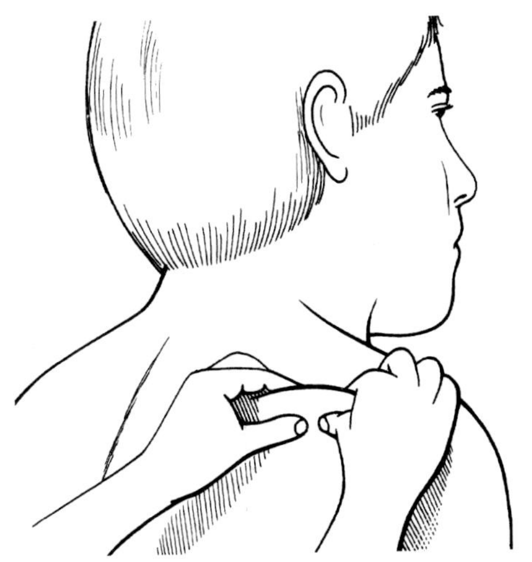

Fig. 20-2 Skin rolling is a connective tissue technique used for evaluation and treatment.

Tissue turgor evaluation may be accomplished by the following two methods of palpation: (1) *Skin rolling* (Fig. 20-2) involves lifting the skin off the muscles, opposing the index finger and thumb, and then rolling the skin in all directions for the purpose of eliciting pain over the trigger point. (2) *Light palpation* is accomplished by use of the index finger pulp with the middle finger lying atop the index fingernail. This latter technique is employed to sense the depth of the trigger point as well as to detect for palpable bands, that is, rope-like structures lying parallel with the muscle fibers.[17] These palpable bands may undergo a local twitch response when the trigger point is stimulated with a snapping palpation.[11,21]

11. What is the rationale for the referral of pain several segmental levels caudad or cephalad?

The neuroanatomic pathway that can be traced from the trigger point to the spinal cord provides a possible rationale for referred pain several segments caudad or cephalad to the actual level of the culprit muscle. When noxious stimuli from trigger points are strong enough, action potentials will propagate along the axon to synapse in the spinal cord. The fibers bifurcate, with most remaining in the same spinal level but some spreading cephalocaudad in the lateral section of dorsal white matter, including Lissauer's tract. A spread of only two or three segments is believed to occur in man.[13]

12. With MFP, is the precipitating injury chronic or acute?

The precipitating injury inciting the onset of MFP may be either acute or chronic in nature,[21] and the patient's presentation may be quite diverse. This malady may occur in patients as diverse as a dental hygienist referred for treatment of a wrist tendinitis, to a middle aged man referred with a diagnosis of hand arthritis and who sustained a hyperextension wrist injury in an automobile accident 3 months earlier, or to a 24-year-old individual referred with a diagnosis of reflex sympathetic dystrophy after a closed forearm crush involving no fractures some 2½ years previously.

13. What therapeutic intervention is appropriate in the treatment of MFP?

Myofascial pain patients offer an exciting challenge to the clinician. The key to successfully treating the patient with MFP is to realize that simply treating the painful area will not correct the patient's condition.

Physical therapy must be directed to the locus of the patient's pain. It is recommended that the therapist refer to dermatome and myotome charts and to *Travell's Trigger Point Manual.* One then solves the emerging clinical puzzle one piece at a time by palpating those muscles that have the potential for referring pain, given the clinical presentation. Therapy may be directed at more than one source when the evaluation includes all those muscles innervated by the same level as the myotome and dermatome of the pain presentation or several spinal levels above or below that level.

Treatments directed at the loci of pain include spray and stretch, phonophoresis and iontophoresis, heat modalities, electrotherapy, ultrasound, connective tissue technique, ischemic pressure technique, splinting, and exercise. Medical management may also include injection and dry needling. Selection of treatment is based on tissue response to given treatment (such as changes in trigger point irritability). If the treatment does not relieve the patient's pain, then reidentification of the pain locus or a change in the treatment technique is necessary. Treatment frequency is dependent on the patient's response, since resolution of the trigger point or movement of referred pain proximally is proof of a successful treatment.

Confirmation of treatment success is accomplished by the patient completing another body chart and the therapist comparing initial findings to subsequent findings. More conventional methods include quantitative passive and active range of motion exercises as well as muscle strength grading.

Treatment in the chronic case of MFP must not be directed only toward alleviating the trigger point irritability but also toward strengthening the involved muscles so that joint balance and posture may be reestablished. Without these important factors being addressed, trigger point activation may recur.

14. What is the spray and stretch treatment?

Spray and stretch refers to the use of vapor coolant spray, typically Fluori-Methane, over the muscle's referred zone of pain. The spray is administered at least 18 inches away from the skin surface parallel to the involved muscle fibers (Fig. 20-3). The vapor coolant provides a barrage of cutaneous impulses over the irritated muscle and the referred zone that reflexively inhibits the muscle, thus permitting the therapist to stretch the muscle to its normal length.[17] The barrage of skin impulses block the pain impulses from the trigger point[8,25] within the muscle that would prevent stretching under normal circumstances. This is followed by application of a hot pack for 5 to 10 minutes and then active exercises.[17]

15. What is injection treatment, and is there a less invasive alternative in the treatment of MFP?

Trigger point injection with either procaine, xylocaine, or corticosteroid is a common treatment for trigger point pain in MFP. This treatment has proved to be effective in both acute and chronic cases of MFP.

Phonophoresis or *iontophoresis* may be used in the delivery of corticosteroids and analgesics in lieu of injection,[1,10,11] and are more comfortable for the patient. After iontophoresis, the trigger point may be massaged or receive heat to facilitate disbursement of the medication. Phonophoresis treatment interfaces well with ischemic pressure technique and interferential current.[17]

16. What forms of electrotherapy are appropriate in the treatment of MFP?

Several forms of *electrotherapy* have been advocated in the treatment of MFP and include high volt electrical stimulation, transcutaneous electrical stimulation (TENS), interferential current, and electroacupuncture.[12,14-16,19,20] Interferential current is applied by use of both channels so that channel crossing occurs at the trigger point; the mode may be *fixed or sweep.* With TENS, electrodes are sized appropriately when one is treating the trigger points (TrPs) of the small hand muscles. Use of a probe is also helpful in such cases. TENS electrodes ought to bracket the TrP so that stretching of the involved muscle may occur during treatment without irritating the TrP.[17]

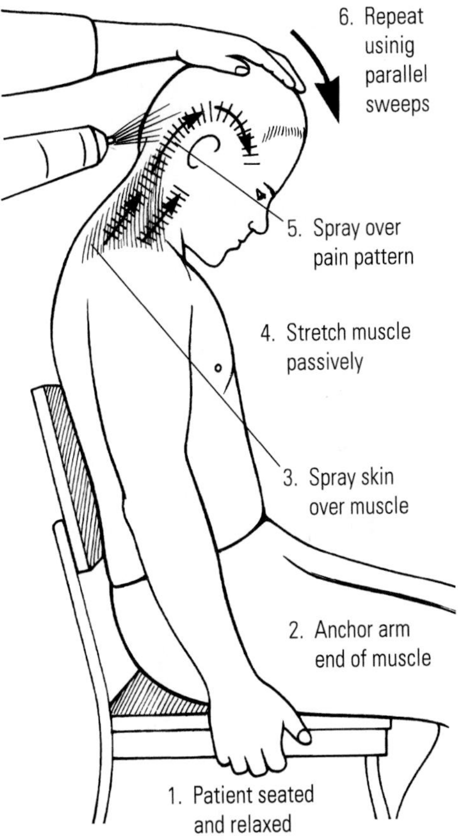
6. Repeat
usinig
parallel
sweeps
5. Spray over
pain pattern
4. Stretch muscle
passively
3. Spray skin
over muscle
2. Anchor arm
end of muscle
1. Patient seated
and relaxed

Fig. 20-3 Application scheme of use of vapor coolant spray followed by stretch of involved muscle. (Redrawn from Hunter JM, Schneider LH, Mackin EJ, Callahan AD, editors: *Rehabilitation of the hand: surgery and therapy,* ed 3, St. Louis, 1990, Mosby.)

17. What connective-tissue techniques are appropriate in the treatment of MFP?

Deep transverse friction technique introduced by Cyriax involves constant application of heavy pressure across the trigger point for the purpose of breaking up adhesions[4,5] (Fig. 20-4).

Skin rolling is a painful technique that involves release of fascia from underlying muscle or overlying skin. Employed by the therapist both during the evaluation (see Fig. 20-2) as well as during treatment, this technique is applied during the latter for approximately 5 or 10 minutes in chronic cases of MFP. Reassessment with palpation follows and identifies those trigger points that are still irritable, which may be treated with ultrasound or interferential current.

Knuckling (Fig. 20-5) is a soft-tissue stretching technique in which the therapist applies stress parallel to muscle fiber. This technique is appropriate with chronic cases where there is adaptive shortening of soft tissue, but it should not be used with the acute patient. During stretching, the therapist uses his or her knuckles to stress, hence stretch, the connective tissue enveloping the muscle fibers.[17]

18. What is the ischemic-pressure technique in the treatment of MFP?

Travell described an *ischemic-pressure technique* in which graded pressure over the trigger point is applied for up to 60 seconds to provide reflex inhibition of the trigger point.[25] The key to this technique is a

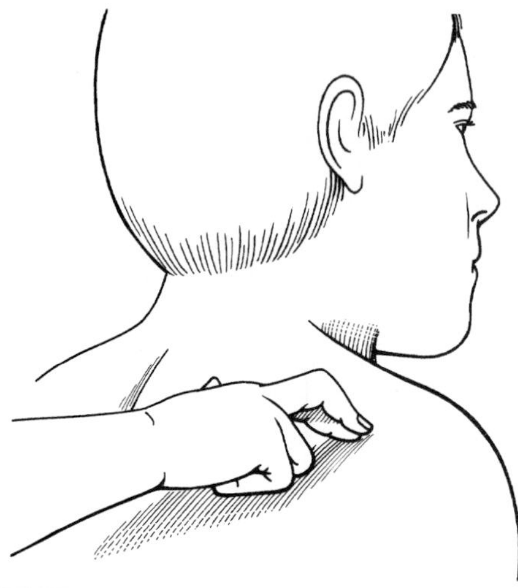

Fig. 20-4 Disruption of trigger point irritation by way of friction massage technique.

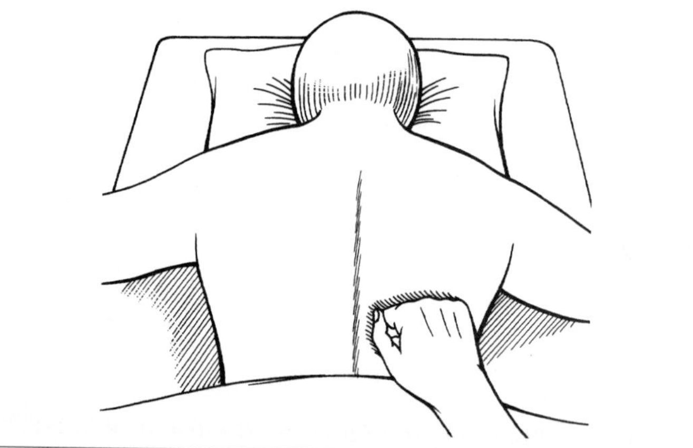

Fig. 20-5 Knuckling is performed parallel to the fibers of the restricted muscle.

gentle, graded pressure (Fig. 20-6). When pressure is applied, the patient will report a graded decrease and resolution of his or her pain during the 60-second interval. An increase of pressure is not applied until the patient feels a decrease in pain. This treatment may be used before TENS or ultrasound treatment.[17]

19. What cold modalities may be used in the treatment of MFP?

Cold modalities aside from the use of vapor coolant spray may aggravate the condition of MFP. The exception to this rule is the use of quick icing for pain relief and the maintenance of hard-won gains in the tissue length in the patient with the chronic disorder. Because these patients require vigorous soft-tissue techniques and multiple treatments, which can yield local erythema and swelling, the application of a plastic bag of slush ice and alcohol may be applied for 5 minutes with a paper towel interposed between the

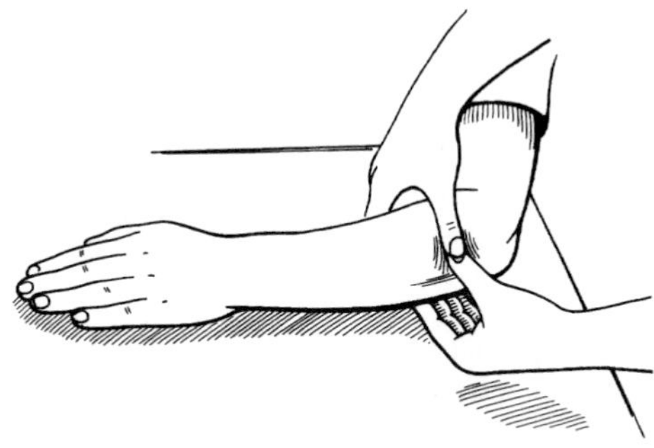

Fig. 20-6 Ischemic pressure technique involves slow and constant application of pressure for the disruption of trigger point irritation.

skin and the bag. Slush may be formed by the mixing of one part of alcohol with three parts of water. Longer application involves chilling to excess, which is a causative factor in MFP.[17]

20. What role does static splinting play in the treatment of MFP?

Splinting use is appropriate during the early stage of treatment when the movement of involved muscles reactivate the trigger point or points before that muscle regains full length and strength. Most commonly, the thumb (adductor pollicis muscle trigger point) and the wrist (wrist flexor and extensor muscle trigger points) are splinted until the trigger point is completely resolved. As the patient begins strengthening, the patient is gradually weaned from usage of the splint.

21. What exercises are helpful in the treatment of MFP?

In many cases the patient's posture at work or leisure provoked the onset of MFP. For example, the glenohumeral joint of the ipsilateral upper extremity is often positioned in a protracted posture. It is important to identify any such alternations in muscle imbalance and restore soft-tissue imbalance about joints by stretching contracted areas and strengthening overstretched muscle. Addressing muscular imbalances is imperative to the prevention of reactivation of trigger points.[17]

22. Describe a hypothetical treatment sequence for the injured fireman's hand.

The initial treatment was addressed toward scar remodeling and not MFP techniques because it was the scar adherence that was provoking the trigger points. Heat, scar massage, and wrist curls were performed while TENS bracketed the scar. The TENS served to dampen the effects of the trigger points during conventional treatment.

During the second visit the patient was able to tolerate an increase of the weight during wrist curls, using approximately 1 kg because of a significant decrease in the pain. An Otoform pad (Alimed, Deedham, Mass.) was fabricated for scar remodeling. Treatment visits 3 and 4 focused on ultrasound and friction massage to both trigger points, followed by ice.

On the sixth visit, TENS bracketed the trigger points while low-resistance work simulation was begun. For the subsequent eighth session, our patient continued to undergo an MFP regimen of friction massage, TENS, and ice while the magnitude of his work simulation was increased. By the twelfth session his trigger points had resolved and work hardening commenced for an additional six sessions. At the end of the work-hardening sequence he was discharged and returned to work full time.

References

1. Antich T: Phonophoresis: the principles of the ultrasonic driving force and efficacy in treatment of common orthopaedic diagnoses, *J Orthop Sports Phys Ther* 4:99, 1982.
2. Bengtsson A, Hendriksson KG, Larsson J: Muscle biopsy in primary fibromyalgia: light microscope and histochemical findings, *Scand J Rheumatol* 15:1, 1986.
3. Bonica J: Management of myofascial pain syndromes in general practice, *JAMA* 164:732, 1957.
4. Chamberlain GJ: Cyriax's friction massage: a review, *J Orthop Sports Phys Ther* 4:16, 1982.
5. Cyriax J: *Textbook of orthopaedic medicine: diagnosis of soft tissue lesions*, vol 1, ed 6, Baltimore, 1975, Williams & Wilkins.
6. Fischer AA: Documentation of myofascial trigger points, *Arch Phys Med Rehabil* 69: 286-291, 1988.
7. Good M: Objective diagnosis and curability of non-articular rheumatism, *Br J Phys Med* 14:1, 1951.
8. Gordon EE, Hass A: A surface analgesic in treatment of musculoskeletal affections, *Ind Med Surg* 28:217, 1959.
9. Gowers W: Lumbago: its lessons and analogies, *Br J Phys Med* 1:117, 1904.
10. Harris P: Iontophoresis: clinical research in musculoskeletal inflammatory conditions, *J Orthop Sports Phys Ther* 4: 109, 1982.
11. Kraft G, Johnson E, Laban M: The fibrositis syndrome, *Arch Phys Med Rehabil* 49:155, 1968.
12. Kraus H: Trigger points and acupuncture, *Acupunct Electrother Res* 2:323, 1977.
13. Lamotte C: Distribution of the tract of Lissauer and the dorsal root fibers in the primate spinal cork, *J Comp Neur* 172:529, 1977.
14. Melzack R: Prolonged relief of pain by brief, intense transcutaneous somatic stimulation, *Pain* 1:357, 1975.
15. Melzack R: Myofascial trigger points: relation to acupuncture and mechanisms of pain, *Arch Phys Med Rehabil* 62:114, 1981.
16. Melzack R, Stillwell K, Fox E: Trigger points and acupuncture points for pain: correlations and implications, *Pain* 3:3, 1977.
17. Moran CA, Saunders SR, Tribuzi SM: Myofascial pain in the upper extremity. In Hunter JM, Schneider LH, Mackin EJ, Callahan AD, editors: *Rehabilitation of the hand: surgery and therapy*, ed 3, St. Louis, 1990, Mosby.
18. Nielson AJ: Case study: myofascial pain of the posterior shoulder relieved by spray and stretch, *J Orthop Sports Phys Ther* 3:21, 1981.
19. Omura Y: Electro-acupuncture: its electrophysiological basis and criteria of effectiveness and safety, part 1, *Acupunct Electrother Res* 1:157, 1975.
20. Procacce P, Zoppi M, Maresca M: Transcutaneous electrical stimulation in low back pain: a critical evaluation, *Acupunct Electrother Res* 7:1, 1982.
21. Simons DG: Myofascial pain syndromes: Where are we? Where are we going? *Arch Phys Med Rehabil* 69:208, 1988.
22. Smith G, Covino B: *Acute pain*, Stoneham, Mass., 1985, Butterworth Publs.
23. Travell J, Rinzler SH: The myofascial genesis of pain, *Postgrad Med* 11:425, 1952.
24. Travell J: *Office hours day and night*, New York, 1968, World Publishing Co.
25. Travell J, Simons DG: *Myofascial pain and dysfunction of the trigger point manual*, Baltimore, 1983, Williams & Wilkins.

Recommended reading

Moran CA, Saunders SR, Tribuzi SM: Myofascial pain in the upper extremity. In Hunter JM, Schneider LH, Mackin EJ, Callahan AD, editors: *Rehabilitation of the hand: surgery and therapy*, ed 3, St. Louis, 1990, Mosby.

Nielson AJ: Case study: myofascial pain of the posterior shoulder relieved by spray and stretch, *J Orthop Sports Phys Ther* 3:21, 1981.

Simons DG: Myofascial pain syndromes: Where are we? Where are we going? *Arch Phys Med Rehabil*, 69:208, 1988.

Travell J, Simons DG: *Myofascial pain and dysfunction of the trigger point manual*, Baltimore, 1983, Williams & Wilkins.

Wolfe F: Fibrositis, fibromyalgia, and musculoskeletal disease: The current status of the fibrositis syndrome. *Archives of Phys Med Rehabil*, 69:527-531, 1988.

21

Chronic and Generalized Aches, Pains, Stiffness at Three Anatomic Sites and Multiple Tender Points as Well as Insomnia and Headache of at Least 3 Months in Duration

A 45-year-old female assistant bank manager presents a prescription from her rheumatologist that reads: "Primary fibromyalgia syndrome—therapy as needed." The patient offers her hand and offers you a limp handshake. It is the winter season.

OBSERVATION The patient is a well-dressed, groomed, and slightly graying individual who conveys the impression of seriousness. She holds herself in a ramrod straight, military type of posture.

SUBJECTIVE The patient complains of a history of diffuse aching pain in her shoulders, hips, and low back lasting for 2 years. Recently, symptoms have become increasingly severe in the early morning and late afternoon. She reports sensitivity to bright lights and loud noises and confided that she was concerned about what she viewed as decreased work productivity, since the onset of her condition. She often wakes up after a night's sleep feeling unrefreshed and often experiences ill-defined headaches in the morning hours. She admits to not having taken a vacation for the past 4 years or taking time out to exercise or relax. She further complains of occasional vague numbness in her fingers, which she could not relate to any particular position or activity. As of late she finds that she needs to urinate quite frequently and has been experiencing a loose bowel more often as well. She does not drink, smoke, or bite her nails.

PALPATION The patient jumps and cries out during palpation over the upper trapezius and low back areas. There is no tenderness in any of her joints.

RANGE OF MOTION Grossly within functional limits.

STRENGTH Grossly within normal limits relative to her age.

FLEXIBILITY Gross tightness is observed in the upper back and shoulders as well as in the lower extremities (manifesting as tight hamstrings, quadriceps, and triceps surae muscle groups).

SENSATION Normal to light touch and pinprick in both upper extremities.

1. **What is primary fibromyalgia syndrome (PFS)?**
2. **What is the clinical presentation of PFS?**
3. **What is the cause of PFS?**
4. **What are the most common sites of tenderness?**
5. **What is the differential diagnosis of fibromyalgia?**
6. **What is the difference between myofascial pain and fibromyalgia (fibrositis)?**
7. **What therapeutic intervention is appropriate for PFS?**

1. What is primary fibromyalgia syndrome (PFS)?

Fibromyalgia is a nonarticular rheumatic disorder that affects approximately 6 million Americans.[5] Of the many forms of nonarticular rheumatic disorders, fibromyalgia is specific to the fibrous white connective tissue[1] components of muscle, tendons, ligaments, and other "white" connective tissue in the large muscles of the shoulders, back, and hips; hence, an appropriate synonym for fibromyalgia is *muscular rheumatism*.[1,3] Women constitute 70% to 90% of all afflicted patients, and the most common age of diagnosis is between 35 and 55 years;[2,8,10] this condition, however, does occur among juveniles and the elderly.[9] Fibromyalgia may be the same disorder as chronic fatigue syndrome, though the etiologic role the Epstein-Barr virus has not been established with either disorder.[5] The term "fibrositis" has historically been associated with fibromyalgia but is actually a misnomer, since no inflammation is present with PFS. Moreover, fibrositis has been also used to describe myofascial pain, and so, because fibrositis means different things to different people, it has been appropriately suggested that this term be abandoned.[1,9]

2. What is the clinical presentation of PFS?

The clinical presentation of PFS includes pain that is widely[4] and even vaguely distributed, an amplified sensation (such as hypersensitivity of pain, weather, cold, humidity,[9] bright lights, and loud noises; stiffness; generalized fatigue or tiredness and exhaustion; and disturbed or nonrestorative sleep). Patients often wake up unrefreshed and more exhausted than the night before with chronic and diffuse headaches, irritable bowel, subjective swelling or numbness, urinary frequency caused by an enhanced perception of bladder fullness,[4] and paresthesia such as numbness that is ill defined over variable areas, implying neurologic disease; however, confirmation of objective neurologic findings in the latter complaint are absent.[5]

Some patients have significant anxiety and stress,[9] are typically hard driving, and are demanding both of themselves and of others. Patients may be emotionally trying but are often very effective at work because of their dedication. Patients may dislike alcohol, drugs, or other emotional or psychologic crutches.[4]

During the examination patients with PFS may give the impression that they are not making a full effort. During palpation, tenderness is not simply reported but may be demonstrated by dramatic twisting leaps. Grip strength (which may be evaluated by shaking the patient's hands) is reduced and poorly sustained. The evaluative encounter is often exhausting for the examiner and the patient and is indicative of the interactive stresses generated between such patients and others.[4]

3. What is the cause of PFS?

The cause of PFS as a system complex is unknown because there is no specific histologic abnormality suggestive of cellular inflammation.[1] Psychologic factors are present in one fourth of all patients. Interestingly the EEG wave patterns during non-rapid eye movement sleep in patients with fibromyalgia are quite similar to non-REM wave patterns of healthy individuals during delta-wave sleep deprivation.[2]

Primary fibromyalgia syndrome may be induced or intensified by physical or mental stress, poor sleep, trauma, or exposure to dampness and cold. A viral infection or toxemia from bacterial infection may also precipitate this syndrome in an otherwise predisposed host.[1] Symptoms may also be exacerbated by emotional stress or by the clinician who does not give proper credence to the patient's concerns and discharges the matter as being "all in your head."

An association between PFS and primary dysmenorrhea, as well as Raynaud's phenomenon, has been established.[9] There may be a constitutional predisposition to this condition.[9]

4. What are the most common sites of tenderness?

Tender points are largely unknown to patients and often not even central to their areas of pain.[4] Areas of point tenderness (Fig. 21-1) include:

- The upper scapular area, particularly the midpoint of the upper trapezius.
- The middle or lower part of the sternocleidomastoid muscle.

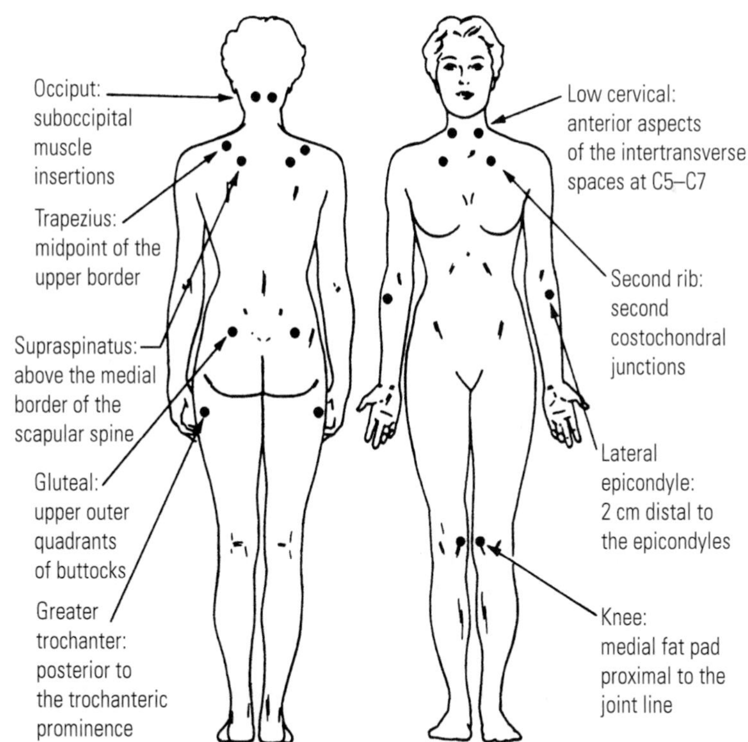

Fig. 21-1 Location of 14 typical sites of deep tenderness in fibromyalgia. (From the Bulletin on the rheumatic diseases, located in Rodan GP, Schumacher HR: *Primer on rheumatic diseases,* ed 8, Atlanta, 1983, The Arthritis Foundation.)

- The lateral portion of the pectoralis major muscle, or the second costochondral junction.
- The midsubstance of the supraspinatus muscle located in the suprascapular fossa.
- The middle to upper and outer quadrant of the buttock at the iliac crest.
- Just distal to the medial or lateral epicondyles of the elbow.
- The medial fat pad at the knee.
- Just posterior to the hip trochanters.[9]

5. What is the differential diagnosis of fibromyalgia?

Fibromyalgia is characterized by chronic generalized aches, pains, and stiffness involving at least three anatomic sites as well as multiple tender points at characteristic locations; persistence of these criteria for at least 3 months must occur, without any other underlying cause or disease to account for pain, before a diagnosis of PFS is confirmed.[5] Additionally, three of the 10 minor criteria must also be met, including variation of symptoms according to weather, physical activities, aggravation of symptoms by stress or anxiety, general fatigue, poor sleep, chronic headache, subjective swelling and numbness, and irritable bowel syndrome.[6]

Whereas PFS specifically refers to signs and symptoms not caused by any underlying disease,[9] secondary fibromyalgia may result from hypothyroidism, polymyalgia rheumatica,[9] systemic lupus erythematosus,[1] early onset of rheumatoid arthritis,[1] depression, anemia, and myopathy.

6. What is the difference between myofascial pain and fibromyalgia (fibrositis)?

Although there appears to be a blurred distinction between the somewhat similar sounding names of myofascial pain and primary fibromyalgia syndrome (PFS), it is erroneous to equate these two conditions. It is essential that practitioners recognize and understand the clear distinction between the two maladies. A lack of differentiation between these two conditions greatly influences the choice of management and thus makes an enormous difference to the patient.

The similarities of PFS and myofascial pain syndrome (MPS) include muscle pain, muscle tenderness on palpation, and the fact that both are very common maladies. However, with MPS, pain may be acute or chronic; there is a referred pain pattern specific to each involved muscle; nonmusculoskeletal symptoms are unusual; myofascial trigger points (TrPs) are found only in muscle, and radiate pain remotely, that is, beyond the site of palpation to a referred zone of pain, whereas the number of trigger points may be confined to one or more; muscles containing trigger points frequently contain taut bands; the twitch response of culprit muscle is present; the psychologic status of patient is usually not a factor; and poor sleep may result from the pain.[9]

On the other hand, the clinical presentation of PFS includes pain that is chronic; there is diffuse pain involving many muscles, ligaments, or bones; nonmusculoskeletal symptoms are common; fibromyalgic tender points (TePs) are found in muscle and other sites such as tendon insertions, fat pads, and bony prominences; TePs do not refer pain remotely on application of pressure; the presence of twitch response taut bands are unusual; TePs are usually more than four within some 14 specified sites; disturbed sleep is a factor in most cases; and psychologic factors are important in about 25% of patients.[9]

There is, however, some speculation as to whether myofascial pain and primary fibromyalgia syndrome are two separate disease entities or somewhat related pathologic conditions. This uncertainty is prompted by the clinical encounter of patients who occasionally present a confusing array of signs and symptoms from both conditions. One cannot help but wonder whether these two conditions are actually related along a range of a similar disease process seen from different points of view. Resolution of this question remains to be discovered.[7]

7. What therapeutic intervention is appropriate for PFS?

Since many patients suffering from PFS are sedentary, symptoms of this malady are frequently relieved by a major effort at physical reconditioning. The following activities and modalities have been found therapeutically beneficial toward relief of the symptoms of PFS: local heat, stretching exercises, strengthening exercises, massage, relaxation techniques, restful sleep, nonsteroidal anti-inflammatory medication, moderate activity, warm, dry weather, posture instruction and exercises, swimming exercises, aerobic prescription of exercise, and a low dosage of tricyclic agents at bedtime to promote deeper sleep.[1,5] Patients should be reassured that they do not have a dangerous, life-threatening illness and PFS does not cause degenerative or deforming illness.[19] The prognosis for PFS is favorable with a comprehensive and supportive program.

References

1. Berkow R: *The Merck manual of diagnosis and therapy*, Rahway, N.J., 1987, Merck, Sharp & Dohme Research Laboratories.
2. Moldofsky H, Scarisbrick P, England R, Smythe HA: Musculoskeletal symptoms of non-REM sleep disturbance in patients with "fibrositis syndrome" and healthy subjects, *Psychosom Med* 37:341-351, 1975.
3. Netter F: *The CIBA collection of medical illustrations*, vol 8: *Musculoskeletal system*, part 2, Summit, N.J., 1990, CIBA-Geigy Corp.
4. Rodan GP, Schumacher HR: *Primer on rheumatic diseases*, ed 8, Atlanta, 1983, The Arthritis Foundation, p 140.
5. Schumacher HR, Bomalski JS: *Case studies in rheumatology for the house officer*, Baltimore, 1990, Williams & Wilkins, p 63.
6. Simons DG: Myofascial pain syndromes: Where are we? Where are we going? *Arch Phys Med Rehabil* 69:209, 1988.
7. Skootsky S: Incidence of myofacial pain in an internal medical group practice. Presented to the American Pain Society, Washington, D.C., Nov 6-9, 1986.
8. Wolfe F, Hawly DJ, Cathey MA, et al: Fibrositis: symptom frequency and criteria for diagnosis: evaluation of 291 rheumatic disease patients and 58 normal individuals, *J Rheumatol* 12:1159-1163, 1985.
9. Yunus MB, Kalyan-Raman UP, Kalyan-Raman K: Primary fibromyalgia syndrome and myofascial pain syndrome: clinical features and muscle pathology, *Arch Phys Med Rehabil* 69:451-454, 1988.
10. Yunus MB, Masi AT, Calabro JJ, et al: Primary fibromyalgia (fibrositis): clinical study of 50 patients with matched normal controls, *Semin Arthritis Rheum* 11:151-171, 1981.

Recommended reading

Goldenberg DL: Fibromyalgia syndrome: an emerging but controversial condition, *JAMA* 257:2782-2787, 1987.

Simons DG: Myofascial pain syndromes: Where are we? Where are we going? *Arch Phys Med Rehabil* 69:209, 1988.

Smythe HA: Fibrositis syndrome. In Conn HF, editor: *Current Therapy*, ed 27, Philadelphia, 1975, Saunders.

Starlanye D, Copeland ME: *Fibromyalgia and chronic myofascial pain syndrome: a survival manual.* New Harbringer Publications Inc. Oakland, CA 1996.

Yunus MB, Kalyan-Raman UP, Kalyan-Raman K: Primary fibromyalgia syndrome and myofascial pain syndrome: clinical features and muscle pathology, *Arch Phys Med Rehabil* 69:451-454, 1988.

Neonate Presenting with Leftward Head Tilt and Rightward Facial Flattening

22

Your clinic receives overflow from the local managed care center and in walks a mother with her infant, presenting a prescription that states "WRYNECK - therapy: TIW for 9 weeks." The baby is male, 7 weeks old, and presents with a slight rightward head tilt and slight leftward facial flattening. There is a history of breech presentation and an initial Apgar score of 8 and then 9, minutes later.

OBSERVATION Both femurs and tibiae appear to be of equal length when viewed from above as well as from the side.

PALPATION There is a firm fusiform swelling in the distal aspect of the right sternocleidomastoid muscle.

RANGE OF MOTION Rightward neck rotation is limited, as is leftward neck tilt. Bilateral hip motion demonstrates greater than 60° of abduction.

MUSCLE STRENGTH Head extension while in prone position to approximately 30°.

SPECIAL TESTS Negative Barlow's and Ortoloni's signs. There is no measurable leg-length discrepancy.

CLUE:

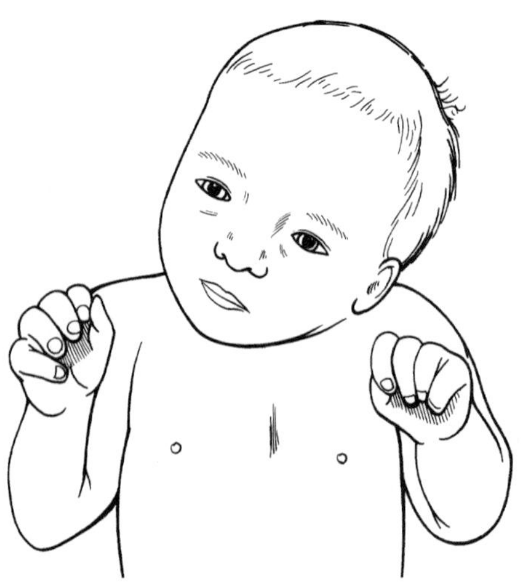

1. **What is wryneck?**
2. **What anatomy is prerequisite to understanding this disorder?**
3. **What are the kinesiologic characteristics of the interesting sternocleidomastoid muscle?**
4. **What is the evolution of this disorder, and what is the clinical presentation?**
5. **What are the cause and pathologic features of this condition?**
6. **What are associated conditions, if any?**
7. **What is the differential diagnosis?**
8. **What acute conditions may be confused with congenital muscular torticollis?**
9. **What osseous lesions are to be ruled out?**
10. **What inflammatory disorders are to be ruled out?**
11. **What neurologic disorders are to be ruled out?**
12. **What is ocular torticollis?**
13. **What trauma may result in torticollis?**
14. **What miscellaneous disorders may be confused with congenital muscular torticollis?**
15. **What cosmetic deformities of the face and skull may result in the untreated condition of this disorder?**
16. **What therapeutic intervention is appropriate in the treatment of this condition?**
17. **What are the criteria for operative management?**
18. **What therapeutic intervention is appropriate after surgery?**

1. What is wryneck?

Wryneck deformity, in this child, is classified as *congenital* or *infantile muscular torticollis*. Wryneck is actually a composite of both *torticollis* and *anterocollis*[1] and is immortalized in the statue of Alexander the Great located in the British Museum, without, however, the accompanying facial distortion.[3] The former designation derives from two Latin words, that is, *tortus*, which means 'twisted', and *collum*, meaning the 'neck'; in effect, *rotation*. Anterocollis refers to the tilt component of this disfigurement. This condition is relatively common, since the incidence of the pathologic condition ranges from 0.3% to 0.5% of the general population.[6] Contracture typically occurs on the right side.[2]

2. What anatomy is prerequisite to understanding this disorder?

The sternocleidomastoid muscle is composed of two major divisions known as the sternal and clavicular heads, each of which has its own subdivisions. Although each division possesses a separate head of origin distally, all subdivisions merge to insert proximally as a composite head (Fig. 22-1). The proper or full name of this interesting muscle, that is, the sternocleidomastoid, bespeaks the two distal origins of that muscle, namely, the sternum and the clavicle, as well as the proximal insertion located at the tip of the mastoid process. The main motor supply is from the spinal accessory nerve, which itself is composed of the vagus nerve and segments of the upper five cervical nerves.

3. What are the kinesiologic characteristics of the interesting sternocleidomastoid muscle?

Contraction of one side of the sternomastoid turns the head to the opposite side; this is equivalent to saying that turning one's head to the right is accomplished by contraction of the left sternomastoid muscle. Simultaneous contraction of both muscles extends the head on the neck. In both instances, this superficial muscle boldly stands out, clearly defining the neck's contour. Unilateral sternomastoid contraction is opposed by contralateral trapezius activity, so that rightward head turning is opposed by the left trapezius.

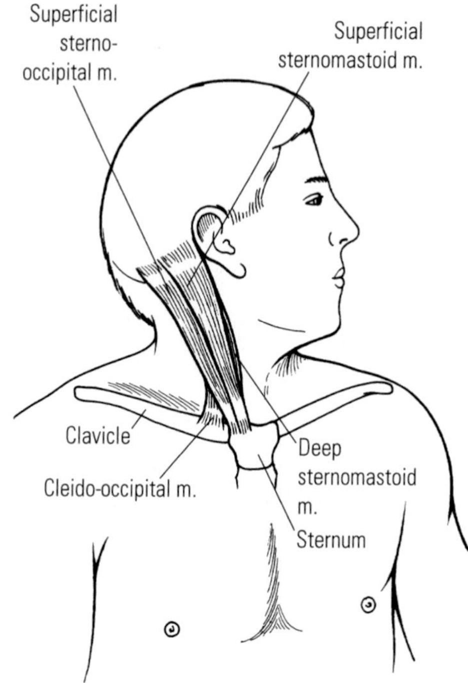

Fig. 22-1 External view of right sternocleidomastoid muscle. Unilateral contraction of this muscle permits ipsilateral lateral cervical flexion and contralateral head rotation. Bilateral sternomastoid contraction permits neck flexion. (Redrawn from Rockwood CA, Matsen FA, editors: *The shoulder*, vol 2, ed 2, Philadelphia, 1990, Saunders.)

If both muscles contract, the face and head will extend on the cervical spine. Sternocleidomastoid secondarily aids respiration by virtue of elevating the thoracic cage.

4. What is the evolution of this disorder, and what is the clinical presentation?

Although minimal at birth, wryneck deformity is usually discovered in the first 6 to 8 weeks of life[4] as a unilateral, firm, nontender, and enlarging swelling, eventually reaching the size of the distal phalanx of the adult thumb. The site of this mass is just beneath the skin and is attached to or embedded within the body of the sternomastoid muscle.[2] This mass attains maximum size within the first month of life and then gradually regresses over a subsequent period of 6 to 12 weeks.[2]

The temporary growth and regression of this mass interferes with unilateral longitudinal muscular growth, thus leaving in its wake an imbalance between the neck's two sternomastoid muscles. Contracture follows and is accompanied by head tilt toward the affected side with rotation of the chin contralaterally (Fig. 22-2). As a result, rotation of the neck to the side of the deformity is limited, as is lateral tilt to the opposite side. If untreated, craniofacial disfigurement will ensue during the first year.[2]

5. What are the cause and pathologic features of this condition?

The pathologic characteristic of this condition is simply the replacement of muscle with fibrous tissue. The exact cause of fibrosis is unknown. A multifactorial theory is postulated attributing the fibrotic mass to ischemia of the sternomastoid muscle,[6] particularly the sternal head, because of intrauterine malposition or increased pressure otherwise resulting during passage through the birth canal.[2]

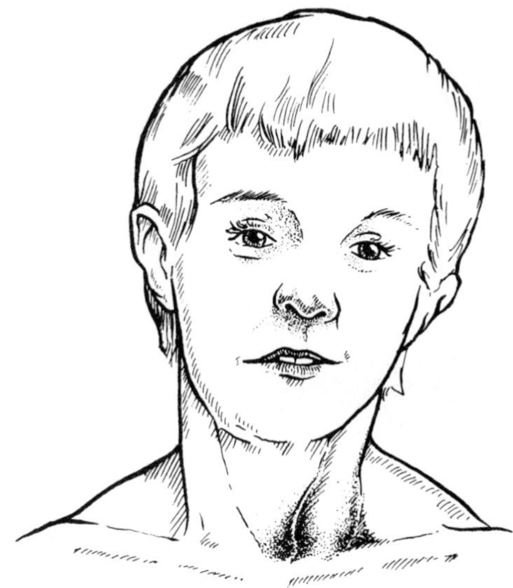

Fig. 22-2 Untreated left congenital muscular torticollis in a 14-year-old boy. Notice the asymmetry of the face. On the affected side the face is shortened from above downwards. The levels of the eyes and ears are asymmetrical. (From Dandy DJ: *Essential orthopaedics and trauma*, Edinburgh, 1989, Churchill Livingstone.)

6. What are associated conditions, if any?

As many as 20%[2] of all infants who have congenital muscular torticollis also have congenital dysplasia, that is, dislocation of one or both hips.[4] As such, a high index of suspicion is appropriate to justify clinical examination for hip dislocation.[6] Additionally the hips of suspected infants must therefore be imaged by ultrasound or a single anteroposterior pelvic radiograph even if the clinical exam is normal (Fig. 22-3). Bear in mind that the radiograph is not a reliable image until 10 weeks when the hip has completely ossified.[5] The aforementioned epidemiology supports the hypothesis that both wryneck and hip dysplasia are related to intrauterine malposition or presentation.[5]

7. What is the differential diagnosis?

The differential diagnoses of congenital muscular torticollis may be divided into seven categories: acute torticollis, osseous causes, inflammatory causes, neurologic disorders, ocular torticollis, trauma, and miscellaneous.

8. What acute conditions may be confused with congenital muscular torticollis?

Acute calcification of the intervertebral cervical disk of unknown cause that produces neck pain and spasm often results in torticollis postures. This rare and idiopathic condition[5] most commonly involves the C6-C7 disk space. Calcification occurs only after an abrupt onset of symptoms that include fever (in about one fourth of all patients),[2] neck pain and stiffness, and torticollis. Management includes rest, use of a cervical collar, and nonsteroidal antiinflammatory medication.[5] Two thirds of afflicted children are symptom free within 3 weeks of onset, whereas others may require up to 6 months.[2]

Acute rotary displacement of the atlantoaxial joint, either from acute rotational injury or from upper respiratory infection[2] (such as acute pharyngitis), may cause fixed head tilt. In this case there is a characteristic radiographic appearance of the dens in relation to the lateral masses. Both these conditions occur in the older child and are very rare in the infant.

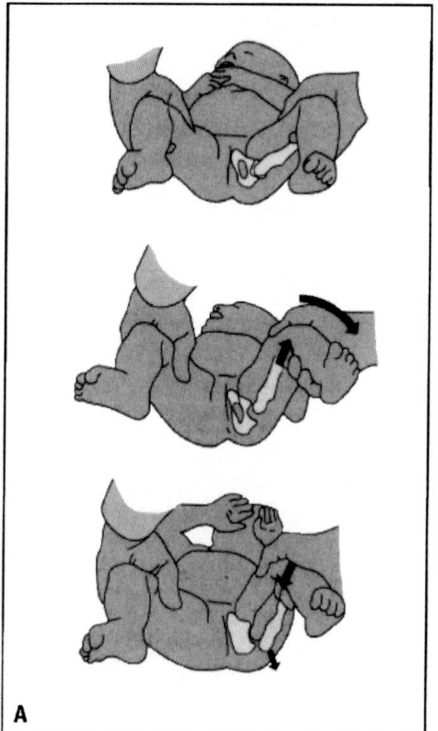

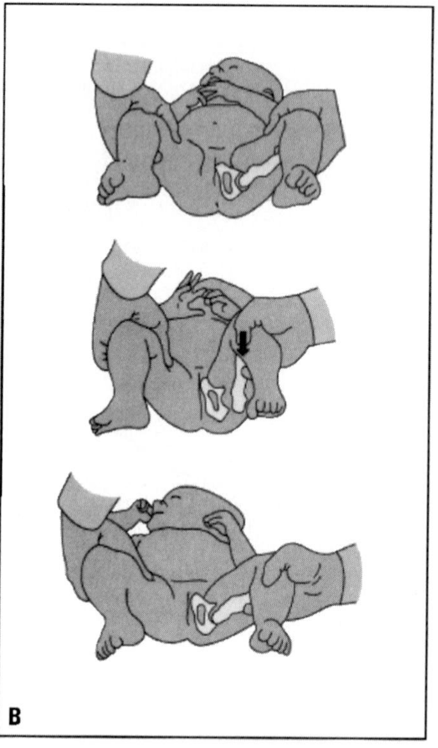

Fig. 22-3 **A,** Barlow's sign. Hip instability is demonstrated when one attempts to gently displace the hip out of the socket over the posterior acetabular rim. **B,** Ortolani's sign. The hip is first adducted and the thigh is depressed to subluxate or dislocate the hip. The thigh is then abducted. The reduction of the displaced hip causes a palpable "clunk" as the femoral head reenters the socket. (From Staheli LT: *Fundamentals of pediatric orthopedics*, New York, 1993, Raven Press.)

9. What osseous lesions are to be ruled out?

Every patient should have radiographs of the cervical site to exclude congenital bony anomalies. *Osseous lesions* manifest in two types:

Hemivertebra in the cervical spine is confirmed by radiographs and is technically defined as a pure lateral tilt without a rotary component. Essentially a lateral kink in the spine, a hemivertebra causes compensatory scoliosis above and below, which may cause root irritation and strain the small joints of the spine. When occurring in the cervical region of the spine, the caudal compensation may manifest as torticollis.

Klippel-Feil syndrome is an uncorrectable bony neck malformation attributable to congenital fusion of two or more cervical vertebrae.[2] The characteristic appearance in severe cases is that of a short, broad, "webbed" neck, low posterior hairline, thoracic kyphosis deformity, and gross restriction of motion[5] (Fig. 22-4). Because of natural cervical fusions, motion is often concentrated at one or more levels and is frequently associated with instability, thus placing the cervical cord at risk for injury. For this reason, children with this syndrome should not participate in activities such as diving, contact sports, gymnastics, or use of the trampoline. Renal ultrasound is essential to rule out internal congenital defects. Despite its being unsightly, the concomitant deformity is not amenable to correction.[5]

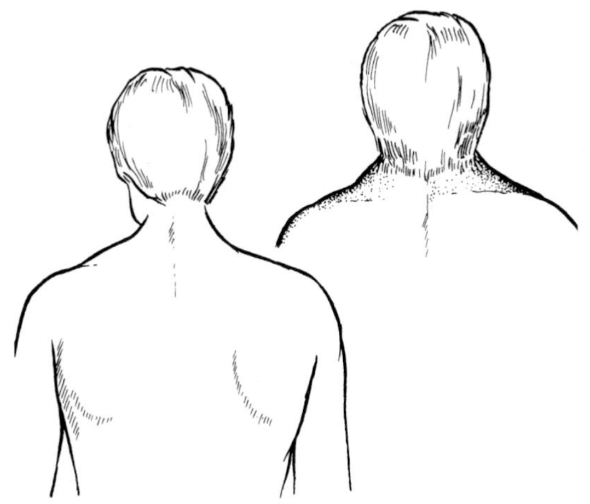

Fig. 22-4 Klippel-Feil syndrome. A short webbed neck with a low hairline. (From Dandy DJ: *Essential orthopaedics and trauma*, Edinburgh, 1989, Churchill Livingstone.)

10. What inflammatory disorders are to be ruled out?

Inflammatory causes

Inflammatory disorders. A major cause of torticollis in older children is *bacterial or viral pharyngitis* of the cervical nodes. Children typically between 5 and 10 years of age may suddenly develop a painless, stiff, and torticollis neck after a sore throat. Resisted neck movements may be slightly painful but are not weak. This condition most probably results from a swollen gland lying under and therefore irritating the sternomastoid muscle; resolution is approximately within 2 weeks from onset.

- *Juvenile rheumatoid arthritis*, causing erosion of the waist of the dens in those patients with systemic or polyarticular onset during the first 1 or 2 years after onset; this predisposes the odontoid to becoming more susceptible to fracture and displacement.
- *Cervical adenitis*, caused by retrophalangeal or tonsil infection that often appears as a conspicuous unilateral upper palate bulge on the same side as the torticollis.
- Tuberculosis

11. What neurologic disorders are to be ruled out?

Neurologic causes

- *Paroxysmal torticollis* is seen in infants 2 to 8 months of age and manifests as recurrent attacks of head tilt lasting from a few hours to a few days. This occurs as a result of a variety of neurologic causes including drug intoxication.[2]
- *Dystonia musculorum deformans* is a rare progressive syndrome usually beginning in childhood and is characterized by dystonic movements that result in sustained and often bizarre postures. Symptoms usually begin with torticollis, or inversion and plantar flexion of the foot while walking. Two hereditary patterns are described for this condition: autosomal dominant in families on northern European extraction and recessive in some Ashkenazi Jewish families. In advanced stages the body may become twisted "like a pretzel." Mentation is usually preserved, and treatment is usually unsatisfactory.
- *Cerebellar tumors* may result in torticollis, though onset is gradual; other peripheral neurologic signs are usually present.
- *Cervical spinal cord tumor*
- *Syringomyelia*

12. What is ocular torticollis?

Ocular torticollis, such as *rotary strabismus*, is usually the result of an imbalance of either the superior or inferior oblique eye muscles, or occurring after fourth cranial nerve dysfunction. Torticollis does not begin to manifest until 4 to 6 months of age, that is, when the infant begins to focus on objects. This form differs from muscular torticollis in two ways: (1) there is full neck range of motion, and (2) with muscular torticollis the face is turned *away* from the side of the head tilt and angled upwards, whereas with the ocular type the face is slightly turned *toward* the side of the head tilt.[6]

13. What trauma may result in torticollis?

Torticollis commonly occurs after an injury to the C1-C2 articulation, or fracture or dislocation of the dens (C2). Similarly, children with Down's syndrome, Morquio's syndrome, skeletal dysplasia, and spondyloepiphyseal dysplasia commonly suffer from C1-C2 instability and accompanying torticollis.[2]

14. What miscellaneous disorders may be confused with congenital muscular torticollis?

- *Sandifer's syndrome* is sudden posturing of the neck and trunk because of esophagitis caused by gastroesophageal reflux with or without hiatal hernia that may not always be accompanied by vomiting. Abnormal posturing is believed to be attributable to the discomfort felt by reflux.
- *Fibrodysplasia ossificans progressiva* is enlargement of the sternocleidomastoid and other neck muscles that is accompanied by areas of soft-tissue calcification in the cervical musculature.
- *Surgery of the upper pharynx*, such as *tonsillectomy*, may result in inflammation and local edema, which in turn causes local ligamentous laxity; as a result of this, a greater motion of C1 on C2 than normal is allowed and may precipitate rotary subluxation.[2]

15. What cosmetic deformities of the face and skull may result in the untreated condition of this disorder?

Muscle contracture prevents bilateral even longitudinal muscle growth and therefore, as the spine grows, the involved muscle and soft tissue fail to keep pace and their relative shortness is reinforced.[6] If the contracture is left untreated, secondary deformities of the face and skull (plagiocephaly) can develop in the first year. Flattening of the face or back of the head occurs as a function of the sleeping posture[2] while one is afflicted with this condition. Children who sleep prone will be more comfortable with the affected side down; ergo, that ipsilateral side of the face becomes distorted. In children who sleep supine, reverse modeling of the contralateral posterior skull may occur.

If the condition continues to remain untreated during the years of skeletal growth, considerable cosmetic deformity will commence. The relative levels of the eyes and ears change but may be compensated for and made less noticeable when the head is slightly tilted to one side but made more obvious when the head and neck are straight in midline. Eye strain may result from an ocular imbalance, whereas a lower cervical–upper dorsal scoliosis with concavity toward the affected side may develop. As growth proceeds, the soft tissue on the affected side, including the scalenus anterior and scalenus medius muscles, and the carotid vessel and adjacent soft tissue undergo adaptive shortening. Thick, fibrotic, and tendon-like bands eventually replace the sternomastoid muscle, which, along with the thickened and contracted deep cervical fascia, make the head appear to be tethered to the clavicle.[2]

16. What therapeutic intervention is appropriate in the treatment of this condition?

Eighty-five to ninety percent of patients yield good results after conservative intervention of range-of-motion and stretching exercises.[2] Intensive[4] therapy is essential and ought to begin as soon as possible for a duration of at least 1 year.[1] From a practical standpoint, however, it is very difficult to perform adequate stretching on an infant more than six months of age because of resistance. Because of this, aggressive yet gentle stretching is appropriately initiated early on and continued for as long as the child will tolerate it or until the condition resolves.

- Give gentle, nonsudden, slow, and passive stretching of contracted muscle and related soft tissue, such as tilting of the head so that the higher ear approximates or touches its adjacent shoulder. This is followed by rotation of the head so that the chin approaches or touches the shoulder on the side of the affected muscle (Fig. 22-5).
- When adequate stretching has been obtained with head in neutral, these maneuvers should be repeated with the head in hyperextension, while countertraction is applied when the ipsilateral shoulder and chest

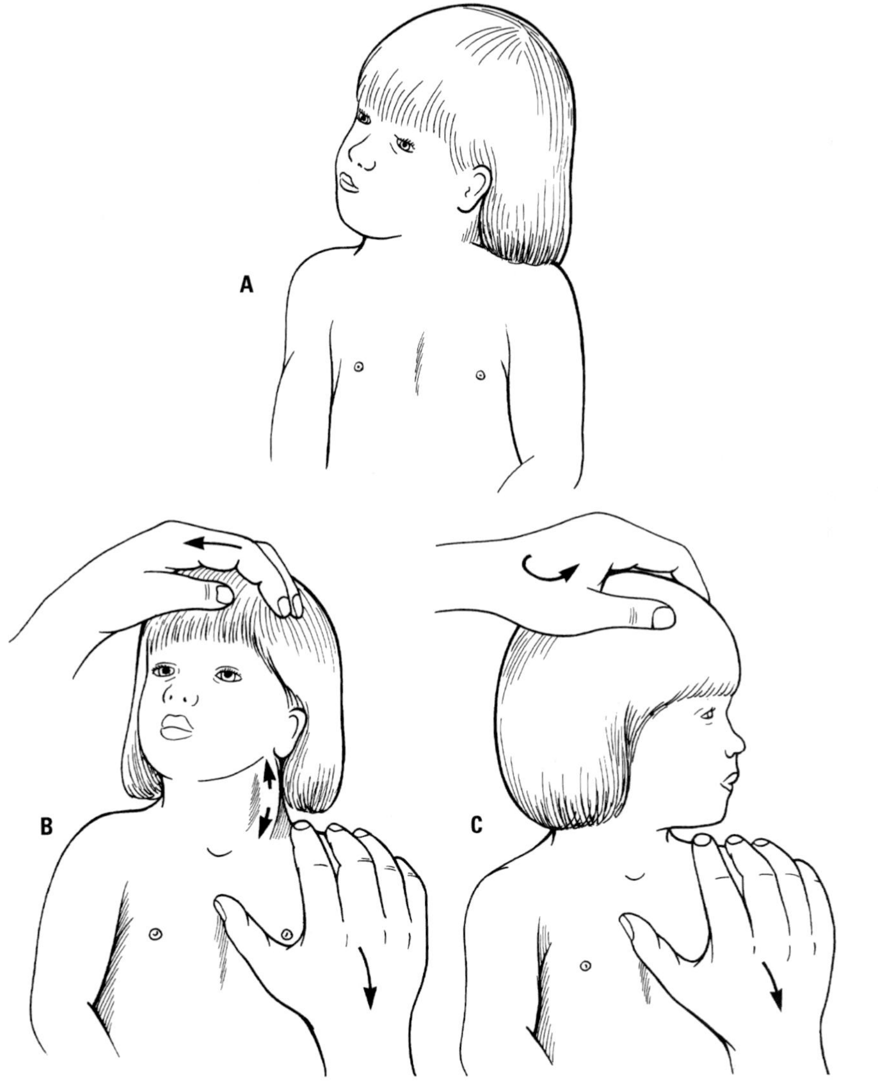

Fig. 22-5 Sequence of passive stretching exercises to the contracted left sternomastoid muscle in congenital muscular torticollis.

are held. Gravity assists when the infant is positioned supine in the mother's lap with the head lolling in hyperextension.

- Conscientiously stretch at least 3 or 4 times per day for 10 times per session and hold the involved muscle in the stretched position for a count of 10 seconds.
- Position the crib so that the infant's affected side is to the wall, so that he or she will rotate his head toward the uninvolved side when his attention is distracted. The infant will then actively stretch the involved soft tissue when reaching and grasping for toys.
- Massage[1] to the contracted sternomastoid muscle while taking care to avoid the area over the carotid artery.
- Teach appropriate range-of-motion and stretching techniques to parents, while stressing the need for consistent adherence to the treatment regimen. Parents must be cautioned not to use excessive force or speed in their desire to "get better quicker."

17. What are the criteria for operative management?

In those children who go untreated during the early months of life, the developing deformity becomes progressively resistant to stretching.[4] Established facial asymmetry and limitation of normal motion beyond 30° usually precludes a good result. In this patient population and approximately 10% to 15% of cases resistant to conservative treatment, surgical release of the contracted muscle is appropriate. Removal of the mass in early infancy is inappropriate.

18. What therapeutic intervention is appropriate after surgery?

A postoperative therapeutic regimen includes passive stretching exercises of the same kind performed preoperatively and should begin as soon as the patient can tolerate handling of the neck. The patient, with time, is eventually progressed to active exercises. The surgeon may prescribe a head cast, brace, or helmet to position the head in an overcorrected position for 6 weeks after surgery.[5]

References

1. Berkow R: *The Merck manual of diagnosis and therapy*, ed 15, Rahway, N.J., 1987, Merck, Sharp & Dohme Research Laboratories.
2. Netter FH: *The CIBA collection of medical illustrations*: vol 8: *Musculoskeletal system*, part 2, Summit, N.J., 1990, CIBA-Geigy Corp.
3. Pineyro JR, Yoel J, Rocco M: Congenital torticollis, *J Int Coll Surg* 34:495-505, 1960.
4. Salter RB: *Textbook of disorders and injuries of the musculoskeletal system*, ed 2, Baltimore, 1983, Williams & Wilkins.
5. Staheli LT: *Fundamentals of pediatric orthopedics*, New York, 1992, Raven Press.
6. Wilkins KE: Special problems with the child's shoulder. In Rockwood CA, Matsen FA, editors: *The shoulder*, vol 2, Philadelphia, 1990, Saunders.

Recommended reading

Staheli LT: *Fundamentals of pediatric orthopedics*, New York, 1992, Raven Press.

Wilkins KE: Special problems with the child's shoulder. In Rockwood CA, Matsen FA, editors: *The shoulder*, vol 2, Philadelphia, 1990, Saunders.

Part Five

Nerve and Muscle Lesions

Acute Hemiparalysis of All Facial Muscles after Cold Exposure

23

A 32-year-old female participated in a human rights protest during a cold evening that brought on the first frost of the winter season. A candlelight vigil was held until the wee hours of the morning during which the wind intensified the cold. She wore no scarf or earmuffs. At dawn she went home to sleep for 5 hours and woke up with a pain in her left cheek. Upon looking in the mirror she was horrified to view her face grossly misshapen on one side. She immediately went to the emergency room at the local hospital. The neurologist on staff diagnosed her as having Bell's palsy and referred her to therapy. When asked, the patient admits to waking up in the morning and finding her pillow wet from saliva having drooled out of the left side of her mouth during sleep. Obvious facial asymmetry is observed, and the ipsilateral forehead appears flattened and lacking normal skin creases. Muscle testing revealed less than fair strength in the following muscles: occipitofrontalis, frontalis, orbicularis oculi, zygomaticus major, corrugator, buccinator, mentalis, and platysma. Sensory testing revealed loss of sweet and salty taste in the anterior two thirds of the tongue. There is a positive Bell's sign.

CLUE:

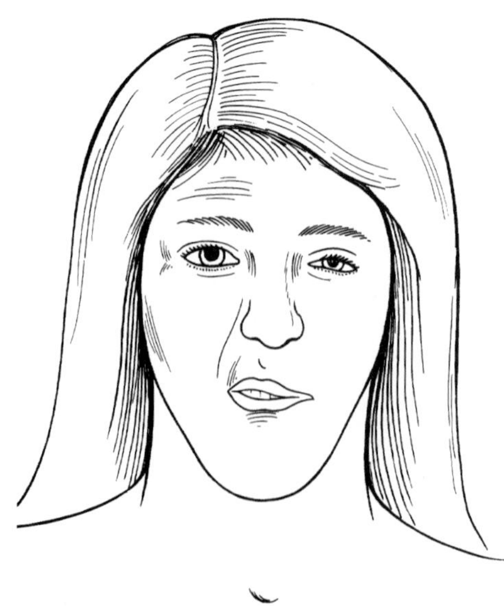

1. **What is acute idiopathic facial palsy?**
2. **What relevant microbiology is appropriate to an understanding of the herpes simplex virus?**
3. **What method of entry do viruses employ when entering the human nervous system?**
4. **Is there a relationship between the acute onset of Bell's palsy and exposure to cold?**
5. **What are the signs and symptoms at clinical presentation?**
6. **What is the anatomy of the facial nerve?**
7. **What is the topographic paradigm in understanding facial palsy?**
8. **How does a lesion at the internal auditory meatus manifest?**
9. **How does a lesion proximal to the geniculate ganglion manifest?**
10. **How does a lesion of the geniculate ganglion manifest?**
11. **What is the manifestation of a high facial canal lesion?**
12. **What is the function of the stapedius muscle?**
13. **What is the manifestation of a more distal facial canal lesion?**
14. **What is the manifestation of a lesion at the stylomastoid foramen?**
15. **How does facial palsy of the upper motor neuron type differ from Bell's palsy, which is of the lower motor neuron type?**
16. **What is the corneal blink test?**
17. **What is the differential diagnosis?**
18. **What is the prognosis for recovery?**
19. **What is the medical management of Bell's palsy?**
20. **What is the traditional therapeutic management of Bell's palsy?**
21. **Why are nonspecific gross facial exercises inadequate to the management repertoire of Bell's palsy?**
22. **What are the psychologic ramifications to the patient's being afflicted with facial palsy?**
23. **What neuromuscular training (NMR) techniques are available to the patient after facial paralysis?**
24. **What is the premise of NMR, and for what population is it appropriate?**
25. **What is the role of therapy in NMR?**
26. **What is the role of the home exercise program in NMR?**
27. **When is NMR management not appropriate?**
28. **What is the optimal time for referral?**
29. **What are the essential components to neuromuscular retraining?**
30. **What is the method of NMR?**
31. **What are the two categories of motor disturbance that facial paralysis is classified into?**
32. **What NMR treatment strategy addresses the patient with flaccid paralysis or paresis?**
33. **What NMR treatment strategy addresses the patient with synkinesis or mass action?**
34. **What is the rationale behind electrical stimulation as a treatment modality?**
35. **When is surgery appropriate?**

1. What is acute idiopathic facial palsy?

Clinical, epidemiologic, and laboratory data suggest that what was once referred to as idiopathic facial palsy, better known as Bell's palsy, is actually an acute, benign, cranial polyneuritis that is most likely caused by the *herpes simplex virus.*[1] Named after the Scottish anatomist and surgeon John Bell, Bell's palsy occurs unilaterally and with *sudden onset,* often overnight, and reaches peak flaccidity with resultant paresis or paralysis within a few hours. For all its shocking and horrible insult to its victim, this malady is a nonprogressive, non–life threatening, and often spontaneously remitting process. A large proportion of sufferers experience a premonitory symptom, referred to as a *prodrome,* which is actually a symptom indicating that onset of this pathologic condition is imminent. Similar to carpal tunnel syndrome, there is an increased incidence of Bell's palsy during pregnancy,[17] as well as an increased incidence of diabetes mellitus in patients afflicted with Bell's palsy. Some evidence exists for a genetic predisposition to Bell's palsy. The incidence of Bell's palsy has been estimated at between 15 to 40 cases per 100,000 population with no age, sex type, or racial predilections.[24]

2. What relevant microbiology is appropriate to an understanding of the herpes simplex virus?

Although nearly 80 known Herpesviridae infest animals, only six of these are known to infect humans. Three of the more famous of these include the herpes simplex virus, the Epstein-Barr virus, and the varicella-zoster virus, which causes herpes zoster, which is responsible for chickenpox during a primary infection and for shingles neuralgia in the aged after a period of dormancy and reactivation. Herpesviruses are ubiquitous in the sense of their having worldwide distribution, since few humans escape becoming infected by them during their lifetime. Because herpesviruses are fragile and do not survive long periods in the environment, transmission is principally through direct contact by bodily secretions at susceptible sites, such as oral, ocular, genital, or anal mucosa, the tympanic membrane, the bloodstream by injection, or the respiratory tract by someone else's sneeze. The virus does not penetrate keratinized skin.[26]

Herpes simplex viruses (HSV) are among the most common troublesome and annoying maladies affecting humans. Occasionally, they may be life threatening, as when they progress to herpes simplex encephalitis, in which the cerebrospinal fluid is bloody in the absence of any trauma. Known as the most common sporadic disease of the brain in the United States today, this pathogen carries a 70% mortality.[26]

Herpes simplex virus is subdivided into HSV-1, commonly known as oral herpes, and HSV-2, or genital herpes. Whereas the former infection spreads by oral secretions and is identified as the occupational hazard of dentists, dental hygienists, respiratory care unit personnel, and wrestlers, the latter infection is spread through sexual contact. With both herpes strains, recurrent infections occur frequently by reactivation of the endogenous virus, despite the presence of circulating antiviral antibodies. Precipitating factors include emotional stress, menstruation, fever, sunlight, and other factors. Thus all herpesviruses induce a lifelong latent infection in their natural hosts.[26]

3. What method of entry do viruses employ when entering the human nervous system?

Viruses enter the nervous system by either one of two routes: (1) through blood, or (2) directly through the nervous system. In the latter, the virus requires a specific receptor to interface with to gain access. For example, the poliovirus enters via the anterior horn cell, whereas the viruses causing viral meningitis interfaces upon a specific receptor on the meninges of the nervous system. The herpes simplex virus, as in rabies, gains entry through a peripheral nerve or nerves and moves proximally to the central nervous system by retrograde axoplasmic flow.[26]

Transmission and primary infection by herpes simplex is similar to that of all herpesvirus infections, except for herpes zoster, in that all are mostly asymptomatic. As the patient recovers from the primary infection, HSV travels up the sensory nerve pathways to reside latently in sensory cranial nerve ganglia such as the trigeminal, vagal, and perhaps the facial nuclei as well.[1]

4. Is there a relationship between the acute onset of Bell's palsy and exposure to cold?

The virus is somehow reactivated and replicates within the ganglion cells where it is protected from circulating antibodies. Reactivation may be related to cold exposure, since circumstantial evidence seems to link the onset of Bell's palsy after recent exposure to cold. Proximal damage is caused by the virus traveling up the nerve to the brainstem where it may induce a localized meningoencephalitis (as evidenced by increased protein in the cerebrospinal fluid). Distally the virus travels down the axon or axons to induce a radiculitis of the facial nucleus nerve cells, manifesting the signs and symptoms of Bell's palsy. This radiculitis is in fact caused by autoimmune demyelinization[1] rather than ischemic compression of the facial nucleus nerve cells. Inflammation (neuritis) and concomitant edema leading to ischemic constriction of the nerve axon may play a contributory role within the narrow unyielding bony confines of the more distal facial canal, located in the vicinity of the middle ear cavity within the temporal bone.[1]

5. What are the signs and symptoms at clinical presentation?

Some but not necessarily all of the following characteristics are present in typical Bell's palsy (Fig. 23-1):

- Ipsilateral muscle sagging with ironed-out appearance of normal folds and lines about the lips, nose, eyes (crow's feet), and forehead; there is a widened palpebral fissure present.
- Inability to fully or even partially puff cheeks, whistle, or wrinkle one's forehead.
- Miosis (of the eyelid).
- Ipsilateral numbness or pain of ear, face, neck, or tongue, occurs in approximately half of all patients.
- When asked to squeeze one's eyes tightly shut, the patient, in attempting to comply, demonstrates a positive Bell's sign: the eyeball rolls upward and inward, exposing the white sclera (Fig. 23-2). This movement on attempted closure is an involuntary synkinetic movement that usually but not invariably occurs when we close our eyes or sleep. With Bell's palsy, this movement may now be viewed because the levator superioris palpebrae (cranial nerve III) is unopposed by the orbicularis oculi (cranial nerve VII). This inability to close the eyelid is called *lagophthalmos.*

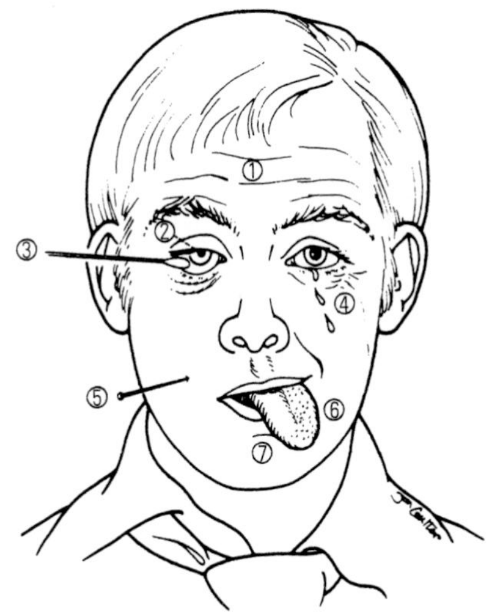

Fig. 23-1 Some common neurologic signs in patients diagnosed with Bell's palsy: *1,* flattening of the ipsilateral forehead; *2,* miosis; *3,* loss of corneal sensation; *4,* normal tearing on the uninvolved side only; *5,* diminished nasolabial fold, ipsilateral facial laxity, and drooping of the ipsilateral mouth; *6,* tongue deviation if unilateral hypoglossal paralysis is also suspected; *7,* loss of taste papillae on the anterior two thirds of the tongue. (From May M: *The facial nerve,* New York, 1986, Thieme-Stratton.)

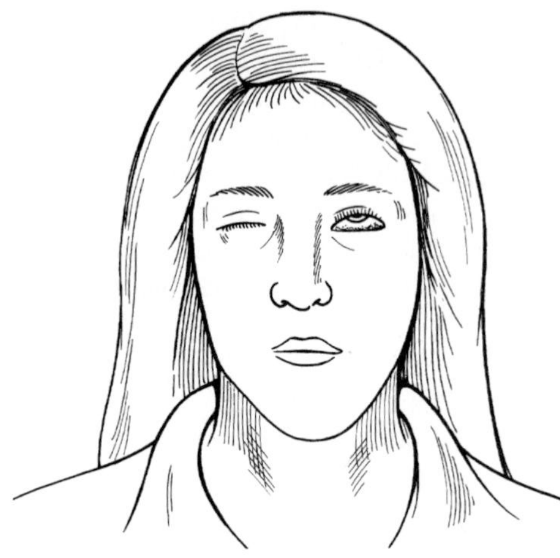

Fig. 23-2 Positive Bell's sign of left eye.

- The patient will report in the affirmative when asked about food becoming lodged between his or her teeth and cheek because of paralysis of the buccinator muscle, saliva and drink dribbling out of the mouth, or noticing upon his or her waking from sleep how the pillow had become wet from saliva.
- Diminished submandibular salivary flow or ipsilateral tearing.
- Speech, particularly labial sounds, are affected.
- Decrease in or loss of ipsilateral stapes reflex.
- An absent ipsilateral blink reflex.
- When the patient attempts to smile or bear teeth, the lower facial muscles are pulled to the opposite side by the intact contralateral muscles, giving the impression of a sneer. Normally, this would not occur because the facial muscles, akin to many muscles elsewhere on the body, are arranged so that a balance exists and provides for symmetry of expression. This imbalance may lead to facial muscle contracture on the normal side, with muscle lengthening or stretching on the flaccid side.
- Loss of (sweet, sour, and salty) taste in the anterior two thirds of the tongue and decreased salivation on the affected side. Taste alterations may also occur with trauma or tumors.
- Hyperacusis caused by affectation of the nerve branch supplying the stapedius muscle; the patient may complain of holding the telephone away from the ear.
- Examination may show an area of decreased pinprick sensation along the distribution of Arnold's nerve behind the involved ear.
- Red appearance of the chorda tympani nerve in somewhat less than half of all patients evaluated within the first 10 days after onset in whom this nerve could be visualized.

6. What is the anatomy of the facial nerve?

The facial nerve is a mixed nerve consisting of motor, sensory, and autonomic fibers. The motor and sensory roots of the facial nerve emerge from a small fissure in the posterior area of the skull to enter the *internal auditory meatus* located in the petrous portion of the temporal bone (which also contains the middle and inner ear).

Having emerged from the meatus, the two roots, now called the "facial nerve" because they are now encased within the facial canal, proceed distally, to the vicinity of the inner ear, where the sensory nerves synapse with the cell bodies of the sensory neurons of the facial nerve collectively known as the *geniculate ganglion*. Beyond this point, axons responsible for different functions are routed either anterior (autonomic and sensory components) or posterior (motor) to the ganglion, the latter coursing toward the stylomastoid foramen.

Once emerging from the stylomastoid foramen behind the earlobe, the facial nerve (with its motor component) enters the parotid salivary gland to bifurcate into two main divisions (Fig. 23-3). The upper division divides into temporal and zygomatic branches, whereas the lower division gives rise to the buccal, mandibular, and cervical branches. These branches have been listed in cephalic to caudal order and serve to innervate the muscles of facial expression and those of the scalp and neck; additionally, two muscles at the floor of the mouth, namely, the stylohyoid and the posterior belly of the digastric muscle, are also innervated by the facial nerve. The muscles of the jaw not supplied by the facial nerve are the masseter, temporalis, and pterygoid muscles, which are innervated by the trigeminal nerve (V).

The *occipitofrontalis* controls the muscles of the scalp, the frontal belly of the *epicranius* raises the eyebrows and wrinkles the forehead as in surprise or fright, the *corrugator supercilii* draws the eyebrows together "tightly knit" and is associated with frowning, the *orbicularis oculi* controls the sphincter muscles of the eyelids, the *buccinator* controls the muscles of the cheek, nose, and mouth. One can test the latter by asking the patient to "pull back the corners of your mouth." The alar position of the *nasalis* permits nostril flaring, the transverse portion of the *nasalis* permits narrowing of the nostrils, the *procerus* allows scrunching up of the face, as may occur when smelling something offensive, the *orbicularis oris* puckers the lips as in whistling, the *mentalis* scrunches up the chin and protrudes the lower lip as in pouting, whereas the *pterygoideus medialis* and *pterygoideus lateralis* permit protrusion of the lower jaw that occurs when one bares the lower teeth. Additionally, the *zygomaticus major* is the principal muscle used in laughing, whereas the *risorius* permits that facial expression associated with a nongenuine, lame, or half-attempted smile. The *platysma* is tested when one asks the patient to "wrinkle up the skin on your neck" or "pull down the corners of your mouth."

7. What is the topographic paradigm in understanding facial palsy?

The topographic paradigm in diagnosis of facial paralysis is classic in the otolaryngologic study of Bell's palsy. This idea is based on the idea that loss of function has a one-to-one correspondence with given portions of nerve that have undergone disorder. There is nothing mystifying about this. An analogy may be made of the median nerve of the upper extremity. The median nerve courses down along the shaft of the humerus and, at the cubital fossa, branches off to supply the majority of muscles of the flexor compartment of the forearm. In the event of a knife or bullet wound immediately before that branch supplying the flexor carpi radialis, preservation of function to the pronator teres would be maintained, and partial or total loss of function would manifest distal to that location.

In the same manner, a focal lesion to the facial nerve anywhere along its route would spare sensory and motor function up until but not beyond that point (Fig. 23-4). The questions that follow present the sites of lesions and their manifestations in an order that begins with the proximal and hence more severe manifestations of facial palsy and work their way to less severe manifestations as the lesion site manifests more distally.

8. How does a lesion at the internal auditory meatus manifest?

Having passed only a short distance through the posterior cranial fossa, the motor and sensory roots of the facial nerve, accompanied by the vestibulocochlearis nerve (VIII), enter the internal auditory meatus. A lesion at the entrance to the internal auditory meatus may occur from tumor of the vestibulocochlearis nerve or its nerve sheath and manifests in a full-blown facial palsy that is accompanied by deafness and possibly balance problems.[27]

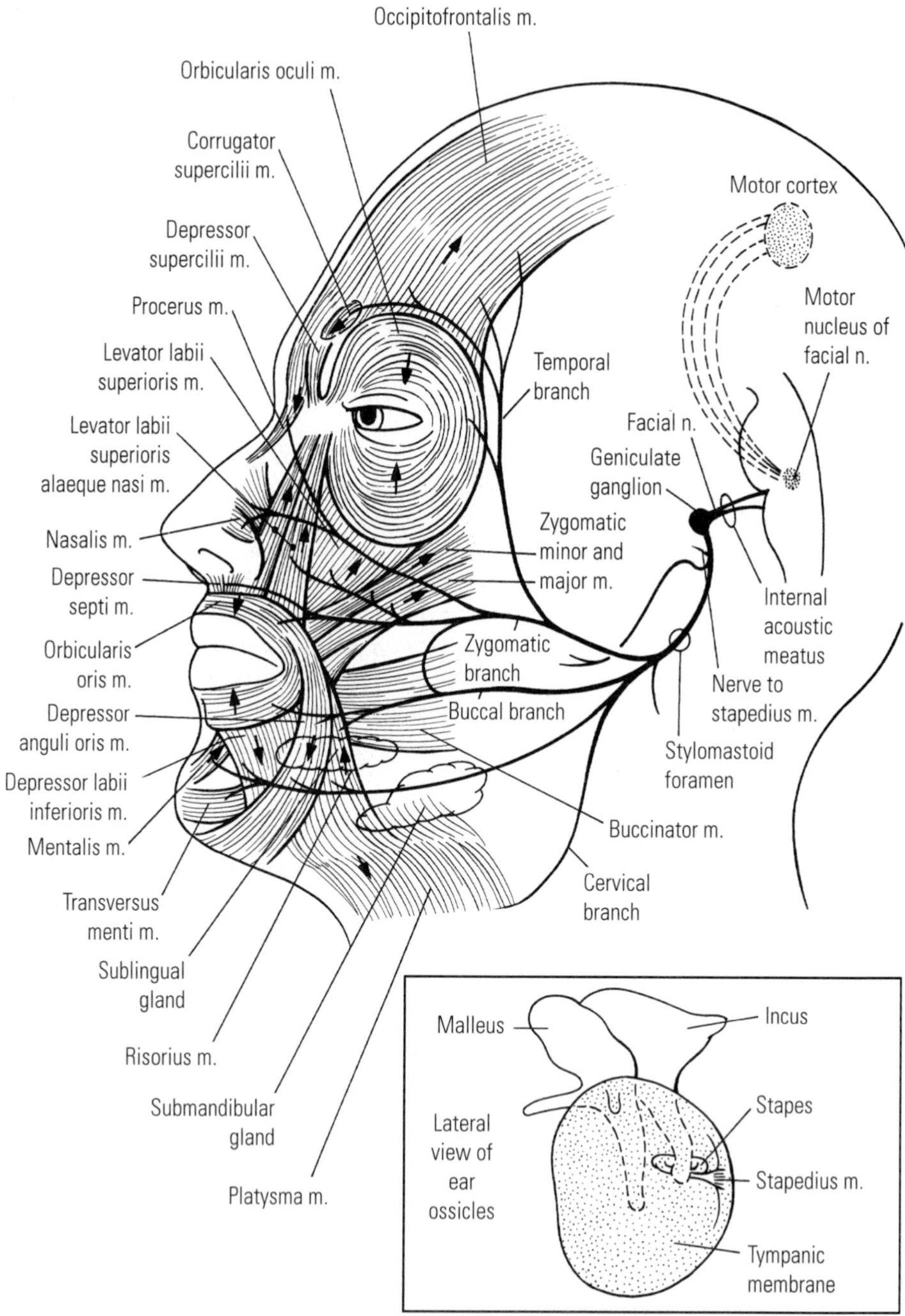

Fig. 23-3 Course and distribution of the facial nerve. *Arrows* demonstrate direction and angle of pull for respective muscles.

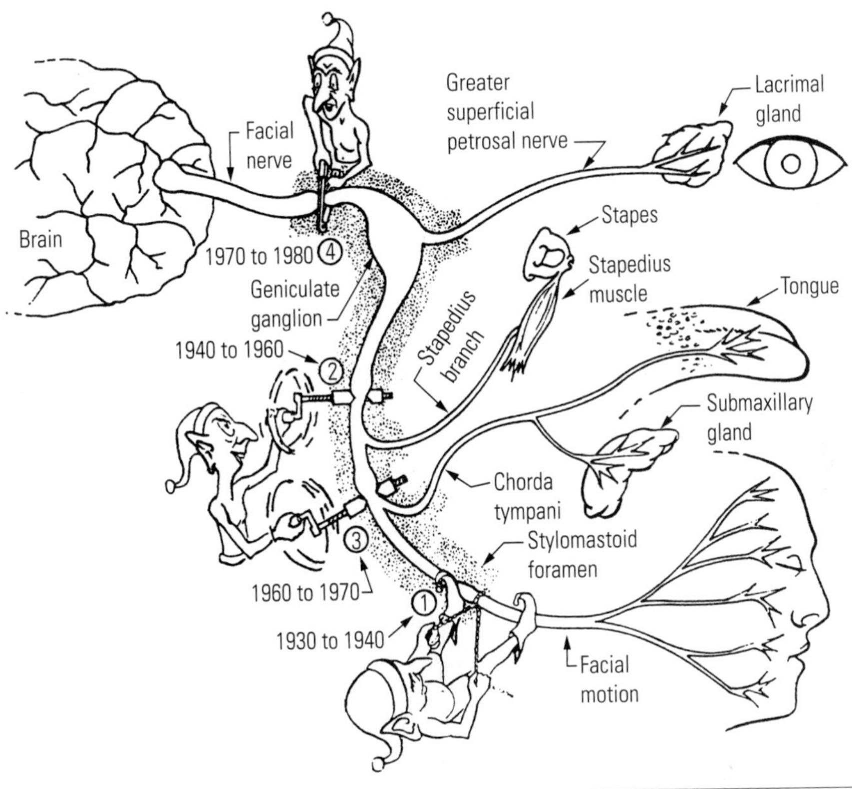

Fig. 23-4 This illustration portrays the decades-old controversy between otolaryngologists and head and neck surgeons. The latter have maintained that idiopathic facial palsy was attributable to inflammation resulting in ischemic *compression*, whereas the former correctly maintained that the operative mechanism was *autoimmune demyelinization*. Over time, head and neck surgeons slowly capitulated but nevertheless maintained that decompression was the appropriate management as specific sites were abandoned and other sites more proximal were targeted for surgery. Currently, the stalemate centers about the locale of the internal auditory meatus. This illustration may be conveniently referred to as charting the sites of lesion locales. (From Adour KK: *Otolaryngol Clin North Am* 24(3):664, 1991.)

9. How does a lesion proximal to the geniculate ganglion manifest?

A lesion proximal to the geniculate ganglion will result in diminished or lack of tear secretion and consequent eye drying, since the greater superficial petrosal nerve is blocked from transmitting parasympathetic impulses to the spinopalatine ganglion. The net result is a full-blown facial palsy accompanied by dry, red, and swollen eye.

10. How does a lesion of the geniculate ganglion manifest?

A lesion at the geniculate ganglion results in a full-blown facial palsy but with normal tear secretion, since the lacrimal fibers have been spared. In fact, it may appear as if there is an overproduction of tears, though this is actually not the case. The eye may still dry out because of weakness of the orbicularis oris. Weakness of this muscle causes the lacrimal puncta to no longer contact the glove to collect tears into the conjunctival sac. These wasted tears will then uselessly pour over the cheek rather than bathe the eye. Additionally, pain is often felt behind the ear.[27]

11. What is the manifestation of a high facial canal lesion?

A lesion high up in the facial canal refers to that area just distally beyond the geniculate ganglion and manifests with *hyperacusia* (that is, normal sounds heard abnormally loud) because of the effect of ischemia to that nerve branch supplying the stapedius muscle. Full-blown facial palsy will occur without the preceding manifestations of more proximal lesions. On examination, a decrease in or loss of the ipsilateral stapes reflex will manifest.

12. What is the function of the stapedius muscle?

The middle ear chamber is a cavity within the skull that contains the smallest bones in the body, the malleus (hammer), incus (anvil), and stapes (stirrup). These bones are suspended within the cavity by ligaments in a mechanically significant order: the distal malleus, rigidly attached to the eardrum, covers greater than one half the drum area, but the footplate of the stirrup covers the oval window, the entrance to the inner ear. These auditory ossicles form a mechanical linkage that interestingly perform a twofold antagonistic function:

- The ossicles together function as a lever mechanism to amplify pressure from sound waves imparted to the eardrum and deliver them to the oval window and are amplified considerably. This lever system enables us to hear sounds the energies of which are some 1,000 times weaker than we would otherwise hear.
- The middle ear's second function engages this same ossicle linkage to protect the inner ear from excessively loud sounds. Sound-intensity dampening is accomplished by two small muscles; one, the tensor tympani (cranial nerve V), is connected to the eardrum, the other, the *stapedius* (cranial nerve VII), inserts on the stapes (see Fig. 23-3). In the event of an intensely loud sound, these muscles contract and, in doing so, momentarily dismantle this amplifying system by drawing in the eardrum and drawing the stapes away from the oval window. Unfortunately, because this protective mechanism does not work instantaneously, sudden, intensely loud sounds can wreak permanent damage in the form of hearing loss.

13. What is the manifestation of a more distal facial canal lesion?

A lower facial canal lesion will spare the nerve to the stapedius muscle but will involve the chorda tympani, thereby causing interruption of fibers that permit normal salivation and normal taste in the anterior two thirds of the tongue. This will result in a dry mouth and an unpleasant or distorted sense of taste. These manifestations are accompanied by ipsilateral loss of facial muscle tone. There is preservation of these functions associated with more distal lesions.

14. What is the manifestation of a lesion at the stylomastoid foramen?

A lesion at the styloid foramen or at that locale where the facial nerve superficially emerges from under the earlobe results in paralysis of the entire ipsilateral facial musculature. These are most obvious as a loss of the ability to wrinkle the forehead, whistle, or wink.

15. How does facial palsy of the upper motor neuron type differ from Bell's palsy, which is of the lower motor neuron type?

Supranuclear lesions by definition involve the upper motor neuron that traverses between the cerebral cortex, through the internal capsule, and terminates on the sensory or motor facial nuclei located in the brainstem. Clinically differentiating between a Bell's palsy and a facial palsy that occurred after a focal cerebrovascular accident is made easy by understanding the following neuroanatomy. The rostral portion of the motor nucleus is responsible for supplying nerve fibers to the superior facial muscles, that is, the area around the forehead and around the eyes. Unlike other portions of the nucleus, the rostral portion innervates its assigned area by both crossed *and* uncrossed corticobulbar tract collaterals. Because of this anomaly, facial paralysis after a stroke affects only the lower two thirds of the face while sparing the eyes and forehead. This bilateral innervation does not occur in the lower motor neuron, and therefore facial paralysis of the intranuclear kind, of which Bell's palsy is but one type, will involve the entire face and is only unilaterally innervated[27] (Fig. 23-5). A stroke above the level of the brainstem would also spare taste and hearing.

Additionally, with palsy resulting from an upper motor neuron lesion, the patient can partially often hide his palsy by smiling, since there is preservation of emotionally motivated movement. This fact implies that

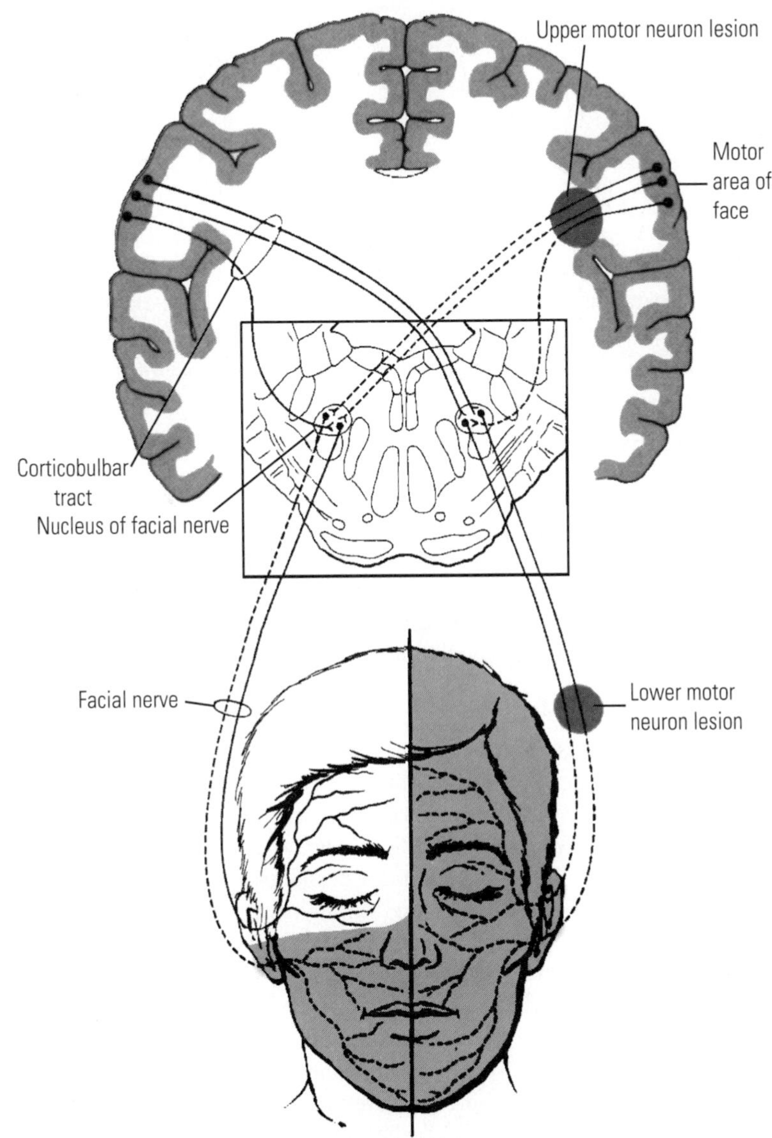

Fig. 23-5 Bell's palsy involves the lower motor neuron (infranuclear lesion) and manifests as a global facial asymmetry involving the ipsilateral upper and lower quadrants. Supranuclear lesions involving the primary (that is, upper) motor neuron result in facial asymmetry in the lower two thirds of the face. The shaded areas of the face show the distribution of paralyzed facial muscles. (From Gilman S, Winans S: *Essentials of clincial neuroanatomy and neurophysiology*, ed 6, Philadelphia, 1982, FA Davis.)

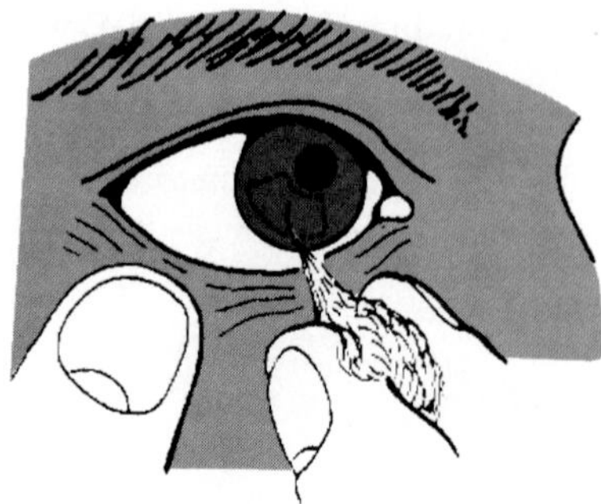

Fig. 23-6 The correct way to elicit the corneal blink test. (From Patten J: *Neurological differential diagnosis,* ed 2, London, 1996, Springer-Verlag.)

emotionally motivated output to the facial nucleus follows a pathway other than the corticospinal tract.

Finally, the degree of paralysis of facial musculature differs, depending on whether the lesion is of the upper or lower motor neuron type. An upper motor neuron lesion will result in contralateral *spastic* paralysis of the lower two thirds of the face, whereas a lower motor neuron lesion will result in ipsilateral *flaccid* paralysis to the entire face on one side.

16. What is the corneal blink test?

The corneal blink reflex is mediated by an afferent (sensory) component by cranial nerve V and an efferent (motor) component controlled by cranial nerve VII. The correct way to elicit the corneal reflex is to touch a tiny swab of cotton to the *unilateral* colored cornea and not the white sclera (Fig. 23-6). The felt sensation is transmitted to the brain by the trigeminal nerve, whereas the efferent blinking response normally manifests in blinking of *both* eyelids. In true Bell's palsy, touching the cornea of the affected side will consensually cause the contralateral eye to close. This is not the case with upper motor neuron lesions.

17. What is the differential diagnosis?

Bell's palsy has a diagnosis of exclusion. Diagnosis is reserved for patients in which an exhaustive search for a cause has proved fruitless. The following conditions also cause facial hemiparalysis.

- *Melkerson-Rosenthal syndrome*, perhaps a form of sarcoidosis, is distinguished from idiopathic facial palsy, since it also includes recurrent facial swelling (edema) particularly of the lip and eyelid that is nonpitting, painless, and short lived (that is, lasting several days). Cheilitis (chapping and swelling of edematous lips) as well as fissuring of the tongue,[24] though the latter is the least common component of this syndrome, present in approximately one third of all cases. Additionally, contralateral unilateral *facial palsy* characteristically accompanies this condition.[32]
- *Otitis media* is a bacterial or viral middle ear infection secondary to an upper respiratory infection that travels from the nasopharynx to the middle ear via the eustachian tube. Disease onset may occur at any age but is most common in young children. The very first complaint is severe earache with or without hearing loss. With time, the tympanic membrane may bulge and eventually rupture, releasing built-up exudate. Symptoms of impending complications include headache, sudden profound hearing loss, vertigo, chills, and fever. Among the complications of this unfortunate condition are *facial paralysis* and brain abscess.[9]
- *Ramsey-Hunt syndrome* (synonym: herpes zoster oticus or cephalicus, or geniculate herpes) is a condition that involves invasion of the eighth cranial nerve ganglion and the geniculate ganglion of the seventh cranial nerve by the same culprit responsible for shingles, chickenpox, and Bell's palsy. Clinical

signs include ipsilateral hearing loss, vertigo or ataxia, and pain. The latter sign is almost always present and more severe when compared to Bell's palsy, and is accompanied by vesicle eruption developing over the four divisions of the facial nerve, that is, those sensory fibers supplying the posteromedial pinna and external auditory canal. Vesicles may be noticed before the onset of facial paralysis but may also appear up to 10 days later. *Facial paralysis* may be either transient or permanent. Because of involvement at the level of the geniculate ganglion, decreased taste, diminished salivary flow, and dry mouth will also manifest.[9]

- *Lyme disease* is a spirochete disorder spread by a deer tick and, in addition to facial palsy, is accompanied by a skin lesion characterized by a red macule or papule, usually on the proximal portion of the extremity or trunk, such as the thigh, buttock, or axilla. Malaise, fatigue, chills and fever, headache, stiff neck, myalgias, arthalgias, nausea and vomiting, as well as a sore throat also occur. The hallmark of this disease, however, is the skin lesion that is erythematous and macular with a pale center. *Facial palsy* is the commonest neurologic manifestation of mild meningitis that is characteristic of stage II of Lyme disease. The problem with definitive diagnosis is that there is no *good* test for Lyme disease. Unless treatment with broad-spectrum antibiotics or tetracycline is initiated early on, the disease may, in some instances, progress undetected to stage III, which is characterized by chronic fatigue syndrome and multiple sclerosis–like symptoms. One must be especially suspicious in cases of children diagnosed with juvenile rheumatoid arthritis who live in endemic areas.[9]
- *Botulism* caused facial palsy is bilateral and includes red (and parched) tongue, oropharynx, nasopharynx, and larynx. Botulism is a form of neuromuscular poisoning that decreases release of acetylcholine from presynaptic terminals. Neurologic symptoms are bilateral and symmetrical, and involvement begins with the cranial nerves and descends caudally. Neurologic symptoms are commonly preceded by nausea, vomiting, abdominal cramps, and diarrhea. Diagnosis is established by toxin isolation from stool specimen.[9]
- *Leprosy* (synonym: Hansen's disease) is a chronic infectious disease caused by a bacillus that has a predilection for cooler body areas, namely, skin, mucous membranes, and those peripheral nerves coursing closest to the surface of the body. Terminal cutaneous branches of the *facial nerve* typically become involved, including those branches to the orbicularis oculi, the orbicularis oris, and the medial parts of the corrugator supercilii muscles, manifesting in an inability to completely close one's eyes (lagophthalmos).[9]
- *Malignancies*. Neoplasms are suggested by a slowly progressing palsy that may spare some branches of the facial nerve but may culminate in complete involvement of that nerve (cerebellopontine angle tumor). Especially suspect are patients having a history of cancer, particularly of the breast, lung, thyroid, kidney, ovary, or prostate. Tumor is to be suspected when there is no recovery of *facial palsy* after 6 months. It is appropriate to palpate for masses in the parotid, submandibular gland, or neck. If the latter are found, referral is promptly made to a physician for skull imaging by radiographs or CT scan.[24]
- *Birth trauma*. Forceps injury can injure the nerve in the face or in the soft petrous bone, especially in light of the lack of a well-developed mastoid process that affords protection of the facial nerve. This is normally absent or poorly developed in the infant, although these children have a high incidence of recovery (approximately 90%). In the adult, injury to the facial nerve may occur after trauma either at the stylomastoid foramen, penetrating injury to the middle ear, facial injury, or fracture of the temporal bone. Such an injury will result in ecchymosis (Battle's sign) around the pinna and mastoid process. Barotrauma is caused by scuba diving and altitude paralysis.
- *Other manifestations*. Other manifestations of facial palsy that must also be ruled out include Guillain-Barré syndrome, poliomyelitis, multiple sclerosis, leukemia, osteomyelitis, Piaget's disease, meningococcal meningitis, infectious mononucleosis (Epstein-Barr virus), syphilis, malaria, cat-scratch disease, herpes zoster cephalicus, otitis media, myasthenia gravis, AIDS, alcoholic neuropathy, vitamin A deficiency, and polyneuritis. Toxic causes include arsenic, carbon monoxide, thalidomide, and ethylene glycol. Iatrogenic causes include mandibular block anesthesia; vaccine therapy for rabies, polio, or influenza; parotid surgery or mastoid surgery; or iontophoresis.[24]

18. What is the prognosis for recovery?

Prognosis very much depends on the extent of nerve damage. Generally the more proximal the lesion, the poorer is the prognosis. Complete resolution occurs in 75% to 80% of most patients who have succumbed to partial facial paralysis,[27] whereas the results after total paralysis are variable. The likelihood of complete recovery is 90% if the nerve proximal in the face retains normal excitability to supramaximal stimulation diminishes to 20% in the event that electrical excitability is absent.[9] Recovery, when it occurs, ordinarily begins within 1 to 4 weeks, may take longer than 8 months, but is always achieved by 12 months after onset.[24] Relapses are uncommon but occur in a minority of patients.

Ten to fifteen percent of all patients have incomplete or inappropriate reinnervation.[27] In the latter scenario, as the nerve regenerates, its sprouting branches may mistakenly innervate muscles not previously supplied by the facial nerve. This misdirected and aberrant growth may innervate lower facial muscles with periocular fibers or vice versa, resulting in contraction of unexpected facial movement on voluntary facial movement *(synkinesia)*. For example, a patient may inadvertently smile when attempting a volitional blink. In contrast, the patient may cry *crocodile tears* instead of salivating when tasting or chewing (but not smelling) food.[9]

19. What is the medical management of Bell's palsy?

- Treatment with prednisone is not of proved benefit but seems to decrease acute pain and therefore ought to be administered soon (as with the first 72 hours) after onset.[2]
- Prevention of corneal ulceration caused by drying out of the exposed eye is mandatory. This is accomplished by use of methyl cellulose drops or use of an eye patch, especially at night.[9]

20. What is the traditional therapeutic management of Bell's palsy?

- Iontophoresis with hydrocortisone to decrease inflammation is appropriately applied before electrical stimulation. Treatment ought to be performed over the ipsilateral cheek, where that nerve runs subcutaneously, and not focally at the stylomastoid foramen. Phonophoresis may also be used.[21]
- Interrupted direct current and negative polarity, with the positive electrode on the ipsilateral forearm. Some 10 to 20 stimuli, repeated three times per session, are applied to the motor points of muscles of the facial nerve distribution.[21] The rationale behind electric stimulation is not that it will cause healing of the nerve; rather it simply maintains the involved muscles' tone until such time that reinnervation occurs. Thus electric stimulation prevents the muscles from becoming fibrotic or fatty after disuse.[9]
- Application of cold laser to the acupuncture points that relate to facial nerve distribution.[21]
- Massage to both involved and noninvolved facial musculature.
- Regimen of facial exercises.
- Of prime importance is psychologic support provided to the patient throughout the ordeal.

21. Why are nonspecific gross facial exercises inadequate to the management repertoire of Bell's palsy?

The efficacy of Craig's "face-saving exercises"[12] is questioned when we consider that gross exercises tend to reinforce abnormal movement patterns.[6] Asking a patient to open his or her mouth widely or move the lower lip from side to side does little but train compensatory movements by way of the masseter muscle or muscles. Asking the patient to move his or her eyes up, down, to the right, and to the left only trains eye movements. Requests such as close the eyes tightly, puff out the cheeks, or broadly laugh, may serve only to promote mass movement and synkinesis,[5] since the maximum effort needed to express these gross movements recruits excessive numbers of motor units.[14]

Because the ratio of muscle fibers to motor neurons is approximately 25 to 1, the facial muscles possess a high index for refinement of movement (compared to the 2000-to-1 ratio in the gastrocnemius).[23] As such, the intricacy and complexity of movement precludes the use of maximum-effort exercises, since motor units other than those targeted may be recruited because of overflow.[22]

22. What are the psychologic ramifications to the patient's being afflicted with facial palsy?

Our face is usually the first and often lasting impression and memory we have on others. How we look deeply affects our self-esteem. This sentiment was eloquently expressed by the Roman consul Cicero (106-43 B.C.) when he described how "The face is the image of the soul."[11] However, more than simply a cosmetic deformity, facial paralysis is very much a disability of communication. Minute changes in facial expression account primarily for human nonverbal communication. This is reflected in the proportionally large area of the motor homunculus that is associated with control of the facial muscles.

Depression, guilt, anger, hostility, anxiety, rejection, and paranoia have been noted after facial paralysis has occurred.[33] Patients may be considered mentally deficient[19] and experience difficulties with interpersonal relationships, employability, making friends, and coping with looks of disgust or horror in others' faces.[16]

To the patient afflicted with facial paralysis, the psychosocial effect may be devastating. Feeling that they are freaks, patients will develop compensatory strategies that they believe will help hide their newfound deformity. Patients may maintain their faces relatively immobile and expressionless so as not to accentuate their paralysis. Patients may habitually sit with slouched postures, often with their head tilted with a hand covering and hiding the involved side from view.[7] Regrettably the sum total of these compensations may cause inhibition of the patient's natural affect and personality.[5] The therapist must gently work with the patient by providing emotional support by allowing the patient to vent his or her feelings. Suggested topics for discussion include discussing and identifying family and friends who, since the start of the patient's facial paralysis, are (1) no longer their friends, (2) are somewhat negative, (3) have always been supportive, and (4) are newly supportive (such as a facial paralysis support group).[5] With time and progress the patient is taught to reverse this denial and decreased facial awareness by encouraging self-esteem.[5]

23. What neuromuscular training (NMR) techniques are available to the patient after facial paralysis?

Facial neuromuscular retraining is a problem-solving approach to facial paralysis that utilizes specific reeducation techniques to promote symmetrical movement while inhibiting undesired movement patterns. The skilled therapist provides feedback training that is supplemented by mirror or electromyographic feedback tailored to the specific needs of the patient. An essential and key element to this approach is the successful implementation of a structured home program.

NMR emphasizes very small and slow, very symmetrical, and very isolated movements with an emphasis on quality of movement. This is in contrast to traditional gross motor strengthening exercises, which tend to reinforce mass movement and promote synkinesis. Normal facial movements are subtle and never harsh or performed with maximum effort.

Recapturing movement is an early goal of treatment. NMR often begins with an attempt to improve the critical function of eye closure. This is accomplished by having the patient focus on making controlled and small movements, aided by the therapist and a mirror. When the patient can execute a faint closure of the eye without other facial twitches occurring simultaneously, he or she may attempt a more definitive eye closure. For example, the patient learns to close his or her eyes very slowly while trying not to let the corner of the mouth move. With constant repetition, the patient learns to control eye closure with less and less conscious awareness. Over time the patient progresses to learn to perform the movement more quickly and forcefully and eventually automatically access that movement in a variety of different circumstances and settings. Accomplishing this milestone is followed by addressing the patient's own goals, such as having a normal smile, improving speech, and eating and drinking.

24. What is the premise of NMR, and for what population is it appropriate?

The premise behind a facial retraining program is the capacity of the central nervous system to modify its organization so as to engram new motor patterns within the existing motor repertoire. Facial retraining techniques may also be used in postacute patients suffering from facial paralysis caused by accidental injury, congenital reasons, carcinoma, postoperative nerve pain, postsurgical tumor resection, herpes zoster oticus, or Guillain-Barré syndrome.[14] NMR may be tailored to the many kinds of neurologic impairments ranging from spinal cord injury, peripheral neuropathy, and cerebrovascular accident.

25. What is the role of therapy in NMR?

The therapist's role is to formulate very specific goals, monitor progress, and serve as feedback to the patient. For example, the therapist may inform the patient, "The corner of your mouth is closing when you're chewing." Thus the therapist's role is to direct a recovery program rather than perform it.

26. What is the role of the home exercise program in NMR?

The patient with facial paralysis is typically involved in the NMR programs for 1 to 3 years during which time some 90% of treatment is performed by the patient at home.[13] Because no two patients have the same functional profile, no two treatment or home programs will be the same. The challenge to the therapist is that he or she must devise exercises to address very specific goals that the patient can perform a varying number of times throughout the day. A successful home program requires self-discipline on the part of the patient and tenacious persistence and adherence to performance of exercises. When the patient achieves success with a specific goal and replicates it with 75% accuracy, the therapist builds upon that success by slightly modifying the strategy.

Structuring therapy in this manner is cost effective in that it reduces the number of billed clinic hours while maximizing the number of patient participation hours. The demands of successful outcome often require a highly motivated patient who follows through with 30 to 60 minutes of consistent, concentrated practice every day. Patients periodically return to the clinic setting to refine movement patterns, learn new exercises, document progress, and establish new treatment goals.[13]

27. When is NMR management not appropriate?

Typically, two stages of recovery occur after the emergence of facial paralysis. During the first stage of nerve regeneration, healing occurs slowly and corresponds to a lack of any facial movement. Initiating intensive therapy at this early stage is inappropriate and may be detrimental to eventual recovery. Like a broken bone protected from stress by the cast,[13] the nerve must first recover before initiation of therapy. Active attempts at exercise before clinical evidence to reinnervation, that is, active facial movement serves only to exacerbate the condition[29] by causing overactivity in the musculature in the intact side.

Waiting for movement to occur can be frustrating for both patient and therapist, though most patients begin to demonstrate movement in 5 to 12 months.[15] The referral time for Bell's palsy is typically delayed until 3 months after onset because of the high probability of spontaneous recovery before that time. If paralysis persists after 3 months, recovery may be incomplete with the development of synkinesis,[4,25] at which point patients should be referred for NMR. Acoustic neuroma or the subsequent surgery is another common cause for facial paralysis. Since the auditory nerve (VIII) and the facial nerve

(VII) course adjacent to each other, the facial nerve may incur damage by the tumor or operative procedure. Postoperative facial weakness, altered taste sensation, and excessively dry or wet eyes are attributable to the reaction of the nerve to the tumor itself or to separation during surgery. The optimal time for referral of these patients is when minimal facial movement becomes apparent, or as synkinesis begins to develop, or by 12 months after onset if no movement has occurred. Recovery typically begins between 5 and 12 months after surgery.[30]

28. What is the optimal time for referral?

The second stage of recovery is characterized by the emergence of small facial movements. As recovery continues, the patient may notice movements beginning in areas of the face that they are not trying to move. This may manifest as eye closure during speech or pulling upward of the corner of the mouth when one is shutting the eye. The presence of this excess movement is known as *synkinesis* and is defined as abnormal synchronization of muscles that ordinarily do not contract together. These movements may occur with volitional or spontaneous movements. Synkinetic movement may pull antagonistically, like a tug-of-war, against the normal, primary movement. Synkinesis may vary in severity from subtle to severe and, in its worst form, mass action, may result in gross deformity of the affected side during any attempted expression. The involved side of the face may feel tight and even painful as the result of uncontrolled muscle contractions.

Thus patients should be referred to NMR when visible signs of return become apparent or once synkinesis is noted. There is no time limit for when facial retraining may begin. Improvements may even occur years after onset.[15]

29. What are the essential components to neuromuscular retraining?

Proper treatment environment. The proper learning environment is enhanced by a quiet, individual room where therapy may be conducted without distraction. This kind of privacy creates a "safe" setting for the patient embarrassed by his or her appearance. Here, they may work undistracted by social stigma and feelings of self-consciousness.

A thorough initial *evaluation* is imperative and determines the degree of available volitional movement, spontaneous movement, and presence of any synkinesis or mass action. The use of videotape is invaluable in capturing sequential facial movements as they occur. Photographic evaluation is valuable because it allows the patient to notice small changes occurring over time that may otherwise not be readily visible. Patients should view photographs reflected in a mirror to preserve the relative position of the paralyzed side.[14]

Patient *motivation* and *cognition* are necessary components to a successful outcome. Cognitive or attention deficits often associated with cerebrovascular accident or accidental brain injury may preclude participation in an NMR program. Similarly, it is imperative that the patient maintain consistency of practice with intense and disciplined concentration during his or her home program away from the clinic.

30. What is the method of NMR?

Patient education lays the foundation for learning selective movement patterns that lead to improved motor function. The therapist educates the patient in basic facial anatomy, kinesiology, angle of muscle pull (see Fig. 23-4), and physiology needed to understand the procedures and goals of treatment. Patients are made partners in their rehabilitation.

Exploration of facial movement. Most persons are not conscious of the specific movements involved in normal facial expression. The patient is instructed to perform small, specific movements on the contralateral side. The initial treatments are a time of discovery for the patient as he or she learns to identify specific areas of function and dysfunction and begin, with the therapist, to formulate strategies to improve facial movement.[14]

Biofeedback is used as an evaluative and a therapeutic tool. As an evaluative tool, surface electrode electromyography (seEMG) biofeedback is used to detect the presence of any functional return of hypoactive muscles before any visually observed facial movement. Weak electrical impulses may be demonstrated and made accessible to the patient in the form of a tone or visible oscilloscope trace in what appears to be an otherwise flaccid muscle. As a therapeutic tool seEMG may be used to increase activity in weak muscles, decrease activity in hyperactive muscles, and improve coordination of muscle groups.

The purpose of seEMG is to bring the normally unconscious control of specific muscles under conscious control. By correlating information from seEMG feedback with proprioceptive and mirror feedback, the patient slowly learns to reproduce new movement patterns outside the clinical setting in the context of a home exercise program.

31. What are the two categories of motor disturbance that facial paralysis is classified into?

Facial paralysis falls into one of two categories, each of which requires different treatment strategies:

- Flaccid paralysis or paresis in which *hypoactivity* dominates. The goal here is to increase muscle activity.
- Synkinesis or mass action. The goal here is to inhibit excess movement in *hyperactive* muscles so as to stave off abnormal and unsynchronous facial movement.
- Improve coordination of muscle groups.[14]

32. What NMR treatment strategy addresses the patient with flaccid paralysis or paresis?

Retraining strategies are an attempt to produce fine motor control of a single muscle or muscle group (such as the levator anguli oris–zygomaticus) are initially developed on the noninvolved side. This is accomplished by having the patient slowly contract these muscles (as in a broad smile) while observing the corresponding seEMG trace with the setting at a relatively low setting. The patient's task is to make appropriate contractions such that even a trace contraction appears as a ramp on the oscilloscope. This is repeated at even higher sensitivity levels until very small and slow facial contractions yield the same ramp function. The patient must focus on how the movement feels as it is being produced. Thus a base line is created for the normal function of that particular muscle. This is invaluable for the patient as the patient uses his or her newfound awareness of this isolated contraction to facilitate replication of this motor action on the involved side.[7]

Next, the patient is encouraged to "shift" his or her feeling of the fine motor control learned on the uninvolved side to the involved side. This painstaking process is aided by use of seEMG in which the patient sits in a darkened room and observes the EMG oscilloscope. The patient observes ramping produced by the uninvolved side and attempts to replicate that ramp by small facial movement on the involved side. This may be repeated thousands of times over as much as 25 1-hour sessions until a small isolated contraction is voluntarily and consistently performed. To prevent diminishment and extinguishment of this newfound contraction, amplification of this movement is necessary so that the patient may see small movements of the involved side in a mirror. Once visible movement is acquired EMG sensory biofeedback is immediately discontinued for that muscle and specific action exercises (SAE) are implemented with mirror feedback to obtain greater voluntary muscle control.[7] The patient is thus weaned from seEMG when he or she has successfully internalized a movement. The patient and a significant other, if possible, are trained in enhancing this motion by exercising exactly as instructed by the therapist. The therapist trains the patient to train himself or herself. Self-esteem, improved physical function, and satisfaction improve as the patient learns to assume control of his or her recovery.

Movements must be initiated slowly and gradually so that the patient may observe and modify the angle, strength, and speed of the excursion as it occurs. Otherwise, rapidly performed movements may revert to an abnormal motor pattern. Similarly, movements must be small in nature so as to limit motor-unit recruitment to those muscles targeted.[22] Large-scale movements serve only to recruit larger numbers of motor units resulting in overflow and diminished accuracy. Finally, movements must be equal on both sides to achieve symmetrical expression. Allowing the uninvolved side to dominate may possibly shunt excess tone to that side, resulting in diminishment of activity on the involved side.[7]

Approximately 90% of the patient's therapy program is carried out in the home setting. Treatment sessions may range from 2 hours per month (for local patients) to an intensive treatment session of 1 to 12 hours of space over 3 to 4 days every 6 months (for patients traveling a great distance). The entire course of therapy may last 18 months to 3 years.[34] During this time the frequency of clinic visits decreases as the patient becomes increasingly proficient in performing his or her home exercise program. Clinic visits involve identifying new problem areas and establishing new goals.

33. What NMR treatment strategy addresses the patient with synkinesis or mass action?

The first step in the treatment of synkinesis is to decrease hypertonus. Increased facial tone, tightness, or rigidity may be present on the affected side and is most likely caused by increased background muscle activity.[35] This activity may be observed as an increased nasolabial fold (musculus levator, m. zygomaticus), decreased palpebral fissure (m. orbicularis oculi), retraction of the corner of the mouth (m. zygomaticus, m. risorius), dimpling of the chin (m. mentalis or the depressors), drawing down of the corner of the mouth (depressors and platysma), and banding of the neck (platysma). Abnormal tone in the lips may manifest as thinning or "puffiness."[14]

Reduction of resting tone is imperative before the inhibition of synkinesis because normal movement cannot be superimposed on abnormal tone. The patient is taught to become aware that facial tightness or stiffness is caused by increased muscle activity at rest, followed by general relaxation training, and seEMG feedback.[5,10] Relaxation of all muscles of the face is necessary so as to prevent the muscles on the noninvolved side from overacting during attempted voluntary movements. Massage of the affected side is helpful over those areas where thickening and immobility are observed.[8,31]

As an example of synkinesis, consider the patient who demonstrates zygomatic activity on attempted smiling but who also expresses synkinesis of the platysma and limited zygomatic excursion. Instead of the expected upward curl at the angle of the mouth (a smile), he or she demonstrates a drawing down at the angle of the mouth (a grimace). By focusing attention on the precisely correct movement pattern, the patient initiated the primary movement slowly while monitoring the areas of synkinesis vigilantly from the start. As synkinesis becomes visible, the primary movement is maintained while the synkinetic response is reduced. This difficult process requires complete concentration so as to "release" the synkinetic area. The exact timing of this sequence is essential for dissociation of synkinesis from primary movement. By inhibition of synkinesis of the platysma, the zygomaticus gains a more normal range of movement without the antagonistic effect of the platysma, resulting in a more natural smile.

Once achieved, the patient may then relax the primary movement as inhibition of synkinesis requires less concentration, and excursion of the primary movement increases as control is learned. Initially this movement pattern may occur only volitionally, whereas over time these patterns are demonstrated spontaneously.[8,31]

34. What is the rationale behind electrical stimulation as a treatment modality?

Research during the 1960s has shown that electrical stimulation of a denervated muscle actually retards in growth of neurofibrils to the motor end plate.[7] The deinnervated neurofibril has no motivation to grow into the motor end plate if it's being electrically stimulated. In response to this, many insurance companies have since refused payment for a treatment that was deemed unjustified. This, in fact, was proved only during the initial 3 to 4 weeks during which fibrillation manifested. Rather, in deference to the aforementioned study, faradic (that is, direct-current) stimulation is appropriate but should rather begin some 28 to 30 days after onset, since that is the time when fibrillation has decreased.

The clinical use of electrotherapy remains controversial. Although nerve conduction and muscle contraction do occur, the reduction of circulatory stasis, increased muscle and nerve nutrition, and the reduction of muscle atrophy have yet to be proved.[5] Furthermore, because of the small size and proximity of the facial muscles, it is difficult to produce an isolated contraction of a specific muscle using electric stimulation. Such large-scale contractions may cause mass action[14] and possibly contribute to synkinesis,[14] which serve only to reinforce abnormal motor patterns.

35. When is surgery appropriate?

In a small percentage of patients axonal regeneration is ineffective, and hypoglossal facial nerve anastomosis may partially restore facial function if none has returned in 6 to 12 months.[4]

References

1. Adour KK: Medical management of idiopathic (Bell's) palsy, *Otolaryngol Clin North Am* 24(3):664, 1991.
2. Adour KK, Bell DN, Hilsinger RL Jr: Herpes simplex virus in idiopathic facial paralysis (Bell's palsy), *JAMA* 233:527-530, 1975.
3. Adour KK, Byl FM, Hilsinger RL Jr, et al: The true nature of Bell's palsy: analysis of 1000 consecutive patients, *Laryngoscope* 88:787-801, 1978.
4. Anderson RG: Facial nerve disorders, *Select Readings in Plastic Surgery* 6:1-34, 1991.
5. Balliet R: Facial paralysis and other neuromuscular dysfunction of the peripheral nervous system. In Payton OD, DiFabio RP, Paris SV, et al, editors: *Manual of physical therapy*, New York, 1989, Churchill Livingstone.
6. Balliet R, Lewis L: *Hypothesis: Craig's "face saving exercises" may cause facial dysfunction*, Edmonton, Alberta, April 1985, Canadian Acoustic Neuroma Association.
7. Balliet R, Shinn JB, Bach-y-Rita P: Facial paralysis rehabilitation: retraining selective muscle control, *Int Rehabil Med* 4:67-74, 1981.
8. Barat M: Principles of rehabilitation in facial paralysis. In Portmann M, editor: *Facial nerve*, New York, 1985, Masson.
9. Berkow R: *The Merck manual of diagnosis and therapy*, ed 15, Rahway, N.J., 1987, Merck Sharp & Dohme Research Laboratories.
10. Brundy J, Hammerschlag PE, Cohen NL, et al: Electromyographic rehabilitation of facial function and introduction of a facial paralysis grading scale for hypoglossal facial nerve anastomosis, *Laryngoscope* 98:405-410, 1988.
11. Cicero: In Stevenson B, editor: *Macmillan book of proverbs, maxims and famous phrases*, New York, 1948, Macmillan.
12. Craig M: Face saving exercises, New York, 1970, Random House.
13. Diels HJ: *Neuromuscular retraining for facial paralysis*, issue no 55, Sept 1995, Acoustic Neuroma Association, Carlisle, Penna.
14. Diels HJ: New concepts in nonsurgical facial nerve rehabilitation. Myers EN, Bluestone CD, editors: *Advances in otolaryngology—head and neck surgery*, vol 9, St. Louis, 1995, Mosby.
15. Diels HJ: Unpublished data. In endnotes of Ref. 14.
16. Elks MA: Another look at facial disfigurement, *J Rehabil* (Jan to Mar):36-40, 1990.
17. Hause SL, Levitt LP, Weiner HL: *Case studies in neurology for the house officer*, Baltimore, 1986, Williams & Wilkins, p 97.
18. Hause WA, Karnes WE, Annis J, et al : Incidence and prognosis of Bell's palsy in the population of Rochester, Minnesota, *Mayo Clin Proc* 46:258-264, 1971.
19. Hoos L, Devriese PP: The management of psychological problems of patients with facial paralysis. In Portmann M, editor: *Facial nerve*, New York, 1985, Masson.
20. Jansen JKS, Lomo T, Nicolaysen K, et al: Hyperinnervation of skeletal muscle fibers: dependence on muscle activity, *Science*, 181:559-561, 1973.
21. Kahn J: *Principles and practice of electrotherapy*, ed 2, New York, 1991, Churchill Livingstone.
22. Kottke FJ: Therapeutic exercise to develop neuromuscular coordination. In Kottke FJ, Lehmann JF, editors: *Krusen's handbook of physical medicine and rehabilitation*, ed 4, Philadelphia, 1990, Saunders.

23. May J: Microanatomy and pathophysiology of the facial nerve. In May M, editor: *The facial nerve*, New York, 1986, Thieme.
24. May M, Klein SR: Differential diagnosis of facial nerve palsy, *Otolaryngol Clin North Am* 24(3):615-616, 1991.
25. May M, Podvinec M, Ulrich J, et al: Idiopathic (Bell's) palsy, herpes zoster cephalicus and other facial nerve disorders of viral orgin. In May M, editor: *The facial nerve*, New York, 1986, Thieme.
26. Mendel GL, Douglas XX, Bennet XX: *Principles and practice of infectious diseases*, ed 3, New York, 1990, Churchill Livingstone, pp 1139-1147.
27. Netter FH: *The CIBA collection of medical illustrations*, vol 1: *Nervous system*, part 2, Summit, N.J., 1986, CIBA-Geigy Corp.
28. Peitersen E: The nature history of Bell's palsy, *Am J Otol* 4:107-111, 1982.
29. Ross B, Nedzelski JM, McLean JA: Efficacy of feedback training in long-standing facial nerve paresis, *Laryngoscope* 101:744-750, 1991.
30. Sataloff RT, Myers DL, Kremer FB: Management of cranial nerve injury following surgery of the skull base, *Otolaryngol Clin North Am* 17:577-589, 1984.
31. Schram G, Burres S: Nonsurgical rehabilitation after facial paralysis. In Portmann M, editor: *Facial nerve*, New York, 1985, Masson.
32. Stevens H: Melkersson's syndrome, *Neurology*, 15:263-266, 1965.
33. Twerski A, Twerski B: The emotional impact of facial paralysis. In May M, editor: *The facial nerve*, New York, 1986, Thieme.
34. Data compiled from the University of Wisconsin Neuromuscular Retraining Clinic fact sheet.
35. Valls-Sole J, Tolosa ES, Pujol M: Myokymic discharges and enhanced facial nerve reflex responses after recovery from idiopathic facial palsy, *Muscle Nerve* 15:37-42, 1992.

Recommended reading

Adour KK: Medical management of idiopathic (Bell's) palsy, *Otolaryngol Clin North Am* 24(3):663, 1991.

Balliet R: Facial paralysis and other neuromuscular dysfunctions of the peripheral nervous system. In Payton OD, DiFabio RP, Paris, SV, et al: *Manual of physical therapy*, New York, 1989, Churchill Livingstone.

Balliet R, Lewis L: *Hypothesis: Craig's "Face Saving Exercises" may cause facial dysfunction,* Edmonton, Alberta, April 1985, Acoustic Neuroma Association of Canada.

Balliet R, Shinn JB, Bach-Y-Rita P: Facial paralysis rehabilitation: retraining selective muscle control, *Int Rehabil Med* 4:67-74, 1991.

Diels HJ: *Neuromuscular retraining for facial paralysis*, issue no 55, Sept 1995, Acoustic Neuroma Association, Carlisle, Penna.

Diels HJ: New concepts in nonsurgical facial nerve rehabilitation. In Myers EN, Bluestone CD, editors: *Advances in otolaryngology–head and neck surgery*, vol 9, 1995, St. Louis, Mosby.

Hauser SL, Levitt LP, Weiner HL: Case studies in neurology for the house officer, Baltimore, 1986, Williams & Wilkins, pp 94-98.

Kahn J: *Principles and practice of electrotherapy*, ed 2, New York, 1990, Churchill Livingstone, pp 92 and 154.

May M: Differential diagnosis of facial nerve palsy, *Otolaryngol Clin North Am* 24(3):613, 1991.

For more information regarding facial retraining, the reader is referred to: Neuromuscular retraining clinic. University of Wisconsin Hospital & Clinics, 2710 Marshall Court, Madison WI 53705.

24

Right Ape-Hand Deformity and Left Clawhand Deformity after Accident in Which Both Hands Were Thrust through a Glass Window

A 25-year-old man has visited from a third-world country and is referred to your hand clinic for evaluation of hand dysfunction. The hand surgeon, your associate, has not yet arrived but has left instructions asking you to begin the examination. The patient sustained a gunshot wound to the right upper trapezius muscle some 3 months ago while discovering a burglar in his home. He attempted to flee by punching out a glass window with both his hands and fell from a height of 6 feet only to dislocate his left shoulder. He was treated at the local emergency room. The significant results of your evaluation yielded the following data:

OBSERVATION A right-shoulder droop is observed. The patient points to a scar site from the bullet at the superficial midcourse of the right upper trapezius muscle. The patient's hands appear as in Fig. 24-1.

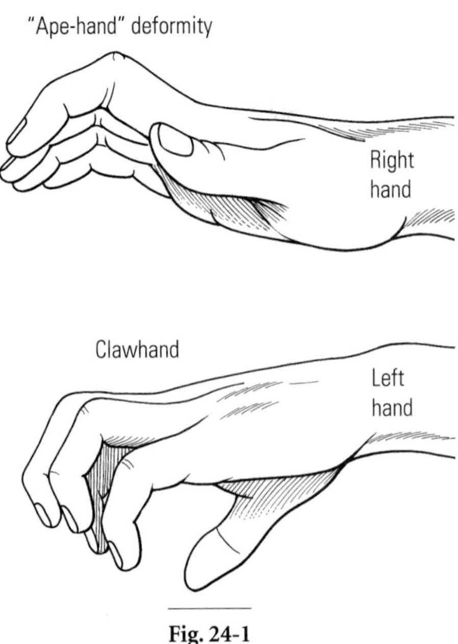

Fig. 24-1

PALPATION When asking the patient to isometrically contract his left deltoid, a soft, noncontractile sensation is imparted to your hands, as compared to the contralateral deltoid.

RANGE OF MOTION Within functional limits throughout the patient's extremities, except to the left shoulder, which demonstrates only 60° of shoulder elevation.

MUSCLE STRENGTH Within normal limits throughout, except to left shoulder flexion, abduction, and extension, which score fair plus. Left external shoulder rotation scores good minus. When asked to shrug his right shoulder, he appears to do so at only half the height of the contralateral shoulder. His left-hand intrinsic muscles exhibit a poor plus grade, and his right hand exhibits an inability to oppose or flex his thumb. There is wasting of the right thenar eminence.

SENSATION The patient is insensate only over a round area over the left middle deltoid muscle (Fig. 24-2).

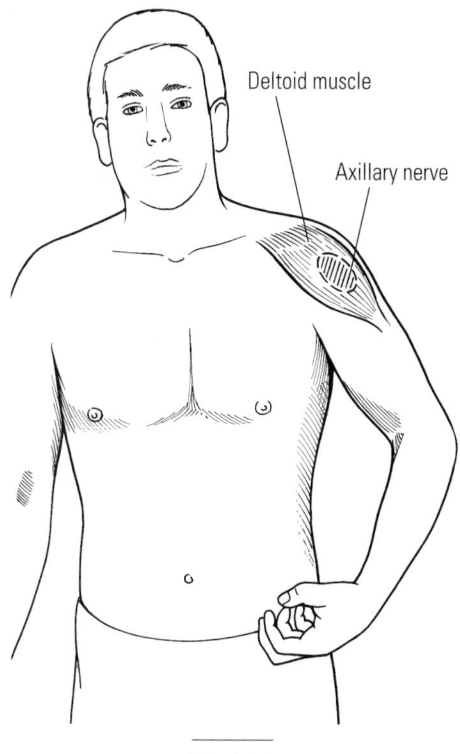

Fig. 24-2

1. **What pattern of nerve injury has occurred to this man's hands?**
2. **What is the anatomy of the peripheral nerve?**
3. **What protective mechanism affords the peripheral nerve protection from compressive force?**
4. **What protective mechanism affords the peripheral nerve protection from tensile force?**
5. **What protective mechanisms are inherent in the vascular supply of the nerves?**

6. **What is the classification of peripheral nerve injury?**
7. **What is a first-degree injury to a peripheral nerve?**
8. **What is a second-degree nerve injury?**
9. **What is a third-degree peripheral nerve injury?**
10. **What are the mechanisms of nerve injury?**
11. **What are clinical examples of the *acute compression* mechanism of nerve injury?**
12. **What are clinical examples of the *chronic compression* mechanism of nerve injury?**
13. **What are clinical examples of the *stretch injury* mechanism of nerve injury?**
14. **What effect does an electrical injury have on the peripheral nerve?**
15. **How common are injection injuries to nerve tissue?**
16. **What happens to a nerve during a partial or complete transection from a knife stabbing?**
17. **What is the sequence of a progressive stretch of nerve resulting in rupture?**
18. **What is the difference between gunshot and shotgun wound injuries to the peripheral nerve?**
19. **What is long thoracic nerve palsy?**
20. **How does the spinal accessory nerve differ from other cranial nerves, and which muscles does it innervate?**
21. **What are the divisions and function of the trapezius muscle?**
22. **What is spinal accessory nerve palsy?**
23. **What is high median nerve entrapment?**
24. **What is the second most frequent upper extremity compressive neuropathy occurring after carpal tunnel syndrome?**
25. **What is the cause of tardy ulnar palsy?**
26. **What compressive neuropathy is associated with Guyon's tunnel?**
27. **What are the causes of injury to the ulnar nerve at Guyon's tunnel?**
28. **How is ulnar nerve compression at the wrist differentiated from a lesion at the elbow region?**
29. **What kind of injury results in radial nerve injury?**
30. **What are the clinical signs and symptoms of musculocutaneous nerve injury in the axilla?**
31. **What is the therapeutic management of nerve injury?**
32. **What is the efficacy of electrical stimulation to denervated musculature?**
33. **What is the faradic electrical stimulation technique to denervated musculature?**
34. **What is *slow-pulse stimulation* to denervated musculature?**
35. **What are four different operative procedures for nerves?**
36. **What are the goals of postoperative rehabilitation?**
37. **What is the role of motor reeducation after peripheral neurosurgery?**
38. **What is the role of sensory reeducation after microneurocoaptation?**

1. **What pattern of nerve injury has occurred to this man's hands?**

- The patient's left-hand deformity is a combination of both median and ulnar nerve palsy with flexion of the proximal and distal interphalangeal joints and hyperextension of the metacarpophalangeal joints in what is known as *clawhand* or *clawfingers* (see Fig. 19-9). This deformity results from the loss of intrinsic muscle action and simultaneous overaction of the extrinsic extensor muscles. This deformity also occurs in syringomyelia.
- This is an *ape-hand deformity* of the right hand in which median nerve palsy causes thenar wasting such that the thumb falls into the plane of the fingers because of the overpull of the extensors. The patient is also unable to oppose or flex the thumb. This deformity may also accompany syringomyelia and amyotrophic lateral sclerosis.

The patient's pattern of proximal muscle weakness implies damage to the axillary nerve, corresponding to paresis of the deltoid muscle as well as the teres minor muscle. Damage to this nerve may have been incurred from a shoulder dislocation as the humeral head pressed upon the posterior cord. This damage is confirmed by loss of sensation over the cutaneous distribution of that nerve. Additionally the droopy right shoulder, decreased ability to shrug the shoulder, and scar presence whose entry and exit sites correspond to the course of the spinal accessory nerve are suggestive of injury to that nerve.

2. What is the anatomy of the peripheral nerve?

Three kinds of nerve fibers are carried in the peripheral nerve—motor, sensory, and autonomic fibers. Several nerve axons running together form a densely packed bundle called a *fascicle.* There are three separate and distinct connective tissue elements serving as supportive tissue sheaths that are associated with nerve fascicles: *endoneurium, perineurium,* and *epineurium* (Fig. 24-3). These connective tissue sheaths facilitate a physiologic and a mechanical function of protecting the axons from excessive tensile force by virtue of their longitudinal collagen fiber orientation.[1]

The innermost viscous *endoneurium* resides between the fibers composing the individual fascicle. The next level of organization is the *perineurium* type of connective tissue that hugs each fascicle providing skeletal support, primarily tensile strength, to the enclosed neural tissue. The final supportive ensheathment is the outermost *epineurium* that surrounds, cushions, protects, and keeps the individual fascicles

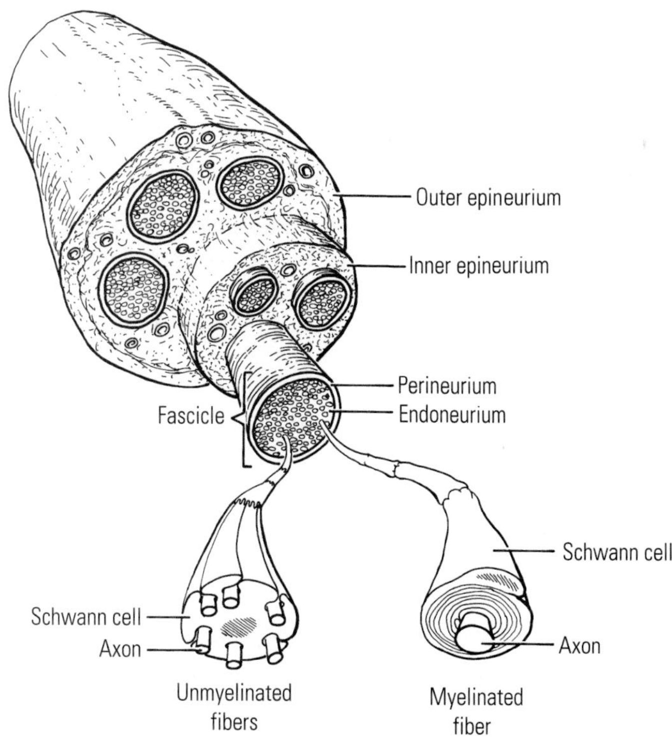

Fig. 24-3 Schema of peripheral nerve architecture. The connective tissue elements consist of the endoneurium, the perineurium, and the inner and outer epineuriums. Individual fascicles contain a heterogeneous mix of myelinated and unmyelinated fibers. (From Terzis JK, Smith KL: *The peripheral nerve: structure, function and reconstruction,* New York, 1990, Raven Press.)

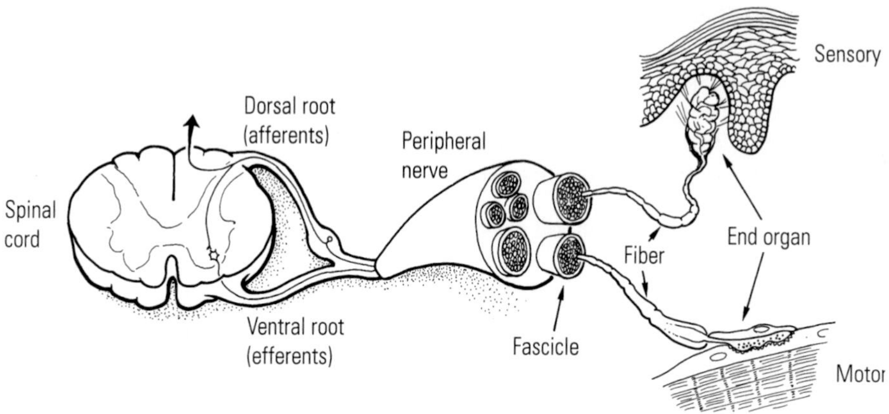

Fig. 24-4 The architecture of the peripheral nerve with central and peripheral connections. (From Terzis JK, Smith KL: *The peripheral nerve: structure, function and reconstruction*, New York, 1990, Raven Press.)

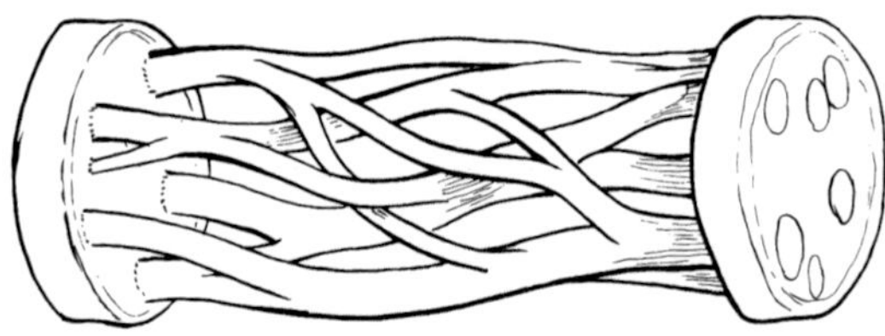

Fig. 24-5 Fascicular organization of the peripheral nerve. (From Terzis JK, Smith KL: *The peripheral nerve: structure, function and reconstruction*, New York, 1990, Raven Press.)

separate while collectively binding them together into a nerve trunk (Fig. 24-4). The outer epineurium facilitates gliding between fascicles, a necessary adaptation to accommodate extremity movement, especially when a peripheral nerve has to bend to an acute angle during limb movement. More epineural tissue is found where nerve trunks cross joints, or in tunnel areas such as the carpal tunnel.[1]

3. What protective mechanism affords the peripheral nerve protection from compressive force?

Fascicles within the *epineurium* run a wavy course and constantly change position within the nerve trunk in what can be described as a fascicular mesh (Fig. 24-5). This arrangement affords both compressive and tensile protection. Furthermore, when a greater number of fascicles are present, a nerve is afforded better protection from compressive force. For example, at the knee crease the common peroneal nerve is composed of approximately eight fascicles, yet only a few centimeters distally at the head of the fibula there are approximately 16 fascicles, since the nerve is more likely to fall subject to external compressive force at that locale.[1]

4. What protective mechanism affords the peripheral nerve protection from tensile force?

The peripheral nerve attenuates applied tension by initially stretching out the undulations that compose the epineurium and the perineurium.[4] The *perineurium's* outer sheath is composed of collagen fibers that lie in three orientations: circumferential, longitudinal, and oblique.[27,28] As tension is applied, the perineurium lengthens because of the oblique perineurial fibers, much in the same way as a "Chinese finger trap."[26] Thus the epineurium lengthens but does so at the expense of creating a compressive force along the length of the nerve by way of increased intrafascicular pressures.[25,29]

5. What protective mechanisms are inherent in the vascular supply of the nerves?

The peripheral nerve relies on continuous aerobic metabolism and is extremely susceptible to ischemia in the event of compression. In compensation of this vulnerability, the peripheral nerve is nourished by two integrated but functionally independent vascular systems referred to as the extrinsic and the intrinsic systems.[26] The arteries and veins composing the extrinsic system additionally possess the added advantage of being coiled in nature. This tortuous appearance in fact serves as a "reserve in length," which allows the nerve significant freedom of movement before the vessels become stretched and suffer traction injury.[17]

6. What is the classification of peripheral nerve injury?

Both Sedon and Sunderland developed classification schemes based on the direct relationship of prognosis for functional return as it correlates with the degree of intraneural disruption (Fig. 24-6). Sedon's triad classification includes neurapraxia, axonotmesis, and neurotmesis in increasing order of nerve injury.[26] Sunderland introduced a fourth- and a fifth-degree injury as part of the spectrum of nerve disorder. These latter types represent gradations of injury necessitating surgical intervention and are based upon integrity of the supporting elements of the nerve.

7. What is a first-degree injury to a peripheral nerve?

The first and most benign gradation of nerve injury is known as *neurapraxia* and describes the least type of injurious injury. Neurapraxia is defined as a *local conduction block* at a singular focal segment along a nerve because of compression or traction of the myelin sheath surrounding that nerve. However, because axonal continuity is maintained, axoplasmic transport is maintained, and the involved nerve remains capable of stimulation distal to the level of the lesion.[26] There is no evidence of wallerian degeneration, and electromyographic examination fails to demonstrate any electrical activity at rest. There will be no evidence of fibrillations or sharp positive waves seen if the patient is still paralyzed 3 weeks from onset.[26] Neurapraxia clinically manifests as motor loss that may be quite profound. Additionally, there is also a partial sensory loss and little or no sympathetic disturbance.[15] Classic neurapraxias include tardy ulnar palsy, Saturday night palsy, crutch palsy, or even one's foot falling asleep, with duration of paralysis from several moments to several weeks depending on how long the myelin sheath was compromised. Complete recovery usually occurs within 10 weeks and often less.[26]

8. What is a second-degree nerve injury?

Axonotmesis injury to the peripheral nerve exhibits all the characteristics of a first-degree injury, in addition to *disruption of the axon and myelin sheath with sparing of the Schwann sheath, endoneurium*, and successively larger subdivisions of the nerve.[15] Axonotmesis occurs from a more severe crush or traction injury or if the compression is severe or of such long-standing duration as to rupture the lamella of the myelin sheath and thus expose the unprotected axon to the direct brunt of compression. The resulting disability manifests as complete loss of motor and sensory function below the level of insult that is indistinguishable from a complete nerve transection. The segment of axon distal to the lesion suffers ischemia and begins to disintegrate some 3 to 5 days after the injury. The aforementioned was initially observed by Waller in the 1850s, hence the term *wallerian degeneration*. Corresponding electrical changes indicating denervation are observed after 3 weeks.[15] Fortunately, because the injury does not involve the endoneurial tube, attempted regrowth of the proximal part of the nerve may be guided back to reattach onto the distal portion of nerve at a growth rate of 1 mm per day, 1 cm per week, or approximately 1 inch per month.[4] The prognosis for recovery from second-degree nerve injury is excellent[15] because the return of function occurs within several months after the injury.

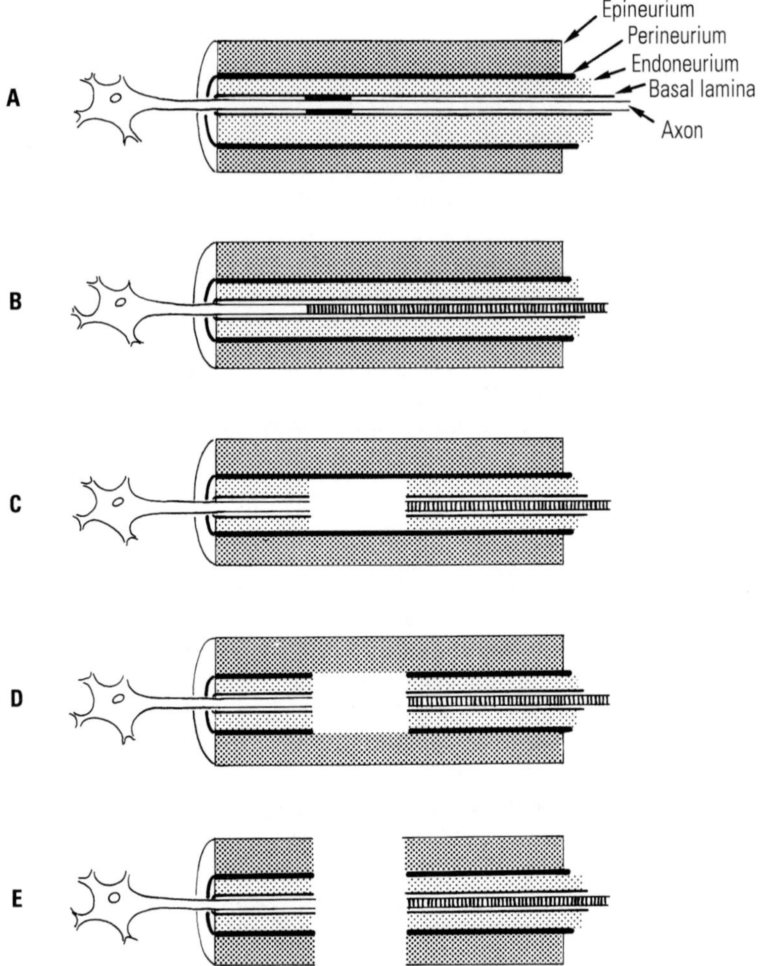

Fig. 24-6 Sunderland's classification of nerve injury. **A,** First-degree injury—local conduction blockade with minimal structural disruption. *Prognosis:* complete recovery within days to months. **B,** Second-degree injury—complete axonal disruption with wallerian degeneration. Basal lamina remains intact. *Prognosis:* complete recovery in months. **C,** Third-degree injury—axonal and endoneurial disruption with interruption of the basal lamina. *Prognosis:* intrafascicular axonal admixture with regeneration yields mild to moderate functional reduction. **D,** Fourth-degree injury—axonal, endoneurial, perineurial disruption. *Prognosis:* moderate to severe functional loss caused by interfascicular axonal admixture. Microsurgical manipulation can improve prognosis. **E,** Fifth-degree injury—complete structural disruption. *Prognosis:* no return without microsurgical manipulation. (From Terzis JK, Smith KL: *The peripheral nerve: structure, function, and reconstruction*, New York, 1990, Raven Press.)

9. What is a third-degree peripheral nerve injury?

Neurotmesis involves complete severance of the axon and of the associated supporting connective tissue. This injury, like a second-degree injury, leads to wallerian degeneration of the axon but differs in that there is little chance for regrowth in the right direction. With a third-degree injury the loss of continuity of the supporting elements leaves the axon without directional guidance and results in misdirected axon growth. Without the benefit of an intact endoneurial tube the likelihood of blind axon sprouts reestablishing continuity

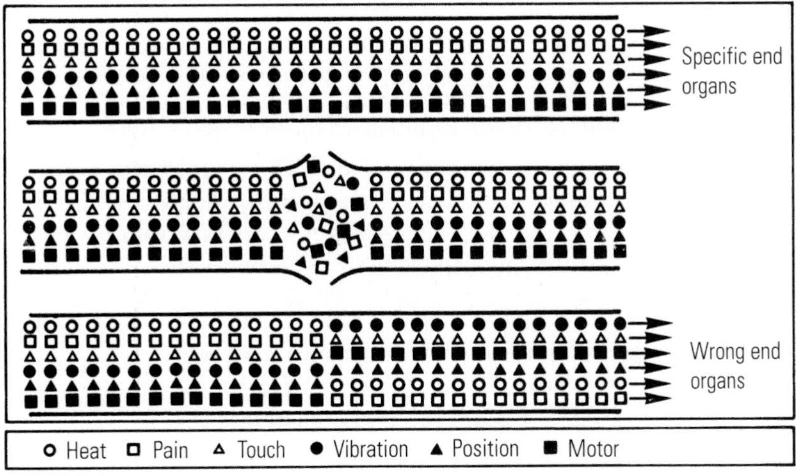

Fig. 24-7 Inappropriate reinnervation as a result of misdirected growth resulting in synkinesis. (From: Dandy D: *Essential orthopaedics and trauma,* Churchill Livingstone, London, 1991.)

with the appropriate end organ is remote.[26] This injury requires microsurgical intervention to reestablish continuity by means of fascicular realignment. Even then, the tips of the axons sprouting from the proximal stump often have little chance of being apposed with their correct endoneurial sheaths.[2] The result is often, at best, only an altered sensibility (Fig. 24-7). For example, heat or light touch may be experienced as pain because the incorrectly innervated patch of skin is hypersensitive.[3] Electromyographic findings after neurotmesis are the same as those observed after a second-degree injury, with additional or no action potentials on attempted voluntary contraction[15] of the denervated muscle.

10. What are the mechanisms of nerve injury?

The various mechanisms of nerve injury include acute and chronic compression, ischemia, traction, x radiation, inadvertent injection injury, or electrical injury. The common pathophysiologic denominator is mechanical deformation or ischemia-induced metabolic failure, or both.[26] An academic debate continues as to which factor contributes to nerve demise in certain mechanisms. Perhaps both factors are operative or even additive in their contribution toward nerve insult. Additionally, each category of injury carries with it a different prognosis. Thus, despite the fact that at the time of acute injury, there are clinical manifestions of numbness, pain, paralysis, or paresthesias, they by themselves shed very little light on the pathophysiologic course and ultimate prognosis. Because of this uncertainty, it is imperative that the examining clinician understand the nature and mechanism of injury.[26]

11. What are clinical examples of the *acute compression* mechanism of nerve injury?

Acute compression of the nerve is defined as any heavy force that compresses a nerve against an unyielding structure. Injury from this mechanism may take the form of internal or external compression. Clinical examples of this class of nerve injury include high-velocity gunshot wounds or blast shrapnel wounds with severe fractures in which bone fragments compress the nerve, inadvertent crush by clamps or forceps during misguided attempts at hemostasis during surgery, and lengthy high-pressure tourniquet application.

12. What are clinical examples of the *chronic compression* mechanism of nerve injury?

Examples of *chronic internal compression* mechanisms of injury include tumors, ganglia, or callus. Carpal tunnel syndrome is another example of an internal chronic compression neuropathy. Whereas an example of a *chronic external compression* mechanism includes the comatose person whose nerve is compromised by pressure against a bed rail, a patient with chronic compression neuropathy rarely reports a history of trauma, and a great many present with complaints of pain, paresthesia, and weakness.

13. What are clinical examples of the *stretch injury* mechanism of nerve injury?

Nerve-stretch injuries are associated with fractures, fracture-dislocations, dislocations, obstetric trauma, and occasionally the state after inadvertent retraction during surgery. Stretch resulting in rupture or avulsion more commonly occurs with obstetrical brachial plexus injury than with peripheral stretch injury because spinal nerve roots lack perineurium. Spinal nerves thus represent a weak link in the peripheral nervous system by not having the protective cover of this middle nerve sheath.[25]

14. What effect does an electrical injury have on the peripheral nerve?

Electrical injury involves complicated and as-yet unelucidated pathophysiologic features that clinically present from minor to life threatening. The most common site of electrical injury is the upper extremity by high-voltage linemen or by the home do-it-yourself handyman who contacts electrical lines with a metal ladder or while attempting to install an antenna.[7,21,22] Lightning stroke injuries are exceedingly rare.[21]

Electrical current follows the path of least resistance, and resistance to flow increases in various tissues in the following order: nerve, blood vessels, muscle, skin, tendon, fat, and bone. Electrical current often follows the paths of existing neurovascular bundles and create extensive deep (that is, subfascial) tissue destruction that is compounded by flash thermal burns at entrance and exit sites. The movement of current often enters peripherally at the neurovascular bundles and moves centrally. Subarachnoid bleeding is common. Patients are at risk for developing ischemic compartment syndrome. This horrible injury is further compounded by the often violent tetanic contractions accompanying electrocution that results in hemorrhage from muscle rupture or bone fracture, as muscles pull too hard on their bones. A major pathologic change is the conversion of electric energy to heat energy, resulting in coagulation necrosis. Electrical injuries are associated with a high percentage of extremity amputations.[7]

The resultant neurologic deficit occurring after electric injury is of immediate onset and typically involves the motor nerves, though the reason for this specificity is unclear. Although most injured nerves show some recovery with time, complete resolution is uncommon.

15. How common are injection injuries to nerve tissue?

Peripheral nerve injection injuries are all too common and are fraught with medicolegal overtones because of their frequent iatrogenic cause. Because of this, the tendency is not to publish such events, and the true incidence and outcome of nerve injection injury is probably unknown.[12] The cause of injury has been shown to be the result of injection of a neurotoxic substance and not the result of mechanical needle injury. This was confirmed in studies where repeated injection with normal saline failed to produce injury.[12,21]

The history of nerve injection injury is typical. The patient often complains of severe pain at the injection site, which radiates along the distribution of that nerve and is associated with neurologic deficit. For the first 3 months after the injury, observation is appropriate, and electrophysiologic studies are obtained approximately 6 weeks after the injury. Careful evaluation for clinical evidence of return is appropriate at 3-week intervals. Repeat electrodiagnostics are appropriate if no clinical evidence of return of function has occurred after 3 months.[12]

Early exploration with irrigation of the offending agent and external neurolysis is neither helpful nor indicated. Surgical exploration is indicated only after 4 months if no clinical recovery has occurred.

16. What happens to a nerve during a partial or complete transection from a knife stabbing?

A laceration of peripheral nerve results in a clearly defined area of motor sensory and autonomic deficit that results from an open wound caused by a low-velocity sharp instrument. Less often, these injuries may occur in a closed wound secondary to a fracture. A gap between the proximal and distal ends of the nerve occurs and is bridged by scar tissue. This situation will not improve without microsurgical intervention.[26]

17. What is the sequence of a progressive stretch of nerve resulting in rupture?

To sustain mechanical injury, the longitudinal stretch imposed upon a nerve must exceed the inherent limits of elasticity of that nerve. The sequence of compromise of the supporting elements of the peripheral nerve and finally of the nerve itself occurs along the following progression. Tension is first resisted by the outermost epineurium by way of stretching out redundant fascicular folds composing this outermost nerve cover. Tension is next withstood by the perineurium directly as a function of the number of fascicles within that middle protective nerve cover. The undulations composing this middle nerve cover similarly lengthen in an attempt to attenuate tensile force. Tensile force is also withstood by the orientation of collagen fibers making up the outer sheath of the perineurium. During the elongation of perineurium, axons begin to break and retract proximally and distally. Once perineurial rupture is complete, the proximal and distal nerve stumps are rapidly separated, since no strength is afforded by the endoneurium, myelin, or axons.[26]

18. What is the difference between gunshot and shotgun wound injuries to the peripheral nerve?

Gunshot wounds often involve "near-misses" of the nerves by *low-velocity* large bullets (200 msec) generating shock waves in soft tissue. These bullets drill a clean hole through soft tissue and occasionally cartwheel, in which case more damage is incurred. The cavitation that occurs here creates oscillation of wounded tissue that results in alternate stretching[15] and relaxation of the peripheral nerve as cavitation proceeds. The resultant nerve injury is of the first-degree type, in which focal conduction block without axon degeneration occurs after local stretching of the nerve.

On the other hand, *shotgun* wounds are a result of a high energy–*high velocity* (1000 msec) weapon, in which smaller projectiles can create massive injuries. When the muzzle velocity of a projectile reaches and exceeds the speed of sound, kinetic energy becomes proportional to the cube of velocity, and tissue damage, in turn, becomes largely dependent on velocity. What this translates into is that a small but high-velocity bullet causes severe intraneural disruption for a span of several centimeters proximal and distal to its path, rather than just focally, by means of *compressive force.* If cavitation follows, the subatmospheric pressures that follow the compressive way only compound the injury. With shotgun wounds, the nerve is frequently transected in close to 50% of cases and, if not, is often partially lacerated from adjacent shards of bone in associated bone fractures or is severely contused.[26]

19. What is long thoracic nerve palsy?

The long thoracic nerve exits from the pre-plexus locale, immediately after the exit of the C5, C6, and C7 nerve roots from the intervertebral foramina. Innervating the serratus anterior, this nerve falls heir to lesions from a variety of mechanisms resulting in paralysis of that muscle. Thus *isolated serratus palsy* may occur after viral illness, stabwounds, as a neuritis sequel to deltoid muscle serum immunization, recumbency for a prolonged period,[8] from infections such as diptheria and infectious mononucleosis, or from prolonged wearing of a knapsack.

Isolated serratus palsy may occur after closed trauma to the upper limb or shoulder girdle by way of a traction lesion of the long thoracic nerve. Open injury of the long thoracic nerve is unusual, except when occurring as a complication of either breast surgery for cancer, or surgery done to relieve thoracic outlet compression.[15]

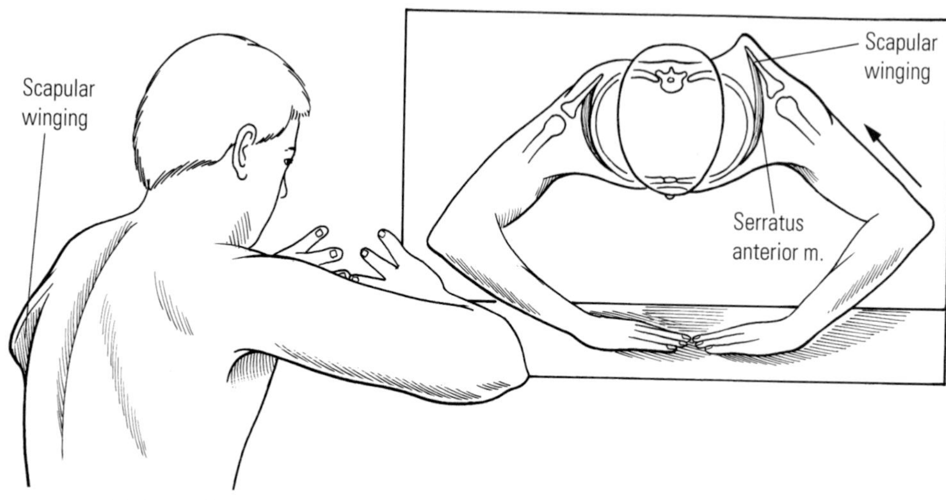

Fig. 24-8 Scapular winging caused by deinnervation of the serratus anterior muscle.

Some patients may become aware of a problem possibly because of significant shoulder pain coupled with difficulty in raising the arm, or they may suddenly realize that their scapula is winging (Fig. 24-8) because of an uncomfortable feeling when sitting in a high-backed chair. The loss of stabilization that the serratus conveys to the scapula alters the precise and interrelated synchrony of balance in those muscles of the shoulder girdle. This altered biomechanical milieu results in less-than-ideal mechanical efficiency to those muscles originating on the scapula and will result in diminished shoulder elevation or even pain.[15]

The prognosis for recovery after closed injury or an atraumatic cause is usually favorable. If paralysis persists for a year, however, without any clinical or electromyographic evidence of recovery, the prognosis is poor. Complete paralysis after an open injury has a poor outlook for recovery. During the time waiting for recovery appropriate therapy includes joint mobilization to the scapulothoracic joint as well as all the major joints of the shoulder girdle to forestall the effects of stiffness, stretching, and strengthening of the muscles of the shoulder girdle so as to prevent their readjustment in length attributable to scapular winging, as well as electric stimulation to the motor point of the serratus anterior to maintain the contractility of the fibers of that muscle. Additionally, some patients experience relief from the dragging, painful feeling in the shoulder by the wearing of a pelvic-support orthosis.[5] There are good surgical options for the patient with poor prognosis that involve tendon transfers of the pectoralis minor or major muscles to the vertebral scapular border. Results of surgery are good in terms of pain relief, loss of winging, and return of function.[13]

20. How does the spinal accessory nerve differ from other cranial nerves, and which muscles does it innervate?

The spinal accessory nerve is only one of the cranial nerves that supplies muscles outside the head region but rather adjacent to the head in the neck and shoulder girdle. The name of this eleventh cranial nerve derives from the close structural continuity of this nerve root with the tenth cranial nerve. In fact, the eleventh cranial nerve has a dual origin from the spinal root contributions of cervical nerves C1 to C4 and a cranial nerve root contribution from the vagus nerve; hence our nerve is said to be an *accessory* to the vagus nerve.

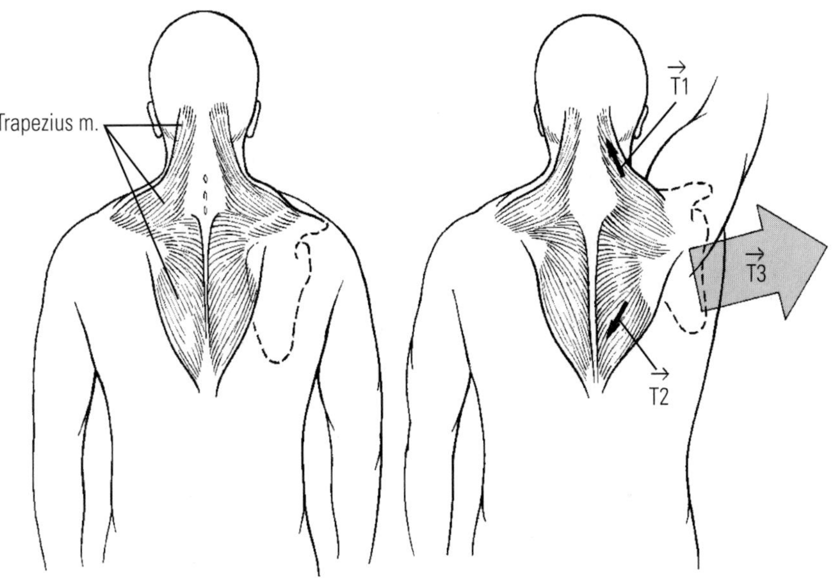

Fig. 24-9 Trapezius as a force couple. Graphical representation of vector subtraction of T_1 and T_2. T_3 represents the resultant displacement.

The spinal accessory nerve is a motor nerve that innervates the sternocleidomastoid muscle and facilitates contraction that tilts the head ipsilaterally and rotates the head contralaterally. It also innervates the powerful trapezius muscle because of the following developmental reason. Embryologically the trapezius starts out as a high neck muscle and descends caudally on the neck and back during fetal elongation; as a result the muscle drags down along its original source of innervation deriving from the head.

21. What are the divisions and function of the trapezius muscle?

The trapezius is a three-part back muscle that is the most superficial of muscles of the shoulder girdle. Although all three divisions of this muscle originate from essentially the same location, they are distinguished one from the other by their different distal attachment. Although the upper fibers of this muscle act to elevate the shoulder girdle by means of their distal attachment on the clavicle, the lower fibers act to depress the shoulder girdle by means of their distal attachment on the scapula. The paradox that emerges from these contradictory anatomic functions is clarified in the context of kinesiologically understanding the function of the trapezius as a *force couple* (Fig. 24-9). A force couple is defined as two forces working in opposite directions but acting on a single object so as to cause a rotational movement of that object. A familiar example is the turning of a steering wheel in an automobile with the driver's hands located at the 9 o'clock and 3 o'clock positions. If only one hand moved in one direction, the car would not turn, whereas the cooperative albeit diametrically opposed simultaneous movement does permit turning. Similarly, despite the seeming antagonism between the upper and lower fibers of this muscle, co-contraction manifests not as a tug of war but rather as rotation of the inferior angle of the scapula. This upward and outward mediolateral scapular rotation, known as *scapular protraction,* is facilitated by kinesiologic synergy between the upper and lower fibers of the trapezius. It is noteworthy to mention that the most important scapular protractor is the serratus anterior muscle.

The middle fibers of the trapezius do not retract the scapula despite their distal attachment on the root of the scapular spine; lateromedial scapular retraction is accomplished by the rhomboid muscles. The middle fibers instead elongate eccentrically to accommodate synergistic protraction.

22. What is spinal accessory nerve palsy?

Because the spinal accessory nerve is superficially located, it is quite vulnerable to injury,[15] as may occur from traction from a tight shoulder harness during a sudden stop from an automobile accident.[6] Because this nerve is so superficially located, it is also vulnerable to injury as a result of surgical operations to the neck. For example, the nerve may be intentionally sacrificed during the course of a radical neck dissection for cancer. Inadvertent transection of this nerve may occur during the course of minor surgery to the neck area as from a lymph node biopsy.[30] Here the patient may not even realize that anything is wrong until several days after the biopsy when the pain of surgery should have receded, yet pain is still felt, especially when trying to elevate the shoulder. If complete paralysis of the trapezius persists both clinically and electromyographically for greater than 3 months, the nerve should be surgically explored. If the nerve is found to be caught up in scar tissue, neurolysis should be performed, whereas if a discontinuity is discovered, a suture or graft is appropriate if the gap cannot be closed without tension.[11]

The functional loss associated with spinal accessory nerve palsy includes torticollis with the head turned to the ipsilateral side and tilted contralaterally along with a drooping shoulder and an inability to shrug the shoulder ipsilaterally. Additionally the delicate balance of necessary length tension so important to normal shoulder kinesiology will have been altered because of injury of a significant scapular muscle. This will translate into a decreased ability of the scapula to glide synchronously and to provide the appropriate length tension to those muscles facilitating shoulder elevation. As a result there will be weakness of the shoulder abductors. Scapular winging may be accentuated by shoulder abduction and not by foreward humeral flexion as seen in serratus anterior palsy.

23. What is high median nerve entrapment?

High median nerve entrapment includes proximal compression of that nerve in the region of the shoulder and proximal humerus as well as in the elbow region (pronator syndrome, see p. 25). The causes of injury at these sites are more often accidental in nature and may occur in the former following anterior shoulder dislocation. This mechanism, however, more often involves injury to the axillary nerve, which, unlike the median nerve, is unprotected by soft tissue. Another cause of high median nerve injury stems from the usage of improperly fitted axillary crutches by means of excessive external compression to that nerve; this mechanism may also injure the radial nerve. Finally, high median nerve compression may also occur alone or accompany radial and ulnar nerve palsies in inebriated individuals who happen to fall asleep while hanging their arms over a chair (Fig. 24-10) or park bench (Saturday night palsy).[28] Another mechanism contributing to high multiple nerve compression is *honeymoon palsy* in which a partner's head presses on the brachial axillary angle or medial aspect of the arm.

The functional deficit associated with high median nerve lesions include significant compromise of forearm pronation as a result of paralysis of the pronator quadratus, though weak pronation can still be initiated by the brachioradialis and aided by gravity. Wrist flexion is weak, and there is weakness or absence of flexion of the interphalangeal joint of the thumb and of the proximal and distal interphalangeal joints of the index finger,[40] since the muscles producing these movements are supplied by the median nerve after it enters the forearm. Median nerve injuries spare flexion of the metacarpophalangeal joints, which are controlled by the ulnar innervated muscles. Proximal median nerve injury also results in a loss of sensation on the lateral portion of the palm, the palmar surface of the thumb, and the lateral two and one-half fingers.[18]

When a Saturday night palsy type of injury involves the median nerve alone, flexion of the distal interphalangeal joints of the ring and little fingers is unaffected, since the medial portion of the flexor digitorum profundus producing these movements is supplied by the ulnar nerve. However, the capacity to flex the

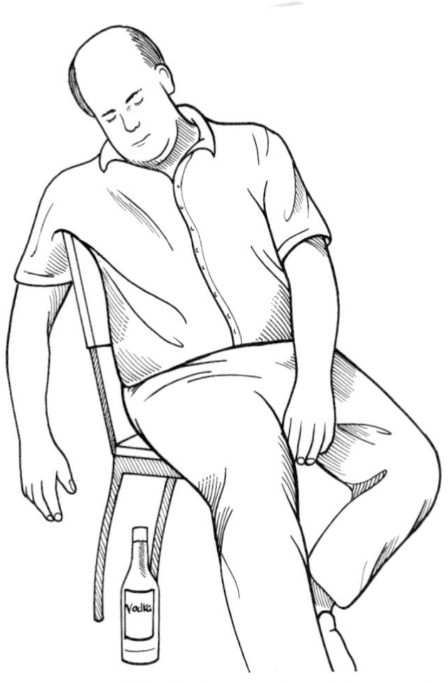

Fig. 24-10 Saturday night palsy: The radial and possibly median and ulnar nerves may be compressed by pressure from the backrest of a chair.

metacarpophalangeal joints of the index and middle fingers will be compromised because the digital branches of the median nerve supply the first and second lumbrical muscles.

A slightly different pattern of injury will manifest from median nerve injury occurring distally to the elbow in the forearm, as may occur from wounds to the forearm. When the median nerve is compromised in the cubital region, there will be loss of flexion of the proximal interphalangeal joints of all the digits as well as a loss of flexion of the distal interphalangeal joints of the index and middle fingers.[18]

The most common site of median nerve injury is distally just proximal to the flexor retinaculum, because of the frequency of wrist slashing from suicide attempts.[18]

24. What is the second most frequent upper extremity compressive neuropathy occurring after carpal tunnel syndrome?

Ulnar nerve entrapment at the elbow is the second most frequent upper extremity compression neuropathy. Whereas carpal tunnel syndrome is characterized by but not confined to sensory impairment, ulnar nerve entrapment results in motor loss that is characterized by considerably more significant disability. In the majority of cases of ulnar nerve lesion, initial symptoms are intermittent hypesthesia in the ulnar nerve distribution that is often associated with elbow flexion, whereas symptoms often abate when the patient extends his or her elbow. Use of the arm, especially in elbow flexion and extension, exacerbates symptoms. Patients are often awakened at night with elbow pain, shooting pain in the hand and fifth digit, and paresthesia and hypesthesia in the ulnar nerve distribution. Symptoms may vary from day to day and may even disappear for a period of time.[4] Signs of injury may include severe motor and sensory loss to the hand that include impaired power of ulnar deviation and impaired wrist flexion in the sense that the hand is drawn radially by the flexor carpi radialis when one is attempting to flex the wrist joint. In the hand there is difficulty in making a fist, since patients cannot flex their fourth and fifth digits at the distal interphalangeal joints. The resultant posture while attempting to make a fist is known as *main en griffe*, or *clawhand*[18] (see Fig. 24-12). The characteristic clinical sign of ulnar nerve damage is inability to adduct or abduct the medial four digits because of the loss of power of the interosseous muscles.[18]

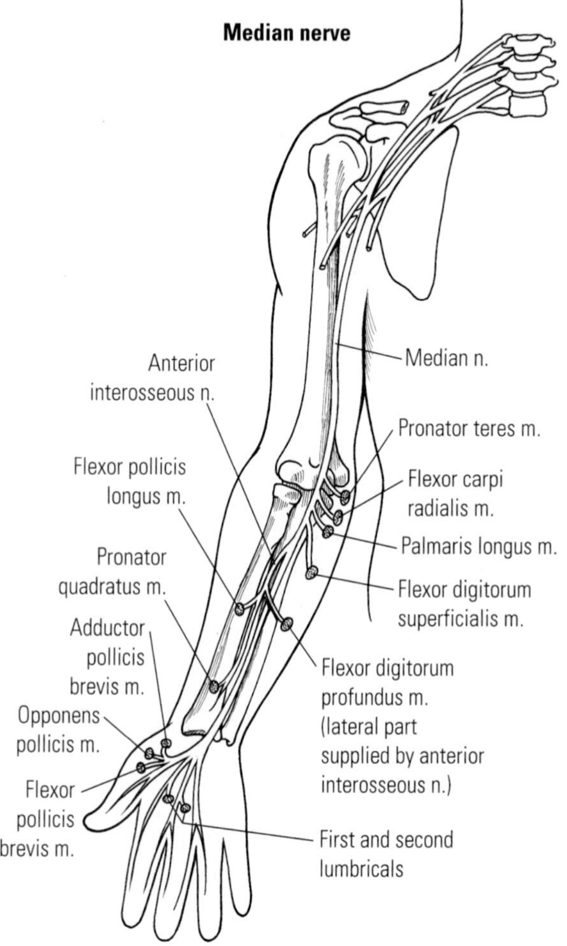

Fig. 24-11 Median nerve distribution and innervated musculature.

The cause of ulnar nerve entrapment may be revealed by a history that includes elbow fracture or dislocation, acute blunt trauma at the medial epicondylar groove, or chronic occupational trauma in workers supporting themselves on their elbows; among such workers the neuropathy is more often seen on the nondominant side because the patient balances with one elbow while using the dominant arm for work.[4] Ulnar nerve trauma may also occur from chronic elbow arthritis in bedridden patients or after periods of unconsciousness as a result of intoxication, anesthesia, or coma caused by illness.[4] The most common site of ulnar nerve injury after insults to the forearm occurs where the nerve passes posteriorly to the medial humeral epicondyle. This most commonly occurs when the elbow hits a hard surface resulting in a medial epicondyle fracture.

More often than not, there is no history suggestive of a cause of compression, in which case the patient is diagnosed as having *cubital tunnel syndrome.* This syndrome is attributable to entrapment of the ulnar nerve between the fibrotic aponeurotic heads of the flexor carpi ulnaris. This aponeurotic band, arising from the medial humeral epicondyle and inserting on the medial border of the olecranon, represents a gateway through which the ulnar nerve enters the cubital tunnel to pass between the two heads of the flexor carpi ulnaris[4]

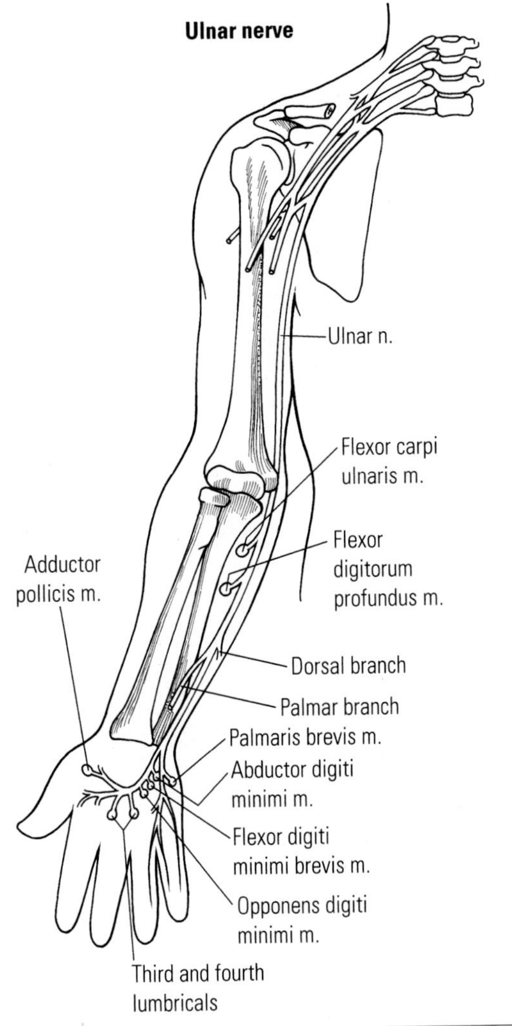

Fig. 24-12 Ulnar nerve distribution and innervated musculature.

(Fig. 24-13). The diameter of this tunnel is narrowly compromised upon elbow flexion for two separate reasons: (1) elbow flexion causes separation of the medial epicondyle and the olecranon; (2) during flexion, the medial collateral ligament bulges medially, causing further narrowing of the cubital tunnel diameter.[4]

Nonsurgical management entails avoidance of repetitive elbow flexion and extension, rest, or splinting the elbow in extension for a period of 2 to 3 months. The elbow flexion test for cubital tunnel syndrome provokes symptoms by placing the ulnar nerve on stretch (Fig. 24-14). Early diagnosis and treatment will result in complete cure.

25. What is the cause of tardy ulnar palsy?

Tardy ulnar palsy results from chronic stretch of that nerve secondary to a cubitus valgus deformity, often after a capitular fracture with arrest of the lateral humeral epiphysis and abnormal growth, or malalignment

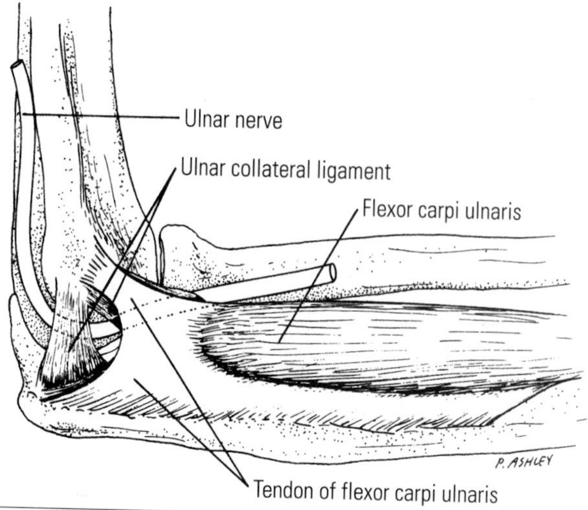

Fig. 24-13 Cubital tunnel. (From Magee DJ: *Orthopaedic physical assessment*, Philadelphia, 1987, Saunders.)

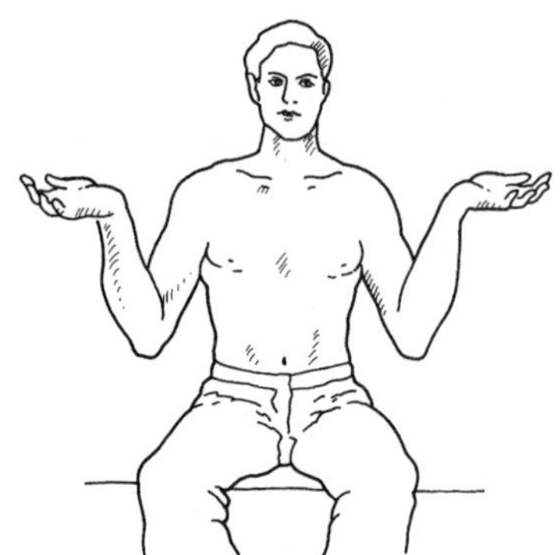

Fig. 24-14 The elbow flexion test for cubital tunnel syndrome. Symptoms may be reproduced or maginified by an upper extremity posture that places the ulner nerve on stretch. Superimposing additional components such as shoulder abduction, depression, and lateral rotation, as well as forearm supination, wrist extension, radial deviation, and contralateral neck flexion may further tense the nerve. (From Beuhler MJ, Thayer DT: The elbow flexion test: a clinical test for the cubital tunnel syndrome, *Clin Orth* 233:213-216, 1988.)

after supracondylar fracture.[4] A common cause of tardy ulnar palsy is chronic elbow arthritis in which the patient, in some cases, may have not noticed any elbow abnormality. When implicated, the patient typically lacks full elbow extension as compared with the contralateral side. Another mechanical cause of palsy is attributed to individuals with too shallow an olecranon fossa. This results in excessive movement of the nerve or even dislocation out of the groove during elbow flexion or extension.[24] Physical findings associated with ulnar nerve palsy include the following:

- Positive Froment's sign.[4] Loss of stability of the metacarpophalangeal joint as a result of ulnar paralysis causes metacarpophalangeal hyperextension with secondary interphalangeal joint flexion, which, together with weakness of the adductor pollicis, the flexor pollicis brevis, and the first dorsal interosseous muscle produces a thumb posture known as *Froment's sign* (Fig. 24-15).

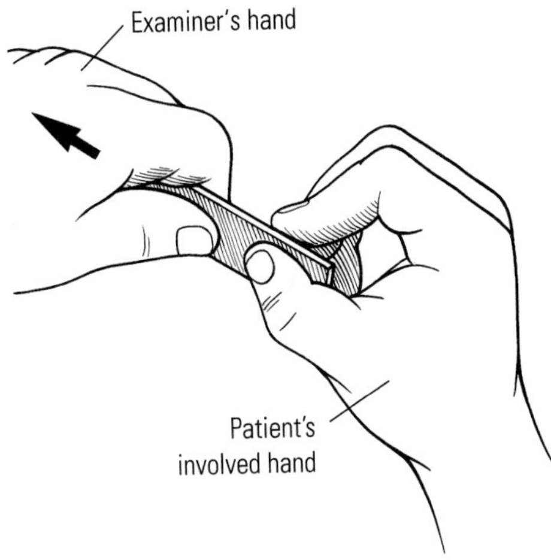

Fig. 24-15 Positive Froment's sign. *1*, Characteristic thumb posture on attempted pulp pinch between the thumb and adjacent digits. *2*, The patient is instructed to hold a sheet of paper between the thumb and index finger while the examiner attempts to pull it away. *3*, Weakness is attributable to diminished or absent innervation of the adductor pollicis, ulnar portion of flexor pollicis brevis, and the first dorsal interosseus. The former two muscles stabilize the metacarpophalangeal joint of the thumb. Weakness of the first dorsal interosseus results in impaired abduction of the index finger, which further impairs the pinch mechanism. The patient tries to retain the paper by flexing the thumb at the interphalangeal joint.

- As the patient tries to pinch harder, the movement becomes less effective while the deformity accentuates.
- The ability to write deteriorates and becomes awkward as muscles weaken.
- Mild clawing and wasting of interosseous muscles.
- Weakness of flexor digitorum profundus of the fourth and fifth digits.
- An inability to adduct the index and pinky finger because of weakness of the volar interossei.
- Insidious onset of numbness and tingling in the little finger and ulnar half of the ring finger.[4]

Electrodiagnostic studies may show a nerve conduction block at the elbow. Nonsurgical management involves explicit instruction to the patient to keep his or her forearm in supination because this position will draw the ulnar nerve away from the site of pressure.[19]

26. What compressive neuropathy is associated with Guyon's tunnel?

Of the different ulnar nerve lesions near the wrist, the most common is compression of the *deep palmar branch* at the base of the palm where the ulnar nerve (and artery) enter the hand at the *ulnar tunnel* known as *canal de Guyon* (Fig. 24-16). Like the carpal tunnel, the ulnar tunnel is a closed space through which the ulnar nerve must pass. Located between the transverse carpal ligament and the volar carpal ligament, the bony parameters of this tunnel are defined by the pisiform medially and hook of the hamate laterally.[4] An ulnar lesion at this site may cause either motor or sensory symptoms, though the latter is less common. When present, sensory symptoms include wrist pain that radiates into the digits or forearm, is often worse at night, and is exacerbated by exercise or wrist motion.[4] Associated signs include Froment's sign, pronounced weakness of the first dorsal interosseous muscle, possible wasting between the thumb and the first finger, and weakened or absent flexion of the fourth and fifth digits.

Ulnar nerve compression associated with Guyon's tunnel may occur at one of two sites. Proximal canal compression results in complete paralysis of all ulnar innervated intrinsic muscles. Long-term proximal

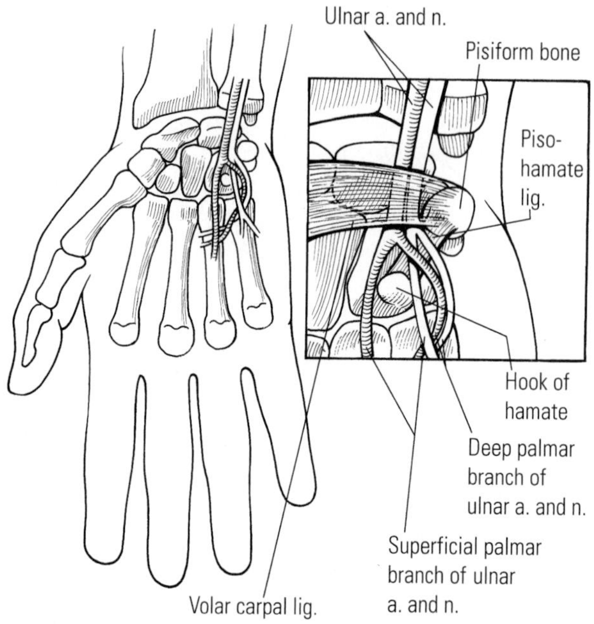

Fig. 24-16 Compression of the deep palmar branch of the ulnar nerve is a shallow trough known as the ulnar tunnel. The walls of this tunnel are the pisiform and the hook of the hamate bone. The floor is bone covered by a carpetlike layer of ligament (pisohamate), and the roof of the trough is the volar carpal ligament and the palmaris brevis muscle.

compression results in the typical *bishop's hand deformity* (Fig. 24-17) because of wasting of the hypothenar, interossei, and medial two lubricale muscles of the hand. Compression occurring distal to or at the level of the hook of the hamate results in the same pattern of muscle loss as before except for hypothenar function, which remains preserved.[4]

27. What are the causes of injury to the ulnar nerve at Guyon's tunnel?

Extrinsic causes of ulnar nerve compression at Guyon's tunnel may result from an acute blow over the hypothenar region, a laceration, or chronic occupational or avocational trauma resulting in a neuritis of that nerve. Injury commonly occurs to professional cyclists, pipe cutters, metal polishers, mechanics, from the repetitive use of pliers and screwdrivers or from using the palm as a hammer to put hubcaps back onto tires.[4] A characteristic callus at the base of the palm is often a good sign confirming such occupationally induced neuropathy. Injury may also occur after wrist fracture involving the pisiform, the body or hook of the hamate, or the metacarpals. Fracture injuries to the hamate are routinely absent on radiographs and are discovered only by oblique views of the hand, lateral tomograms, bone scans, or computerized tomography.[4]

Intrinsic causes of injury include the presence of ganglions, ulnar artery diseases, scar tissue contracture, the presence of aberrant muscles, or pisiform bursitis.

Conservative management of the mild neuropathy includes the avoidance of inciting trauma with or without splinting. This generally results in complete return of function.[4]

28. How is ulnar nerve compression at the wrist differentiated from a lesion at the elbow region?

There are two ways in which elbow and wrist compression of the ulnar nerve are differentiated: (1) sparing of the flexor carpi ulnaris occurs when the nerve lesion originates at the wrist, and (2) there is normal

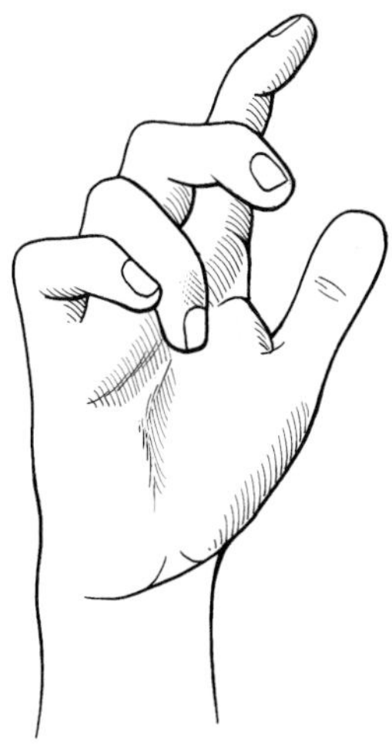

Fig. 24-17 Bishop's-hand deformity is named for its similarity to the ecclesiastical gesture of pronouncing benediction.

dorsal ulnar sensation when the lesion originates at the wrist because the dorsal sensory branch bifurcates off the ulnar nerve some 6 to 8 cm proximal to the wrist.

29. What kind of injury results in radial nerve injury?

Injury to the radial nerve proximal to the origin of the triceps muscle results in paresis or paralysis of the triceps muscle, brachioradialis, supinator, and the extensors of the wrist, thumb, and fingers and is accompanied by sensory loss. The characteristic clinical sign of radial nerve injury is *wristdrop*, defined as the inability to extend or straighten the wrist. This may be confused with wristdrop after a stroke, especially when the onset is acute. Peripheral radial nerve palsy is differentiated from a focal central lesion in that fine movements of muscles innervated by the median and ulnar nerves are not affected with radial nerve lesions. Radial nerve palsy recovers in 8 to 12 weeks, provided that there is little or no axonal damage.

Radial nerve injury may also occur from deep wounds to the forearm, and severance of the deep branch of that nerve produces an inability to extend the thumb and the metacarpophalangeal joints of the fingers. There is no concomitant sensory loss, since the deep branch of this nerve is entirely muscular and articular in distribution. However, when the radial nerve proper or its superficial branch is cut, sensation will be lost on the posterior surface of the forearm, hand, and the proximal phalanges of the lateral three and one-half digits. However, just because there is no sensory loss experienced does not necessarily mean that the radial nerve is intact, because of the considerable overlap between the cutaneous nerves of the hand.[18]

When the radial nerve is injured at the radial groove, the triceps is not completely paralyzed, though other muscles supplied by that nerve distal to that groove suffer paralysis.

30. What are the clinical signs and symptoms of musculocutaneous nerve injury in the axilla?

Musculocutaneous nerve injury in the axilla from, say, a laceration, before its innervation of any musculature will result in paralysis of the coracobrachialis, biceps, and brachialis muscles. Functionally this manifests as significant weakening of elbow joint flexion and forearm supination. Both motions, however, will be somewhat preserved due to brachioradialis and supinator respectively. Additionally, there may also be sensory loss on the lateral surface of the forearm as a result of denervation of the lateral antebrachial cutaneous nerve.[20]

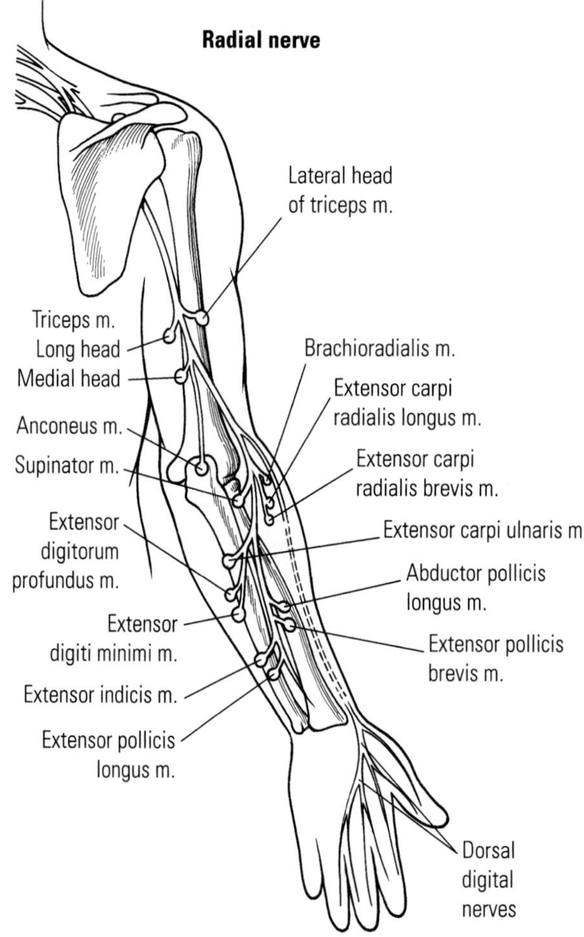

Fig. 24-18 Radial nerve distribution and innervated musculature.

31. What is the therapeutic management of nerve injury?

Therapeutic management for nerve injury must attempt to maintain the appropriate range of the muscle or muscles innervated by the injured nerve, while helping prevent contracture in those muscles antagonistic to the denervated muscle by stretching. Joint mobilization is appropriate to the adjacent joints to stave off the development of joint stiffness. Muscle strengthening is appropriate to those uninjured agonistic and synergistic muscles.

32. What is the efficacy of electrical stimulation to denervated musculature?

There are no rigidly controlled human studies to prove the efficacy of electrotherapy. Animal studies have shown that direct electrical stimulation of denervated muscle was useful in retarding denervation atrophy for both type I and type II muscle fibers.[20] Electrical stimulation is appropriately applied to the motor points of the affected muscle to help maintain the state of contractility of that muscle. The intended strategy of electrical stimulation is artificially to allow the muscle to contract and, in this way, prevent muscle fibrosis until reinnervation permits normal muscle function.

33. What is the faradic electrical stimulation technique to denervated musculature?

One approach to electrical stimulation of denervated musculature is *interrupted direct current*, otherwise known as *galvanic current*. Before electrode placement, the skin site under the electrodes shoulder should be cleansed. The positive ground electrode is placed on the ipsilateral side of the body so as to minimize electrical resistance; however, the ground electrode is not to be placed too distant from the site of stimulation or on an antagonistic muscle group. With the stimulating electrode polarity set on negative the target muscle is stimulated at the motor point or slightly distally at 1-second intervals with about 20 repetitions. After a rest period the above procedure is repeated several times during each treatment session. Treatment is to be discontinued if and when the patient feels pain, skin irritation, or fatigue. After treatment, the skin areas under the electrodes should be massaged with an astringent (such as witch hazel) followed by a light dusting with talcum powder.[14]

Once regeneration has manifested clinically, electrical muscle stimulators may be utilized in lieu of faradic treatment. These units are mostly biphasic in nature (that is, of the alternating current type).

34. What is *slow-pulse stimulation* to denervated musculature?

Liberson developed a "slow-pulse stimulator" that delivers pulses at a rate of approximately 1 pulse every 10 seconds. This stimulator has a timer that limits applications to approximately 20 minutes, and this, unlike galvanic stimulation, has not been found harmful to the intervening skin or soft tissue. Treatment sessions are limited to 20 minutes each hour with an interval of at least an hour between sessions for a total stimulation time of 5 hours for adults and 3 hours for children per day.[16]

35. What are four different operative procedures for nerves? (See Fig. 24-19.)

- *Decompression* is the most commonly performed operation on nerves, such as median nerve decompression at the carpal tunnel.
- *Repair* of transected nerves by microsurgical suture of the perineurium.
- *Neurolysis.* Nerves can become enmeshed in dense scar tissue that tethers the nerve to bone or other tissue to such a degree that interference with function occurs. Neurolysis involves release of the nerve.
- *Grafting.* Large gaps in a nerve can be filled with a cable graft donated by a cutaneous nerve autograft such as the sural nerve. These operations are unreliable but are sometimes an attractive alternative to accepting serious disability.[3]

36. What are the goals of postoperative rehabilitation?

The whole purpose of immediate postoperative rehabilitation is the prevention of factors adverse to a satisfactory outcome.[26] This is accomplished by the maintenance of all involved structures in the best possible condition for reinnervation. The extent of therapy hinges on the magnitude of injury. Obviously, a digital nerve laceration without any concomitant injury requires only little rehabilitation. On the other hand, a major proximal nerve injury will require a substantial amount of rehabilitation. A high degree of patient motivation is required for good therapeutic outcome.[26]

Joint range of motion and tendon excursion are maintained by passive joint motion, active assistive, active, and resistive exercise in that order. Insensate neurotrophic skin should be protected and kept supple by massage and appropriate moisturizers. Edema is appropriately addressed by edema-reducing strategies such as elevations, massage, and exercises.[26]

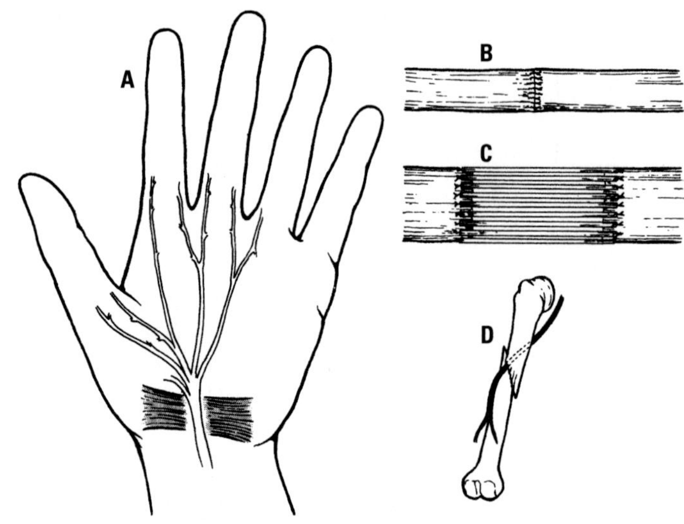

Fig. 24-19 Four different operative procedures for nerves. **A,** Decompression; **B,** Repair; **C,** Neurolysis; **D,** Grafting. (From Dandy DJ: *Essential orthopaedics and trauma,* Edinburgh, 1989, Churchill Livingstone.)

Substitution splinting in the form of passive or dynamic splints or a combination of both kinds of splints addresses the needs of remaining functional muscle groups and permits the gaining of stability so as to allow continued use of the extremity during the recovery period.[26]

37. What is the role of motor reeducation after peripheral neurosurgery?

Biofeedback is an especially important adjunct modality in the patient with a zero or grade 1 muscle function because it may help the patient to more quickly relearn control over those involved muscle groups. Biofeedback is essentially an external circuit that may actually help upgrade the function of denervated or partially denervated muscle function. Functional electrical stimulation is also helpful to the motor relearning process, in which the pattern of stimulation of weak, denervated muscle is included with a functional pattern of motion.[19,23]

38. What is the role of sensory reeducation after microneurocoaptation?

Regeneration of sensory nerve fibers are often imprecise, and the patient is faced with, at the very least, an unfamiliar volley of sensory input after repair. Without appropriate therapy, the patient may remain confused and unable to interpret these new patterns of sensory input leading to false localization and eventually absence of tactile gnosis. Sensory reeducation employs the use of higher cortical functions such as attention, learning, and memory to relearn the locale and identification of normal sensory input. For example, the patient's skin is stroked up and down with a firm, blunt object such as a pencil eraser. The patient sees what is happening and concentrates on the sensory input with his or her eyes closed so as to reconfirm the cause and localization of sensation. In such a fashion, each sensory submodality may be relearned.[26]

Once constant touch and moving submodalities are present in the previously numb area of the fingertips, late-phase sensory reeducation commences. The patient attempts to improve tactile gnosis by concentrating on the recognition of common objects of different shapes, textures, and sizes with his or her eyes open and closed. In such a fashion the patient memorizes the patterns of sensory input.[5]

The most frequently encountered
causes of damage at the
various sites are indicated
C5 and C6 Roots
Most frequently involved roots
in cervical spondylosis.
C7 involved occasionally.
Others very rarely
C7 Root
By far the most frequent "acute cervical
disc lesion" occurs at this level. C6
and C5 less often. Other levels very rarely
Axillary nerve
Fracture of humeral neck
Dislocation of the humerus
Intramuscular injections
Lower trunk of the brachial plexus
Cervical rib syndrome. Altered anatomy
(outlet syndrome). Pancoast tumour of
lung apex
Radial nerve in spiral groove
Direct blow laterally. During
anesthesia medially. While drunk
medially ("Saturday night palsy").
Fractures of the humerus -
immediate or delayed
Radial nerve in the axilla
Incorrect use of a crutch
Radial nerve (Posterior
interosseus nerve)
Nerve enters forearm through
supinator muscle. Occupational
overuse of muscle may damage
nerve. Also occurs idiopathically.
Extensors of thumb and index
finger mainly affected
Ulnar nerve
Damage from repeated minor trauma
Prolonged bed rest
Delayed after fractures
Median nerve
At elbow. Rarely damaged by
direct trauma or fracture
(Anterior interosseus nerve)
Rarely damaged nerve lies very deep
Flexors of thumb and index finger are
affected by damage to nerve
Median nerve (carpal tunnel syndrome)
Nerve damaged by swelling or infiltration
of tunnel it transverses. Transiently seen
in pregnancy. Idiopathically in females.
Complicates rheumatoid arthritis.
Rarely seen in other systemic diseases
Ulnar nerve (deep branch)
Trauma to heel of the hand. Idiopathically
(often a ganglion found on exploration)
No sensory loss in typical cases

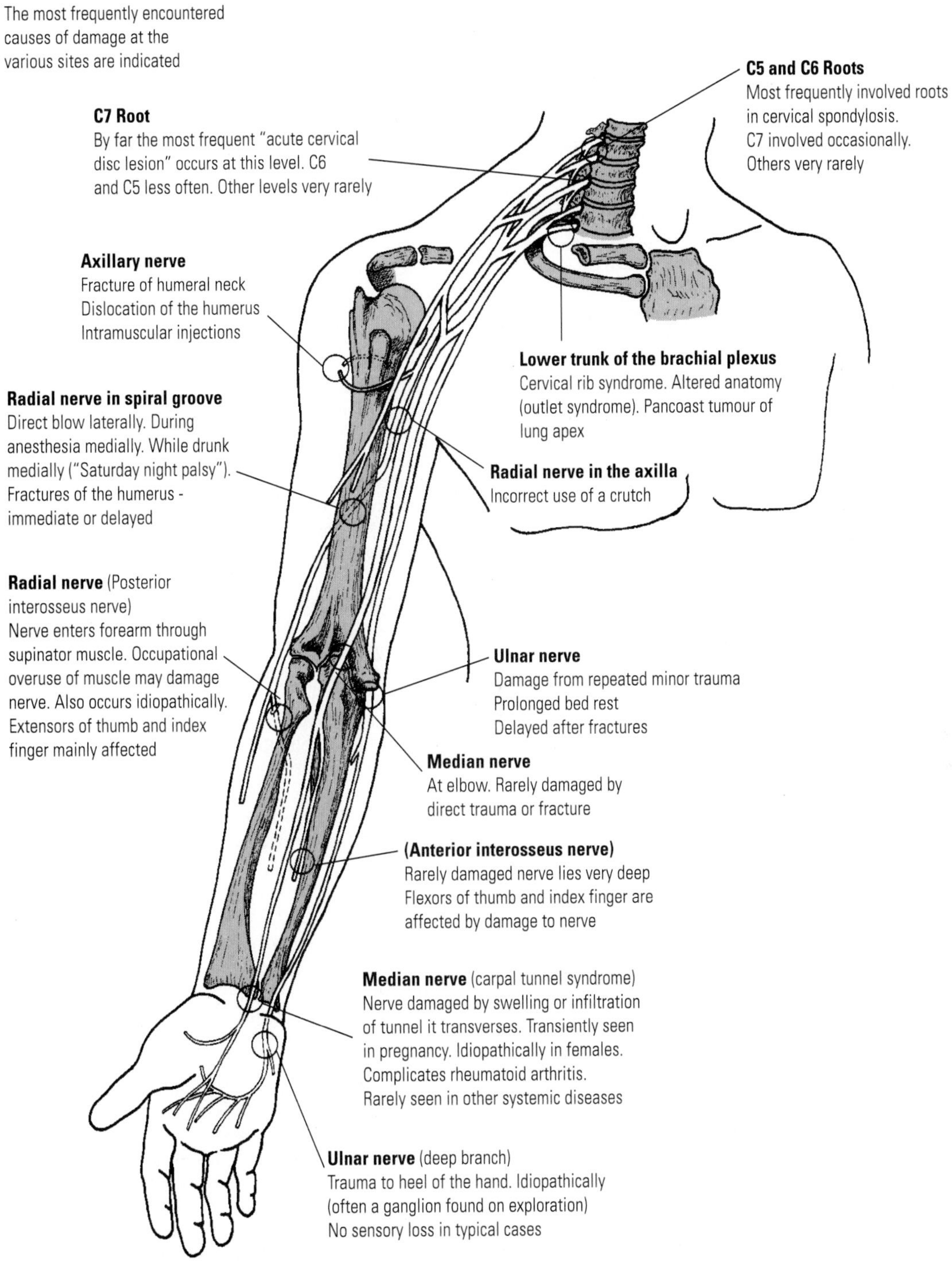

Fig. 24-20 Common sites of nerve injury in the upper extremity. (From: Patten J: *Neurologic differential diagnosis,* London, 1996, Springer-Verlag.)

References

1. Butler DS: *Mobilisation of the nervous system,* Melbourne, 1991, Churchill Livingstone.
2. Cormack DH: *Introduction to histology,* Philadelphia, 1984, Lippincott, p 220.
3. Dandy DJ: *Essential orthopaedics and trauma,* Edinburgh, 1989, Churchill Livingstone, p 49.
4. Dawson DM, Hallet M, Millender LH: *Entrapment neuropathies,* ed 2, Boston, 1990, Little, Brown & Co, p 6.
5. Dellon AL, Curtis RM, Edgerton MT: Reeducation of sensation in the hand after nerve injury and repair, *Plast Reconstr Surg* 53:297-304, 1974.
6. Diamond MC, Scheibel AB, Elson LM: *The human brain coloring book,* New York, 1985, Barnes & Noble.
7. Di Vinceti FC, Moncrief JA, Pruitt BA: Electrical injuries: a review of 65 cases, *J Trauma* 9:497-507, 1969.
8. Foo CL, Swann M: Isolated paralysis of the serratus anterior: a report of 20 cases, *J Bone Joint Surg* 65B:552-556, 1983.
9. Gentili F, Hudson AR, Hunter D, Kline DG: Nerve injection injury with local anesthetic agents: a light and electron microscopic, fluorescent microscopic, and horseradish peroxidase study, *Neurosurgery* 6(3):263-272, 1980.
10. Gentili F, Hudson AR, Kline DG, Hunter D: Peripheral nerve injection injury with steroid agents, *Plast Reconstr Surg* 69(3):482-489, 1982.
11. Harris HH, Dickey JR: Nerve grafting to restore function of the trapezius muscle after radial neck dissection, *Ann Otolaryngol* 74:880, 1965.
12. Hudson AR: Nerve injection injuries. In Terzis JK, editor: *Microreconstruction of nerve injuries,* Philadelphia, 1987, Saunders.
13. Jupiter J, Leffert RD: Non-union of the clavicle: associated complications and surgical management, *J Bone Joint Surg* 69A(5):753-760, 1987.
14. Kahn J: *Principles and practice of electrotherapy,* ed 2, New York, 1991, Churchill Livingstone, pp 91-92.
15. Leffert RD: Neurological problems. In Hunter JM, Schneider LH, Mackin EJ, Callahan AD, editors: *Rehabilitation of the hand: surgery and therapy,* ed 3, St. Louis, 1990, Mosby.
16. Liberson WT, Terzis JK: Contribution of neurophysiology and rehabilitation medicine to the management of brachial plexus palsy. In Terzis JK, editor: *Microreconstruction of nerve injuries,* Philadelphia, 1987, Saunders.
17. Lundborg G: The intrinsic vascularization of human peripheral nerves: structure and functional aspects, J Hand Surg 4(1):34, 1979.
18. Moore KL: *Clinically oriented anatomy,* ed 2, Baltimore, 1985, Williams & Wilkins, p 688.
19. Nelson AJ: Implications of electroneuromyographic examinations for hand therapy. In Hunter JM, Schneider LH, Mackin EJ, Callahan AD, editors: *Rehabilitation of the hand: surgery and therapy,* ed 3, St. Louis, 1990, Mosby.
20. Pachter BR, Eberstein A, Goodgold J: Electrical stimulation effect on denervated muscle in rats: a light and electron microscope study, *Arch Phys Med Rehabil* 67:79-83, 1986.
21. Panse F: Electrical lesions of the nervous system. In Vinken PJ, Bruyn GW, editors: *Handbook of clinical neurology,* New York, 1970, Elsevier, vol 7, pp 344-387.
22. Solem L, Fischer RP, Strate RG: The natural history of electrical injury, *J Trauma* 17(7):487-492, 1977.
23. Solomonow M: Restoration of movement by electrical stimulation: a contemporary view of the basic problems, *Orthopedics* 7(2):245-250, 1984.
24. Spillane JD, Spillane JA: *An atlas of clinical neurology,* ed 3, Oxford, 1982, Oxford University Press, p 195.
25. Sunderland S, Bradley KC: Stress-strain phenomenon in human peripheral trunks, *Brain* 84:102-119, 1961.
26. Terzis JK, Smith KL: *The peripheral nerve: structure, function, and reconstruction,* New York, 1990, Raven Press, p 58.
27. Thomas PK: The connective tissue of peripheral nerve: an electron microscopic study, *J Anat* 97:35, 1963.
28. Thomas PK, Olson Y: Microscopic anatomy and function of the connective tissue components of peripheral nerve. In Dyck PJ, Thomas PK, Lanber EH, Bunge R, editors: *Peripheral neuropathy,* Philadelphia, 1984, Saunders.
29. Wilgis EF, Murphy R: The significance of longitudinal excursion in peripheral nerves, *Hand Clin* 2(4):761-771, 1986.
30. Woodhall B: Trapezius paralysis following minor surgical procedures in the posterior cervical triangle, *Ann Surg* 136:375, 1952.

Recommended reading

Butler D: *Mobilisation of the nervous system,* Melbourne, 1991, Churchill Livingstone.

Dawson DM, Hallet M, Millender LH: *Entrapment neuropathies,* ed 2, Boston, 1990, Little, Brown & Co.

Kahn J: *Principles and practice of electrotherapy,* ed 2, New York, 1991, Churchill Livingstone.

Leffert RD: Neurological problems. In Hunter JM, Schneider LH, Mackin EJ, Callahan AD, editors: *Rehabilitation of the hand: surgery and therapy,* ed 3, St. Louis, 1990, Mosby.

Liveson JA: *Peripheral neurology: case studies in electrodiagnosis,* ed 2, Philadelphia, 1991, FA Davis Co.

Patton J: *Neurological differential diagnosis,* ed 2, London, 1996, Springer-Verlag.

Spillane JD, Spillane JA: *An atlas of clinical neurology,* ed 3, Oxford, 1982, Oxford University Press.

Terzis JK, Smith KL: *The peripheral nerve: structure, function, and reconstruction,* New York, 1990, Raven Press.

25

Momentary Stabbing Pain in Groin and Ipsilateral Buttock and Loss of Ambulation after a Fall That Yanks the Ipsilateral Extended Leg into Excessive Abduction and Flexion

CASE 1

While skiing down an intermediate slope with a ski buddy in the Colorado Rockies, your friend loses control and falls in such a way as to position her left hip in exaggerated flexion and abduction with the knee straight out in extension. She cries out in anguish, and you run to help her as others seek emergency assistance. Before the arrival of the snowmobile that will deliver her to the medic at the first aid lodge, she tells you of a frightening and momentary stabbing pain in the left side of her groin and a pulling sensation near her left buttock at the moment of injury. As you help the ski patrol gently hoist her body out of its entangled posture, the sudden movement causes her to cry out and writhe in pain. Down at the lodge clinic the following clinical picture emerges during the examination.

OBSERVATION The patient cannot walk because of pain and requires the use of crutches. There is slight ecchymosis and swelling over the proximal third of the upper inner and anterior thigh.

PALPATION Moderate tenderness is present both at the left ischial tuberosity and over the upper third of the anterior left thigh within the muscular soft tissue.

PASSIVE RANGE OF MOTION Passive left hip flexion and abduction are painful.

ACTIVE RANGE OF MOTION Pain is elicited on active hip adduction while she is lying supine; active hip extension while in a side-lying or prone position. Antigravity hip extension is not possible.

MUSCLE STRENGTH Judged to be fair plus, though adequate testing is hindered by the patient's pain.

RESISTED TESTS Resisted adductor and knee extension are painful.

SPECIAL TESTS Negative for knee stability. Radiographs taken show no evidence of fracture or avulsion and are otherwise normal appearing.

CASE 2

A 38-year-old male police officer takes his Great Dane out for a walk in the evening after work hours. While stopping at the corner to casually talk to a friend, he begins to feel a considerable tug on the leash held in his left hand. While talking and distracted, he pulls on the leash while widening his base of support by assuming a horse stance so as to counter the pull of his large dog. Eventually, his dog becomes frantic as another dog struts by only several feet past where dog and owner are standing, and the dog's barking culminates in a sideways lunge that forcefully yanks the owner sideways to his left and off balance. He feels an immediate excruciating pain and popping sensation in the left side of his groin and can barely stand. He returns home with great difficulty and only with the help of his friend. Clinical examination reveals the identical signs and symptoms as in *case 1,* minus pain and tenderness to the buttock area; additionally, active hip extension and passive hip flexion are painless and full in range.

1. **What is most likely to have occurred to these patients?**
2. **What are the two categories of injury to which muscle tissue is liable?**
3. **What accounts for distraction injuries often occurring in two joint muscles?**
4. **What are the degrees in the classification of muscle strain?**
5. **Why are distraction strains involving the upper extremity rare as compared to the incidence of these strains in the lower extremity?**
6. **What are eccentric contractions?**
7. **Why is the term "eccentric contraction" a misnomer?**
8. **What are the clinical findings in muscle injury?**
9. **What are differences of clinical presentation between a partial and a total rupture of muscle?**
10. **What is an intramuscular hematoma?**
11. **What is an intermuscular hematoma?**
12. **How are *intra*muscular and *inter*muscular hematomas differentiated?**
13. **What is the medical management of intramuscular hematoma?**
14. **What special problems are unique to the situation of lacerated muscle?**
15. **What common mechanism of injury results in pectoralis major rupture?**
16. **What common mechanism of injury results in a deltoid muscle rupture?**
17. **What common mechanism of injury results in a triceps muscle rupture?**
18. **What common mechanism of injury results in a biceps brachii rupture?**
19. **What common mechanism of injury results in a quadriceps contusion?**
20. **What common mechanism of injury results in a rectus femoris strain?**
21. **What common mechanism of injury results in a gluteus maximus strain?**
22. **What common mechanism of injury results in an adductor strain?**
23. **What is a pulled hamstrings injury?**
24. **What therapeutic management is appropriate for muscle strains?**

1. What is most likely to have occurred to these patients?

The patients have most likely sustained a combined hamstring and adductor *strain* in case 1 and an adductor strain only in case 2. Muscle injuries are among the most common, misunderstood, and inadequately treated conditions in sports physical therapy.[12] The significance of these sorts of injuries is often understated because most patients, having sustained muscle injury, can continue on with their daily activities soon after injury. Chronic problems may develop either because of prolonged self-treatment or continued activity despite pain. The most commonly strained muscles of the lower extremities include the hamstrings, adductor longus, iliopsoas, rectus femoris, and the gastrocnemius muscles.[13]

2. What are the two categories of injury to which muscle tissue is liable?

Distraction ruptures are caused by (1) *overstretching* or (2) *contractile overload*, often occurring in the superficial aspect of muscle or at the origin and insertion. Overload occurs as a result of *intrinsic force*, whether concentric or eccentric, and generated by an individual's own muscle so that the demand made upon a muscle exceeds its innate strength. Examples of how this may occur include sudden deceleration (eccentric), rapid acceleration (concentric), or the potentially dangerous combination of deceleration and acceleration that accompanies sharp cutting movements. The common denominator to this sort of injury is that injury frequently occurs in activities requiring explosive muscular effort over a short period of time, and it occurs in sports such as sprinting, jumping, baseball, football, and soccer.[12] Overstretching of a specific muscle, however, occurs by way of excessive contraction of that muscle's *antagonist*.[3]

Compression ruptures result from direct trauma in which a forceful impact pushes muscle back against unyielding bone.[12] The subsequent contusion and tearing of muscle is generically termed a "charley horse" (possibly after the typical name of old lame horses) and results in the formation of a local mass of blood (hematoma) that escapes into the muscle from damaged vessels. The most common site of a charley horse involves the quadriceps muscle,[11] as may occur from a football tackle, or collision during a soccer game in which one player's knee rams into the anterior area of the thigh of another player.[12] Heavy bleeding may occur from compression injuries *deep* within the muscle, since the momentum imparted from impact may be transmitted to the deep muscular compartment, which bears the brunt of injury by virtue of its being adjacent to bone. Or injury may cause bleeding to the *superficial* portion[12] of the muscle if the injurious force was delivered in a direction other than perpendicular to the surface of that muscle.

3. What accounts for distraction injuries often occurring in two joint muscles?

The hamstring muscle group and rectus femoris from the quadriceps muscle group, as well as the gastrocnemius and the biceps brachii, are all examples of two-joint muscles that are more prone to sustaining distraction injury by virtue of their extended span of length beyond more than one joint.[12] Muscle receptors have the unique task of maintaining an optimal milieu of muscle tone at both ends of the muscle (that is, across each joint) within the narrow confines of the Blix curve. Any deviation from optimum length and optimal tension will place muscle tissue at a greater potential risk for injury, since that muscle will then operate at less than optimum efficiency. Muscles normally operate within relatively narrow margins of length and tension before succumbing to decreased mechanical efficiency by even slightly excessive stretch or swelling of the muscle. Most muscles carry the burden of maintaining this milieu under constantly shifting conditions that move the muscle, lever like, across a single joint. Two-joint muscles are saddled with juggling this same task while moving two separate joints simultaneously! It is no wonder then that two-joint muscles are more likely candidates for injury. The actual site chosen for injury along the muscle's span is governed by the question: Where is the weakest link in the muscle-tendon-bone unit? The answer is that the location differs for each muscle.

4. What are the degrees in the classification of muscle strain?

A strain is a tear in the muscle-tendon complex. Mild to minimal strains are graded first degree, whereas second degree strains involve moderate disruption of the myotendinous unit. There are no clear criteria differentiating a first-degree from a second-degree strain. A designation may be made based on the amount of pain, swelling, and spasm present. Additionally, first-degree injuries tend to heal more readily and allow for an early return to athletic training than do second-degree injuries.[14a]

First-degree, or *mild, strain* represents an overstretching of the muscle or rupture of less than 5% of muscle fibers.[12] There is no significant loss of strength or restriction of movement, though active movement or passive stretching will cause some pain and discomfort. A first-degree strain will often resolve itself without treatment and without residual disability.[6]

Second-degree, or *moderate, strain* is more significant than a mild strain in that it involves greater than 5% of muscle fibers.[12] This kind of muscle injury is the one most frequently seen in the clinic, and must be treated cautiously, inasmuch as it may progress to a third-degree strain. Additionally, a second-degree strain, if untreated, may result in excessive scar formation with delayed healing.[14b]

Third-degree, or *severe, strain* involves total disruption of muscle.[12]

5. Why are distraction strains involving the upper extremity rare as compared to the incidence of these strains in the lower extremity?

Strains involving upper extremity musculature are, barring direct blows, relatively rare as compared to injuries occurring to the lower extremities. The lower extremities act as a transitional point for potentially disruptive forces entering the body by way of ground reaction forces incurred during locomotion. Because of this, the lower extremity evolved a larger bulk and breadth of muscle as well as the frequently recruited protective eccentric contraction as part of a repertoire of strategy that helps fend off disruptive forces. In contradistinction, although the upper extremity possesses the ability to contract eccentrically, it does so at times as a necessity of functioning within a gravitational environment and not additionally, as with the lower extremities, to absorb eccentrically the brunt of impact from normal forces. This, of course, excludes the professional trapeze artist or someone who locomotes by doing cartwheels all day.

For example, in bowling, the volar muscles of the dominant upper extremity eccentrically slow down the ball as it descends just before release across the floor toward the pins. From a functional point of view we can state that the upper extremity, like the lower extremity, contracts eccentrically but does so by choice rather than out of necessity. In other words, the lower extremity must eccentrically contract so that it may successfully cross terrain in a gravitational environment for the purpose of survival, that is, the foraging of food, if nothing else. On the other hand, most if not all tasks of daily living involving the upper extremity are simple open kinetic chain, ballistic movements.

6. What are eccentric contractions?

Whereas concentric contraction involves molecular cross-bridging that approximates the two Z lines composing the sarcomere unit, an eccentric contraction works the muscle such that distraction of the Z lines actually occurs. Eccentric contraction represents the muscular system's coping strategy, recruited to absorb the energy of disruptive forces and deflect potential injury in those situations requiring high velocity or heavy resistive loads. This is not to say that the eccentric mode of muscle contraction is used only when excessive forces are imparted to the musculoskeletal system. Rather, eccentric muscle activity is part of the muscular repertoire of contraction used by the body and especially so for the lower extremities during locomotion. Interestingly, given the fact that humans, before the advent of modernity, have had to walk around quite a bit, it is no wonder that eccentric work costs less energy than concentric work.[1,4]

Eccentric muscle activity involves the voluntary yielding of control in a graded fashion as a direct function of gravity or the opposition of internally generated forces. For example, if you suddenly wanted to

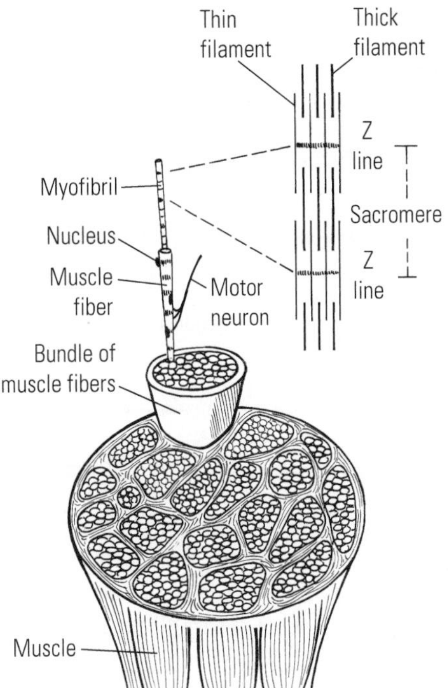

Fig. 25-1 Anatomic organization of skeletal muscle. *Sarcomeres* are arranged end to end, single file, forming a *myofibril.* Bundles of myofibrils make up a syncytial *muscle fiber.* Muscle fibers are grouped together to form *muscle bundles* together in dozens or hundreds to compose a *muscle.* (From Arms K, Camp PS: *Biology,* ed 2, Philadelphia, 1982, Saunders College Publishing.)

squat down to eye level with a toddler, you could do so concentrically but would do so quite abruptly by whipping yourself down to 135° of knee flexion. This motion would be awkward and might cause you to lose balance, or even injure yourself. However, this abruptness and awkwardness is bypassed in the presence of gravity, and so we can easily drop down onto our haunches by means of a "lengthening" contraction of our hip extensor muscles. We become awkward without gravity. The paradox that emerges from this thought experiment highlights the fact that what we normally refer to as flexor or extensor are actually semantically relative terms whose reference point is gravity. Thus, eccentric contractions would not occur to astronauts orbiting Earth who are in a state of weightlessness. What we come away with is that we rather have *agonist* and *antagonist muscles.*

7. Why is the term "eccentric contraction" a misnomer?

The term "contraction" is literally a semantic misnomer because what happens on a microanatomic level is actually a ***distraction*** (elongation) of the myofibril unit. Although the distracted state of the Z lines composing the sarcomere unit conjure up the state of a relaxed myofibril in the concentric framework, cross-bridging of thick (myosin) and thin (actin) molecular filaments presumably still occurs in the eccentric framework. This is precisely the reason the heads of the myosin molecules *do* swivel, albeit in opposite direction, and thus permit the distraction of the Z lines and hence of the myofibril on a larger scale, in a graded controlled fashion (Fig. 25-2). Perhaps "muscle working," or "muscle activity," rather than "muscle contraction," is a more accurate term describing how energy is expended by muscle.

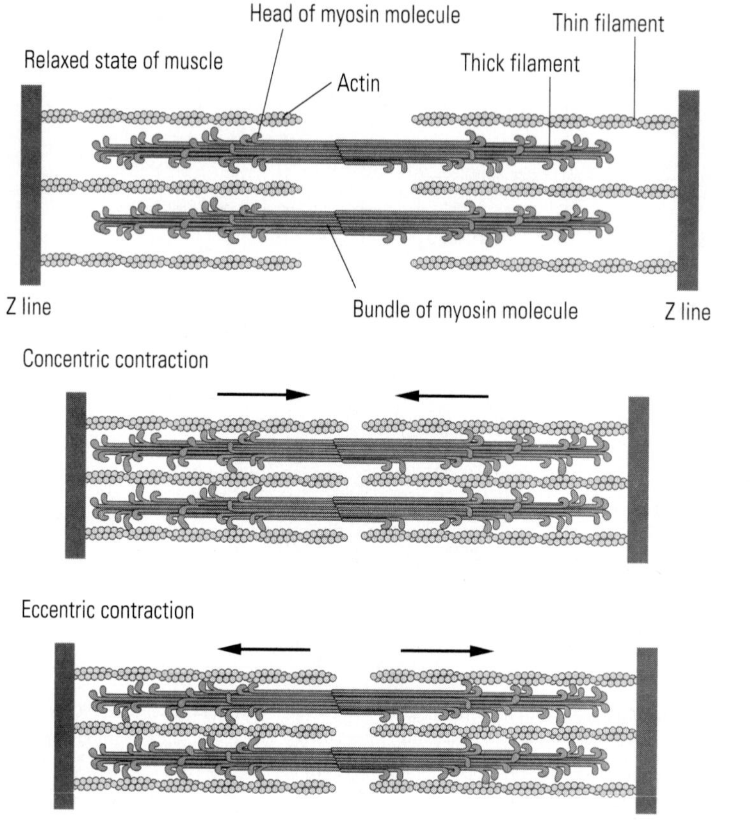

Fig. 25-2 Myosin and actin filaments are actively engaged during concentric and eccentric contraction. In the former, the Z lines approximate; in the latter, they distract. During muscular activity the filaments chemically interact when the heads of the myosin molecules (thick filaments) attach to the molecules (located along the length of the thin actin filaments). This cross-bridging of the filaments results in swiveling of the head of the myosin molecules.

8. What are the clinical findings in muscle injury?

Pain is reported to emanate either from the muscle belly, its origin, or its insertion. Pain and stiffness may decrease during exercise, only to return after exercise with greater intensity. Active or resistive movement in the direction of action of the muscle will reproduce pain as will passive stretch in the opposite direction. Additionally the muscle may demonstrate a decrease in strength. It is not uncommon that there is a history of recurrence of disability in which a person reduces her or his activity level until pain has subsided, only to return to the same activity too soon and incur repeated injury.

9. What are differences of clinical presentation between a partial and a total rupture of muscle?

Although the pain after partial rupture can inhibit muscle contraction, the muscle that sustained a total rupture is unable to contract. In addition, with partial ruptures it is sometimes possible to feel a defect in part of the muscle during examination, whereas with total ruptures one can distinguish a palpable gap or defect across the entire muscle belly. In fact, the muscle may even "bunch up" to form a hump that resembles a local tumor.[12]

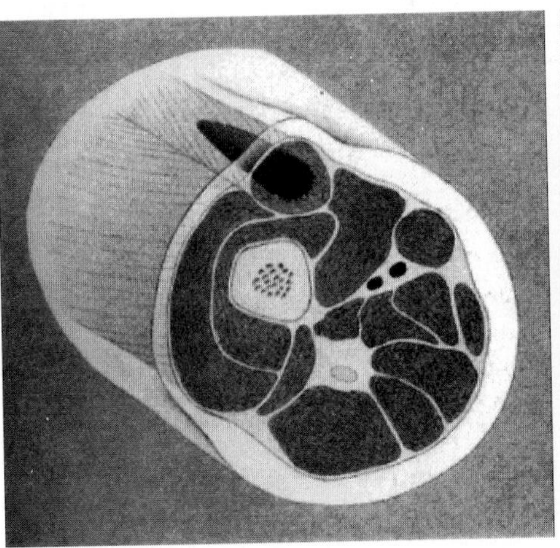

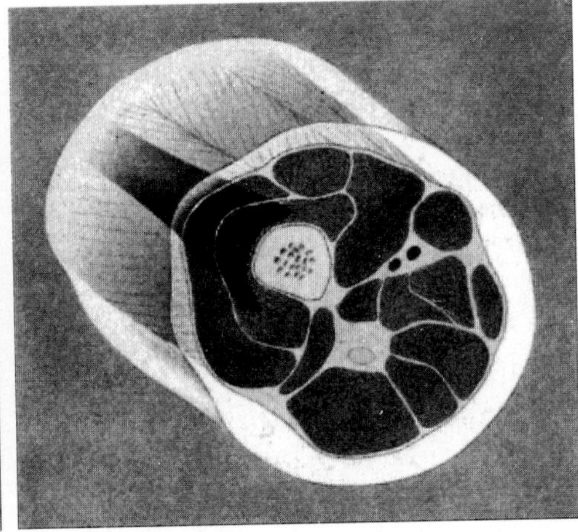

Fig. 25-3 Intramuscular hemotoma. (From Peterson L, Renström P: *Sports injuries: their prevention and treatment,* London, 1986, Martin Dunitz, Ltd.)

10. What is an intramuscular hematoma?

An *intramuscular hematoma* (Fig. 25-3) results from bleeding within the muscle sheath that further results in a *rise of intramuscular pressure.* This is actually a protective measure that counteracts a tendency to any further bleeding by way of compressing the vessels within that muscle. However, the pressure may rise so excessively high as to be counterproductive, leading to an *acute compartment syndrome.*[12]

This dangerous situation results in the occlusion of microcirculation secondary to ischemia or complete loss of blood supply, with potential loss of limb function. For example, after a supracondylar fracture the median nerve and radial artery can both be compressed by swelling within the anterior compartment of the forearm. In the event of paresthesia along the median nerve distribution accompanied by loss of finger extension on clinical examination, an emergency surgical fasciotomy is warranted, despite there being a radial pulse present, so as to avert disastrous loss of limb. Limb loss may occur as the swollen compartment clamps down on the blood vessel or vessels passing through it, thus starving itself of oxygen. The result is muscle necrosis and eventual replacement of muscle tissue in the flexor compartment of the forearm with mats of fibrous tissue. This new tissue will subsequently undergo contracture and pull the limb and its joints into the disabling, permanent, and horrible posture of finger flexion, wrist flexion, and forearm pronation known as *Volkmann's ischemic contracture* (Fig. 25-4) of the forearm.[5]

11. What is an intermuscular hematoma?

An *intermuscular hematoma* (Fig. 25-5) is a relatively more benign situation that involves damage to the muscle sheath in addition to the muscle itself. This allows released blood to flow out of a given compartment and spread into that potential space between muscles, or out amongst the surrounding soft tissue. Thus pressure from the initial injury is not sustained, since there exists an avenue by which any damaging pressure is dissipated. Because of this, swelling is temporary, and muscle function will rapidly return to normal.[12]

12. How are *intra*muscular and *inter*muscular hematomas differentiated?

Rising intramuscular pressure can become dangerous if left unmonitored. Constant reexamination of the injured areas is necessary to distinguish between intermuscular and intramuscular bleeding. It is impera-

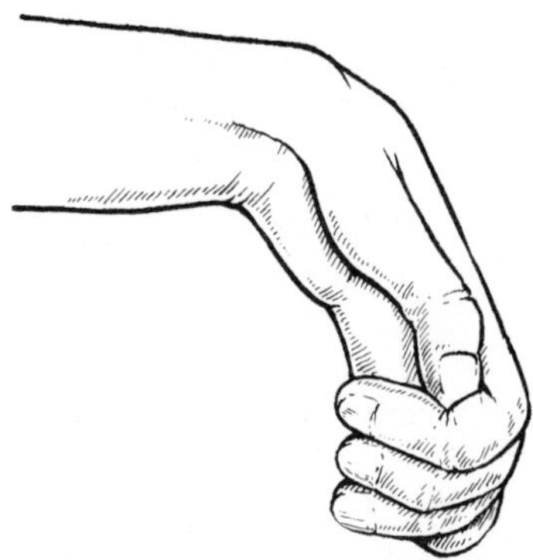

Fig. 25-4 Volkman's ischemic contracture of the forearm. (From Dandy DJ: *Essential orthopaedics and trauma,* Edinburgh, 1989, Churchill Livingstone.)

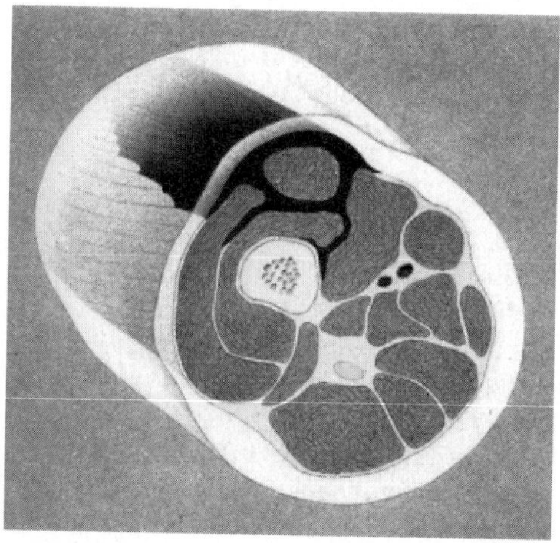

Fig. 25-5 Intermusculer hematoma. (From Peterson L, Renström P: *Sports injuries: their prevention and treatment,* London, 1986, Martin Dunitz, Ltd.)

tive that an accurate diagnosis be made because premature exercise of a muscle affected by extensive intramuscular hematoma or complete rupture can cause complications in the form of further bleeding and sometimes increased scar formation. This in turn is likely to lead to a more protracted healing process and even permanent disability.

Decreased swelling and rapid recovery of function would be suggestive of *inter*muscular injury, whereas increased swelling with sustained poor function are suggestive of *intra*muscular injury. Additionally, if blood has spread and thereby causes bruising some distance from the site of injury, the hematoma is most probably intermuscular. Moreover, if the muscles' contractile ability does not show improvement and if swelling does not resolve itself, an intramuscular bleed is most likely present.[12]

13. What is the medical management of intramuscular hematoma?

If after 72 hours the symptoms caused by the injured muscle fail to improve, the possibility of intramuscular hematoma ought to be considered. The physician may take one or more of the following steps: measure intercompartmental pressure, puncture and aspirate the area with a wide-bore needle if pressure fluctuation is present, request soft-tissue radiographs with or without a contrast medium, administer an ultrasound examination, or undertake surgery. Surgery is especially appropriate if the muscle in question lacks compensatory agonists of equal size and power, as occurs with the pectoralis major. Surgery involves removal of any intervening blood clots, as well as repair of torn muscle by suturing the ends together such that the least possible scar formation will show. This is then followed by a period of immobilization in a plaster cast.[12]

14. What special problems are unique to the situation of lacerated muscle?

Muscle may be lacerated externally by a knife wound or internally from the sharp fragments of broken bone. In the event that muscle tissue is divided transversely, regardless of cause, the muscle will not hold sutures well enough to prevent normal muscle contraction from simply pulling apart the two sutured ends.[5] Another problem with invasive management is that operative insult may cause additional soft-tissue destruction[5] en route as the surgeon attempts to reach the injured area. Therefore, although the fascia surrounding muscle is amenable to repair, the risk of more soft-tissue destruction makes this unwise.[5] These kinds of injury and as well the nontransverse ruptures of a muscle belly cannot be repaired successfully. Healing takes at least 6 weeks, during which sound fibrous scar tissue is laid down to fill the gap.[5]

15. What common mechanism of injury results in pectoralis major rupture?

Pectoralis major rupture is a rare injury that, when occurring, has been reported to occur almost exclusively in males. This major and severe injury is accompanied by significant swelling and ecchymosis typically occurring from weight-lifting activities, particularly the bench press. An attempt to break a fall, resulting in severe force applied to a maximally contracted pectoralis major muscle, is yet another common mechanism of injury. Rupture may occur in that muscle's proximal or distal portion, resulting in immediate shoulder dysfunction, with visible or palpable defect. Partial ruptures are managed conservatively with initial icing and rest in the acute stage, followed by heat, ultrasound, and a program of passive and active assisted exercises of the shoulder subacutely. Although unresisted stretching exercises should be included early in the rehabilitation program, resistive exercises should follow a 6-week recovery period after good shoulder mobility is restored and the pain is resolved. A complete pectoralis rupture requires early surgical treatment in the active athlete.[3]

16. What common mechanism of injury results in a deltoid muscle rupture?

Deltoid muscle rupture is an extremely rare clinical entity, whereas minor strains of this muscle are common in athletic activity, especially in throwing sports. The anterior deltoid may suffer strain during the acceleration phase of throwing, when a forcible contraction and a forward body movement are simultaneously applied to an already stretched musculotendinous unit. The posterior deltoid acts to restrain the shoulder in the followthrough phase at the end of forward arm motion and is thus vulnerable to injury.

Clinical presentation varies with the site of rupture. In the event that the lesion is located near the deltoid's insertion, a defect may be palpable, as well as an associated mass that becomes firmer upon contraction of that muscle. If the deltoid has become avulsed from its origin, there would be a loss of normal contour of the muscle with weakness in flexion, abduction, or extension. If the rotator cuff was also involved, contraction of the spared deltoid will cause the humeral head to protrude in the direction of deltoid deficiency.

Minor strains and partial deltoid lesions are managed conservatively and usually restore the shoulder to full activity with a prescription of local cryotherapy in the acute stage, followed by heat, shoulder range of motion exercises and stretching, and gentle strengthening over a course of 6 weeks.[3]

17. What common mechanism of injury results in a triceps muscle rupture?

A triceps rupture is a rare injury that may result either from indirect injury or from a direct blow. Although the former is characterized by the application of excessive tension to the triceps muscle fibers from, say, a fall onto an outstretched hand, the latter mechanism may result from the elbow striking a fixed object. On examination, a palpable defect of the triceps tendon is usually present and accompanied by pain, swelling, bruising, and weakness of elbow extension. Complete rupture precludes antigravity elbow extension, whereas a false-negative clinical observation may be assessed if extension is allowed to be eccentrically performed by the biceps muscles. Radial head fracture is a common associated finding with tenderness and swelling over the fracture site.[8]

18. What common mechanism of injury results in a biceps brachii rupture?

A *biceps rupture* is ordinarily a rare injury[3] that does occur in greater frequency in military parachutists.[7,15] The mechanism of indirect injury involves the incorrect positioning of the static line in the front of the arm. When the paratrooper jumps, a severe force of 80 pounds per square inch is applied over the biceps, especially if the arm is simultaneously abducted after push-off. The patient will report a tearing or popping sensation at the time of injury, followed by severe pain, swelling, and loss of strength. A visible and palpable muscle defect may be detected if the patient is seen early before the onset of significant hematoma and swelling. Medical management of patients seen acutely after the rupture includes hematoma aspiration and immobilization of the elbow in acute flexion for 6 weeks, whereas subacute ruptures undergo open repair and immobilization in acute elbow flexion for 4 weeks. The angle is then decreased to 90° for an additional 2 weeks.[3]

19. What common mechanism of injury results in a quadriceps contusion?

Quadriceps contusion, otherwise known colloquially as a *charley horse*, is a term for a common injury in contact sports caused by a direct blow to the thigh that compresses the quadriceps muscle into the underlying femur. Examination reveals tenderness, swelling, often a large hematoma on the anterior part of the thigh, and a loss of knee range that may be severe enough to cause a total loss of knee flexion. Radiographic examination is appropriate to rule out the possibility of femoral fracture.[9]

Treatment begins acutely with the application of ice packs for 10 minutes every waking hour for 3 to 5 days after the injury. Knee flexion to the pain barrier is facilitated by the placement of pillows under the knee. The patient may ambulate using crutches, with weight bearing to pain tolerance. Although active range of motion exercise is to be performed within the pain-free range, the patient should avoid passive stretching, which can only increase muscle bleeding. Active hip flexion, though, ought to be encouraged. Once swelling has begun to decrease in the subacute stage, hot and cold contrast applications may be initiated along with quadriceps-strengthening exercises. Active range of motion exercise ought to continue to be performed frequently. Only when regaining 90% of ipsilateral quadriceps length as compared with the uninjured contralateral side, measured in the prone position with both knees actively flexed, may the athlete return to his game.[9]

20. What common mechanism of injury results in a rectus femoris strain?

A *rectus femoris strain* (Fig. 25-6) refers to rupture of the origin, or upper third of this muscle, that is experienced as pain in the groin[12] and anterior area of the thigh.[9] These symptoms are preceded by a sudden stabbing pain or pulling sensation[9] during a vigorous hip-flexion motion that may accompany a sudden fast running start. Injury may also occur after a football tackle or during shooting practice in soccer. Additionally, injury may result from forced hip flexion against resistance or after excessive hip extension, especially when coupled with knee flexion, because this combination placed the two-joint rectus femoris on passive insufficiency and hence at greater risk for distraction strain.

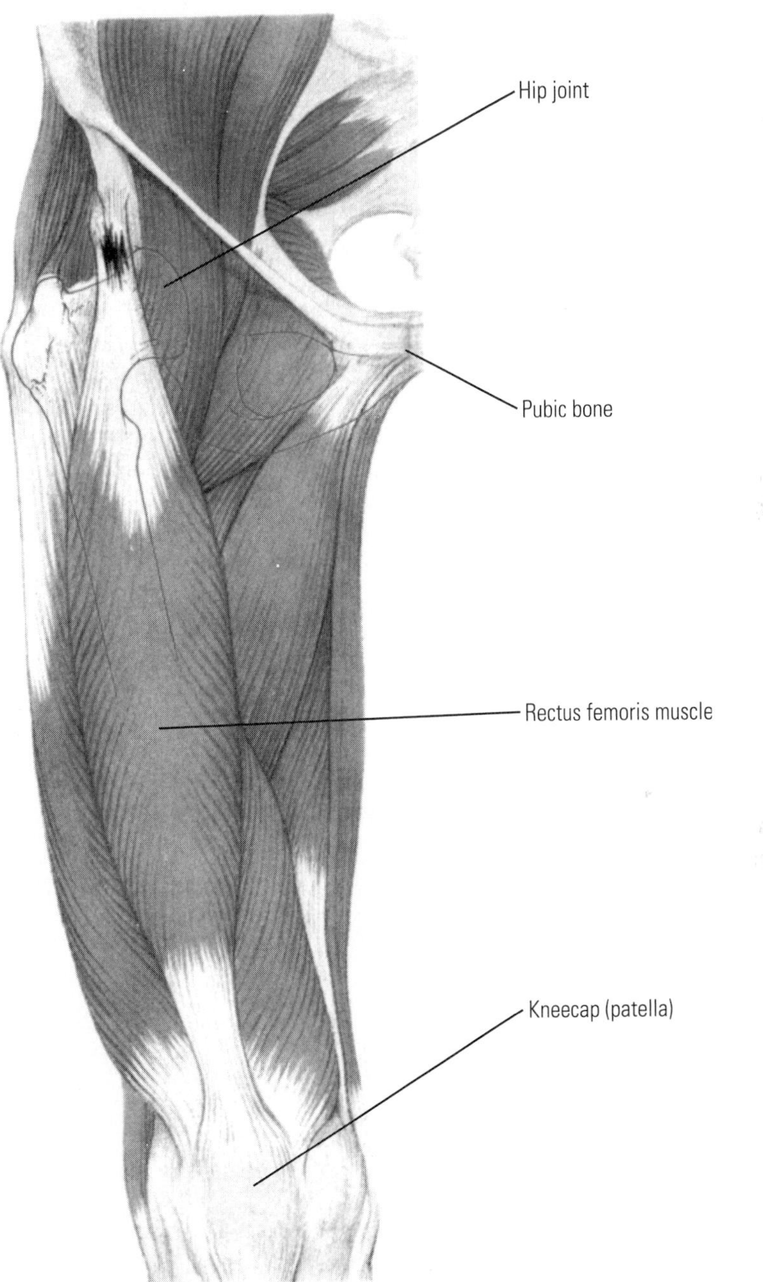

Fig. 25-6 Rectus femoris strain. (From Peterson L, Renström P: *Sports injuries: their prevention and treatment,* London, 1986, Martin Dunitz, Ltd.)

Examination reveals tenderness to palpation that increases during resisted knee extension,[9] or resisted hip flexion as well as from a prone quadriceps stretch. Pain is more likely elicited on resistive knee extension than with resistive hip flexion, since the rectus femoris contributes to hip flexion in a rather minor capacity. Radiographs are indicated if an avulsion off the anterior superior iliac spine is suspected, especially in growing adolescents.[12] Treatment begins with ice massage and then progresses to contrast treatment of alternating ultrasound with cryotherapy. Range of motion and quadriceps setting exercises are appropriate immediately. Strengthening begins with concentric exercises and then progresses to eccentric activities. Backward walking and running is a good concentric workout of the quadriceps, whereas forward locomotion works that muscle eccentrically. The athlete may return to running when the motion shows 80% of range, as compared to the uninvolved side.[9]

Injury to iliopsoas (Fig. 25-7) may occur by way of the same mechanism as that of rectus femoris strain[6] and may occur from strength training with weights and simultaneous performing of deep knee bends, sit-ups, rowing, plowing through the snow for conditioning, running uphill, intensive shooting practice in soccer, badminton, long jump and high jump, hurdling, and steeple chasing. Unlike rectus femoris strain, here symptoms will be elicited from resistive hip flexion but not from resistive knee extension. In a similar vein, the same level of pain is perceived by the patient during the passive prone hip-extension test whether the examiner simultaneously bends the knee. Rupture of the iliopsoas muscle is rare, but when it occurs, it is usually located in the tendon, or tendon insertion on the greater trochanter.[12]

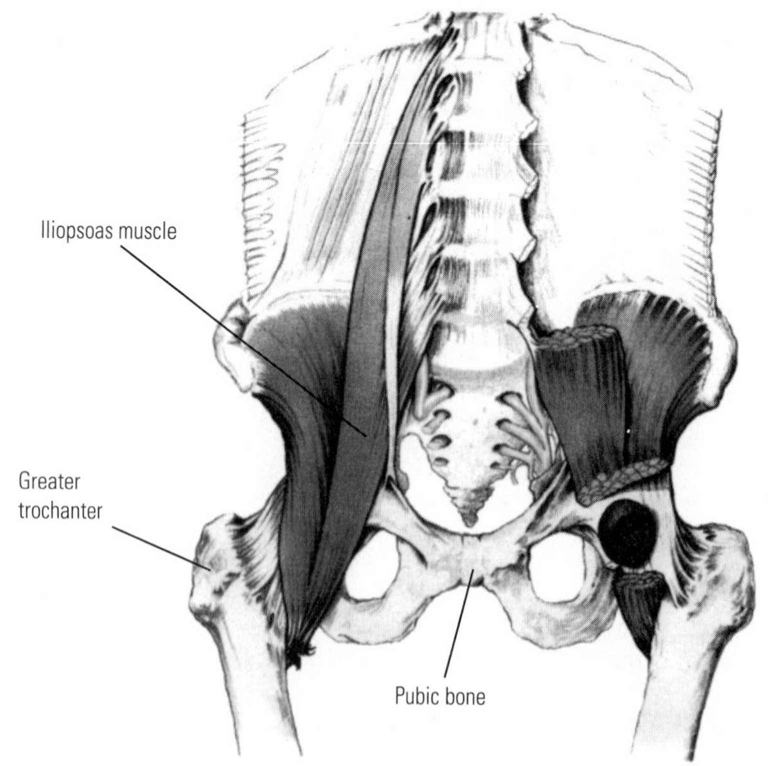

Fig. 25-7 Partial strain of the iliopsoas muscle. (From Peterson L, Renström P: *Sports injuries: their prevention and treatment,* London, 1986, Martin Dunitz, Ltd.)

21. What common mechanism of injury results in a gluteus maximus strain?

An isolated *strain of gluteus maximus* is uncommon but can occur in sprinters. There is often associated sacroiliac joint involvement, and so the examiner must rule out any sacroiliac joint dysfunction, in addition to lumbar involvement or the piriformis syndrome. If the examiner finds tenderness in the muscle bulk of the gluteus maximus but elicits no pain while palpating the sciatic notch, especially during resistive hip external rotation, then, having ruled out the piriformis syndrome, the clinician may suspect a gluteus maximus strain. This is confirmed when the patient reports a history of sudden sharp buttock pain during a burst of speed or sudden directional change.

Acute treatment involves ice massage to the sore area. Subacute treatment (after 72 hours) by deep heating of this thick muscle belly is achieved by means of ultrasound and followed by knee-to-chest exercises to stretch that muscle. As the pain subsides, one should commence a strengthening program that involves stair-climbing activities and the use of leg-press machines to strengthen that muscle.[9]

22. What common mechanism of injury results in an adductor strain?

Adductor strain, otherwise known as a *groin pull* (Fig. 25-8), is a debilitating injury caused by forced external rotation and abduction,[7] as may occur from a sudden directional change during sprinting, or repeated forceful adduction as may occur in soccer, when the ball and an opponent's foot are kicked together,[12] thus causing severe momentary stretching of a contracted adductor muscle. The patient feels a sudden momentary stabbing pain in the groin region that returns when he or she attempts to restart the activity.[12] Although local bleeding causes swelling and bruising, these do not often manifest until several days after the injury. Active or resistive adduction, as well as passive or active abduction, should elicit pain. If the muscle cannot contract, there is reason to suspect total rupture.[12] Complete ruptures occur at that muscle's insertion onto the femur or, less likely, at its origin off the pubic bone. Partial ruptures usually occur in the muscle itself, or at its pubic origin. Radiographs are appropriate here, especially if there is bony tenderness present.[12] If the onset is insidious, the clinician should consider the possibility of proximomedial femoral-shaft stress fracture or periostitis.[9]

23. What is a pulled hamstrings injury?

A *pulled-hamstrings* injury (Fig. 25-9) involves strain rupture of one or more of the three hamstring muscles, usually as a result of excessive overload of those muscles. Sprinters show an especially high incidence of this injury.[10] The often violent muscular exertion[11] that occurs with sprinting or long-distance running[12] may tear or avulse part of the tendinous origin of one of these muscle from their common origin off the ischial tuberosity;[9] injury may also occur in the midthigh region or more distally.[2] Injury will commonly occur during the last half of the swing phase, during which the hamstrings work eccentrically, or during early stance phase, when there is a large concentric boost of energy.[14]

Proposed causes of hamstring strain include an imbalance of strength between the hamstring muscles in each leg and tightness in these muscles. Hamstring strain injury may also occur after long or triple jumping and may occur during a badminton or tennis game,[12] or because of a very hard kick with the knee extended delivered to a football or soccer ball, which inadvertently creates a sudden forceful stretch or eccentric contraction to the hamstrings as the player attempts to decelerate his foot in an effort to control or aim the force delivered to the ball. The resultant injury usually extends longitudinally within the muscle strain, rather than transversely,[9] and the injury is so painful that the runner will often fall and writhe in pain.[11] The athlete may self-diagnose the problem at the time of injury and complain of a "pull" or "pop" sensation. Swelling occurs usually 2 hours[9] after the injury, since the hematoma is initially contained by the dense fascia lata;[11] ecchymosis is observed within 48 hours.[9] Resisted knee flexion will increase symptoms, and the athlete is often unable to straighten the knee during the terminal swing phase of the gait. Avulsion fracture is suspected if the tibial tuberosity is exquisitely tender.[9]

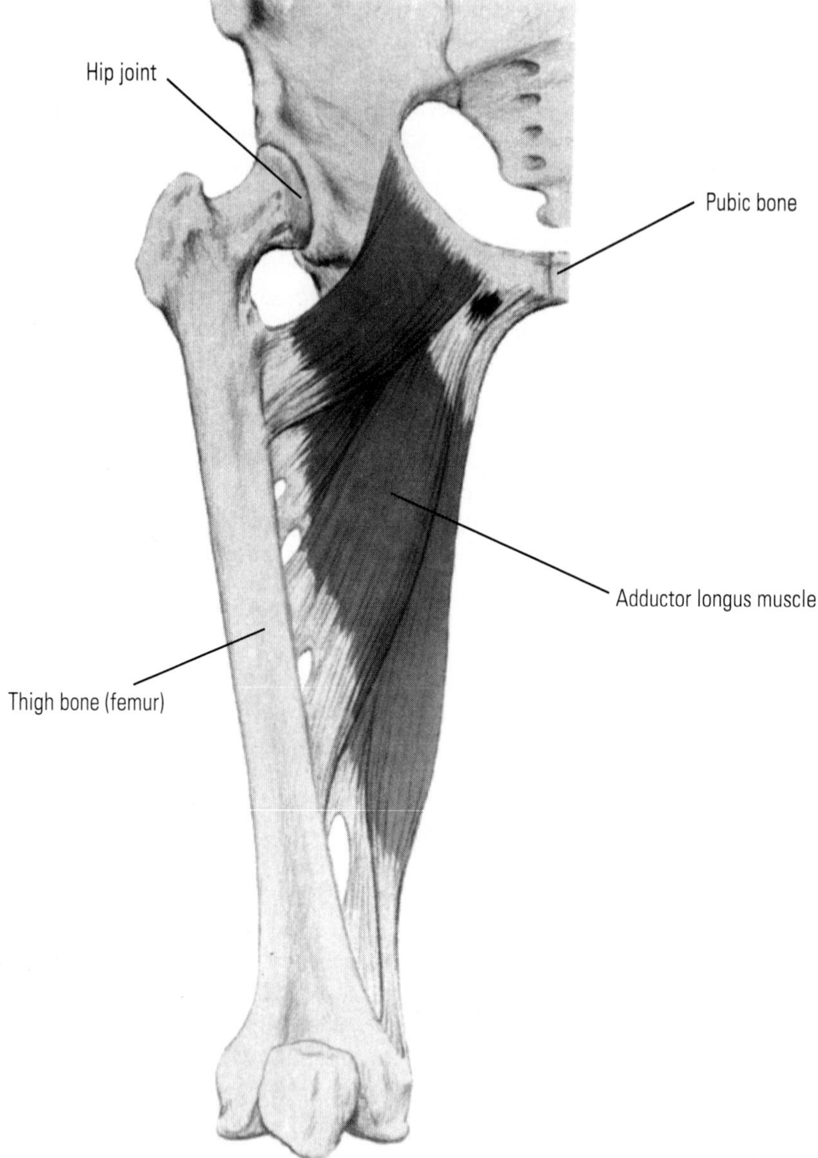

Fig. 25-8 Groin-pull injury. (From Peterson L, Renström P: *Sports injuries: their prevention and treatment,* London, 1986, Martin Dunitz, Ltd.)

The acute stage of management consists in the use of ice packs or ice massage to the site of injury, compression wraps, and possibly crutches. In the subacute phase (after 72 hours), when swelling begins to subside, a program of ice and heat contrasts is appropriate in conjunction with pulsed ultrasound (with or without the use of steroid cream)[2] and is followed by a 30-second passive hamstring stretch in the pain-free range.[9] Progression to active hip and knee hamstring range of motion may be incorporated once symptoms abate.[2] As healing progresses over time, contract-relax techniques to the hamstrings are

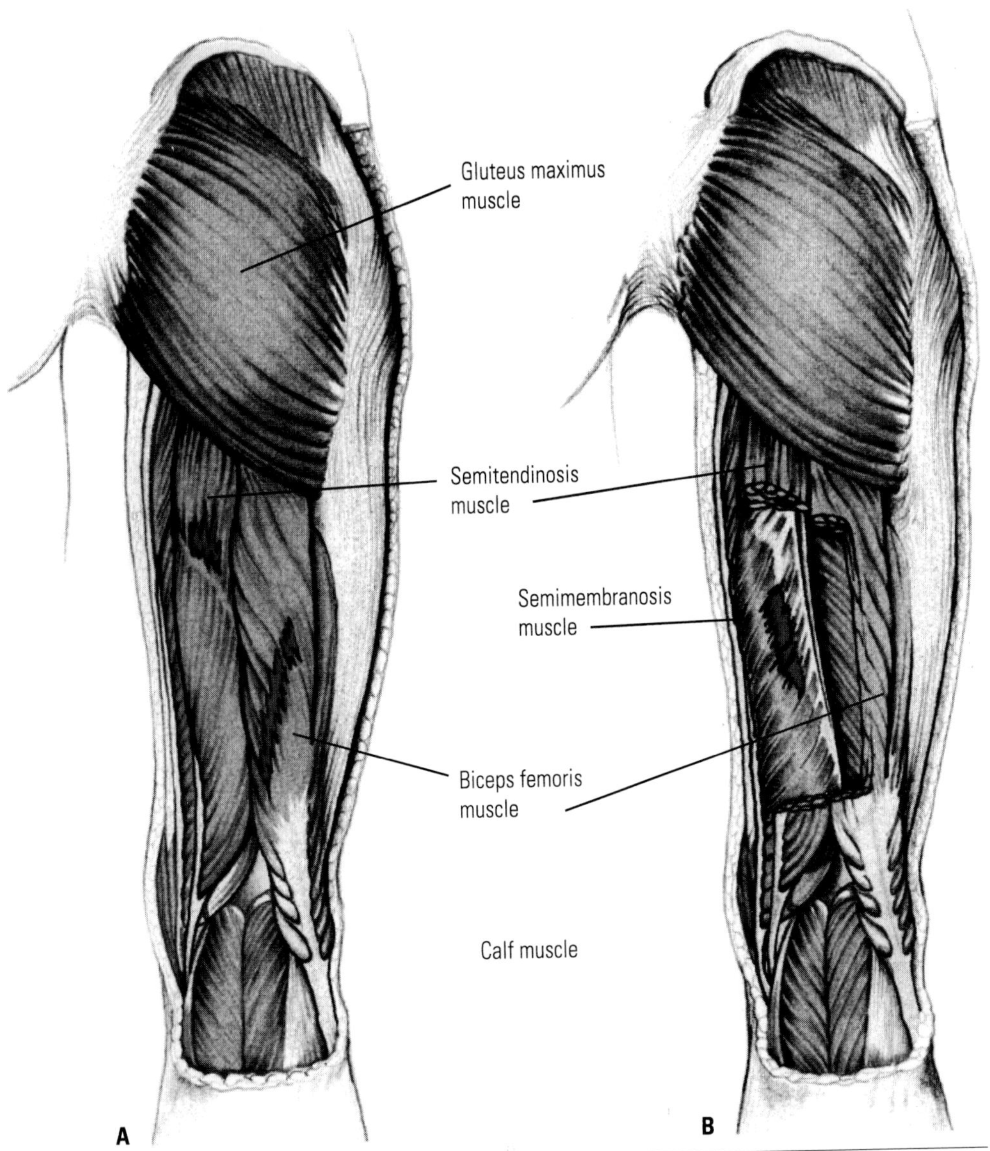

Fig. 25-9 **A,** The injury on the left-hand side of the leg is a rupture of the semitendinosus muscle at the back of the thigh. The injury on the right-hand side of the leg is a rupture of the biceps femoris muscle. **B,** Rupture of the semimembranosus muscle at the back of the thigh. The middle parts of the semitendinosus muscle and the biceps femoris have been removed to show the rupture. (From Peterson L, Renström P: *Sports injuries: their prevention and treatment,* London, 1986, Martin Dunitz, Ltd.)

followed by isometrics to those muscles at varying angles.[2] The final phase of treatment involves active strengthening by means of eccentric activity with gradual increase in both speed and weight. The eccentric-catch exercise is helpful and involves the patient who lowers an ankle weight at successively faster speeds so that he or she eventually progresses to the point of dropping the ankle and catching the weight before the knee reaches full extension[9] (Fig. 25-10).

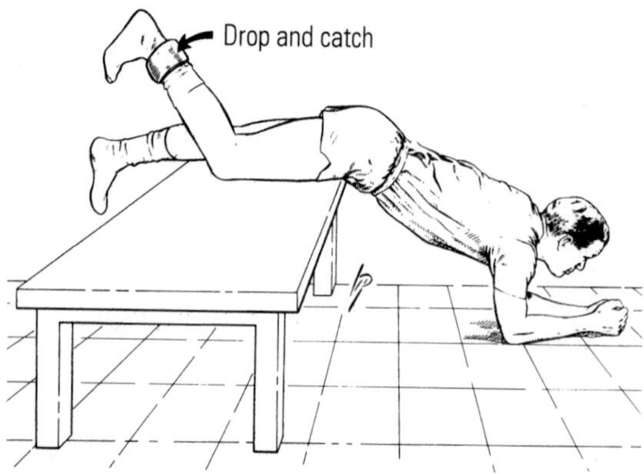

Fig. 25-10 Eccentric "catch" exercise for strengthening the hamstrings. The patient lies prone over the edge of the table so as to approximate the hip and knee angles during the late stance phase. (Modified from Stanton D, Purdham C: *J Orthop Sports Phys Ther* 10:347, 1989.)

Running should begin with a backward-running technique, which will help stretch the hamstrings. Forward running should begin with 60% of speed, with frequent hamstring stretch breaks interspersed throughout the workout.[9] Severe tears, more frequently seen in sprinters than in recreational or long-distance runners, may require immediate surgical repair. Chronic hamstring strain is a nonacute injury that develops slowly and is also implicated in inadequate stretching of these muscles before and after running.[2]

24. What therapeutic management is appropriate for muscle strains?

Studies have shown that healing is more rapid, with restoration of circulation and strength improvement, when rehabilitation is started early. The time required for healing of a third-degree muscle strain varies between 3 and 16 weeks, depending on location and extent of injury.

In the *acute state*

- Ice treatment.
- Elevation.
- Pressure, from an elastic wrap applied from the knee to the groin.
- Rest, though protected weight bearing is generally permitted.
- No active range of motion exercise and no massage. Coagulation, the body's defense against excessive bleeding, springs to action as soon as injury occurs and continues to function for sometime thereafter. This repair mechanism, however, is unstable during the first 24 to 36 hours, and so further bleeding may occur from the impact of new force, vigorous muscle contraction, or unprotected weight bearing. Massage, which is, in effect, repeated minor trauma, should not be used during the first 48 to 72 hours after a muscle injury. After the acute stage, massage is actually beneficial because it can help decrease swelling and stiffness.
- Passive range of motion exercise to the joints of the involved extremity is begun distally and is moved proximally to decrease edema and maintain joint mobility.

In the *subacute stage*

Minor partial ruptures, intermuscular hematomas, and minor intramuscular hematomas are managed by the following progression:

- Heat treatment.
- Ultrasound.

- Deep transverse friction massage serves to prevent adherence of young unwanted fibrous tissue and separate existing adhesions between individual muscle fibers that are restricting movement.
- Pain-free passive stretching facilitates prevention of random alignment of new collagen fibers. Stretching does not, as some think, widen the distance between the muscle fibers; on the contrary, stretching permits muscle fibers to lie more closely together. In a similar vein, pain-free contractile exercises performed early in the rehabilitation process also help structure scar tissue less randomly.
- Submaximal isometric exercises are appropriately begun once resistance to stretching is decreased to the point of achieving full painless range.
- Static (that is, isometric) exercises with light load.
- Pool therapy to encourage active movement.
- Limited dynamic muscle work in the form of short-arc active exercises. At this point, if movement during exercise becomes too painful, the exercises ought to be postponed until they can be performed with minimal pain.
- Dynamic exercises with increasing load.
- Gradually increasing the exercise level to include more aggressive training such as isotonics and isokinetics.
- Eccentric training as part of an injury-sparing strategy.
- Stretching exercises to improve flexibility to all the muscles of that region, including anatomic antagonists to the injured muscle. Stretching should be performed for at least 2 minutes per muscle for optimal results.

References

1. Abbot BC, Bigland B, Ritchie JM: The physiological cost of negative work, *J Physiol* 117:380-390, 1952.
2. Brody DM: Running injuries: prevention and management, *Clin Symp* 39(3):1-36, 1987.
3. Caughey MB, Welsh PW: Muscle ruptures affecting the shoulder girdle. In Rockwood CA, Matsen FA, editors: *The shoulder*, vol 2, Philadelphia, 1990, Saunders.
4. Chauveau MA: La loi de l'équivalence dans les transformations de la force chez les animaux, *Acad* 122:113-126, 1896.
5. Dandy DJ: *Essential orthopaedics and trauma*, Edinburgh, 1989, Churchill Livingstone, p 193.
6. Gould JA: *Orthopaedic and sports physical therapy*, St. Louis, 1990, Mosby, p 385.
7. Heckman JD, Levine MI: Traumatic closed transection of the biceps brachii in the military parachutist, *J Bone Joint Surg* 60A:369-372, 1978.
8. Levy M, Godberg I, Meir I: Fracture of the head of the radius with a tear or avulsion of the triceps tendon, *J Bone Joint Surg* 64B(1):70-72, 1982.
9. Lillegard WA, Rucker KS: *Handbook of sport medicine: a system-oriented approach*, Boston, 1993, Andover Medical Publishers, p 128.
10. Lysholm J, Wiklander J: Injuries in runners, *Am J Sports Med* 15:168-171, 1987.
11. Moore KL: *Clinically oriented anatomy*, ed 2, Baltimore, 1984, Williams & Wilkins, p 419.
12. Peterson L, Renström P: *Sports injuries: their prevention and treatment*, London, Martin Dunitz, Ltd, 1986.
13. Renström P, Peterson L: Groin injuries in athletes, *Br J Sports Med* 14:30, 1980.
14. Stanton D, Purdam C: Hamstring injuries in sprinting—the role of eccentric exercise, *J Orthop Sports Phys Ther* 10:343-348, 1989.

14a. Subotnick SI: *Podiatric Sports Medicine*, Futural Publishing Company. 1979, Mount Kisco, New York.

14b. Subotnick SI, editor: *Athlete's Feet*, Runner's World Publications.

15. Tobin WJ, Cohen LJ, Vandover JT: Parachute injuries, *JAMA* 117(16):1318-1321, 1941.

Recommended reading

Brody DM: Running injuries: prevention and management, *Clin Symp* 39(3):1-36, 1987.

Lillegard WA, Rucker KS: *Handbook of sport medicine: a system-oriented approach*, Boston, 1993, Andover Medical Publishers.

Peterson L, Renström P: *Sports injuries: their prevention and treatment*, London, 1986, Martin Dunitz, Ltd.

Index

"Books are properly compared to tools of which the index is a handle."

John Shaw Billings

C

D

T

U

V

W

Y